PRINCIPLES OF PULMONARY
MEDICINE

Principles of Pulmonary Medicine

Fourth Edition

Steven E. Weinberger, M.D.
Executive Vice Chair, Department of Medicine
Beth Israel Deaconess Medical Center
Professor of Medicine and Faculty Associate Dean for Education
Harvard Medical School
Boston, Massachusetts

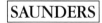

An Imprint of Elsevier

SAUNDERS
An Imprint of Elsevier

The Curtis Center
Independence Square West
Philadelphia, Pennsylvania 19106

NOTICE

Pulmonary medicine is an ever-changing field. Standard safety precautions must be followed, but as new research and clinical experience broaden our knowledge, changes in treatment and drug therapy may become necessary or appropriate. Readers are advised to check the most current product information provided by the manufacturer of each drug to be administered to verify the recommended dose, the method and duration of administration, and contraindications. It is the responsibility of the licensed prescriber, relying on experience and knowledge of the patient, to determine dosages and the best treatment for each individual patient. Neither the publisher nor the author assumes any liability for any injury and/or damage to persons or property arising from this publication.

Previous editions copyrighted 1998, 1992, 1986

Library of Congress Cataloging-in-Publication Data
Weinberger, Steven E.
    Principles of pulmonary medicine / Steven E. Weinberger.—4th ed.
      p. ; cm.
    Includes bibliographical references and index.
    ISBN-13: 978-0-7216-9548-8   ISBN-10: 0-7216-9548-5
    1. Lungs—Diseases.   I. Title.
    [DNLM: 1. Lung Diseases. WF 600 W423p 2004]
    RC756.W45 2004
    616.2′4—dc21

                                  2003041529

Acquisitions Editor: Todd Hummel

Printed in the United States of America
ISBN-13: 978-0-7216-9548-8
ISBN-10: 0-7216-9548-5
Last digit is the print number: 9 8 7 6 5 4

To Janet, Eric, and Mark

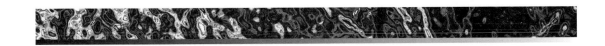

Introduction
to the Fourth Edition

When I was initially asked to write the First Edition of *Principles of Pulmonary Medicine* in the early to mid-1980s, the challenge of preparing a textbook for medical students that provided a pathophysiologic approach—correlating abnormalities in structure and resulting changes in function with clinical manifestations of disease—seemed particularly appealing. At the same time, I wanted the style and the length of the book to be "user friendly," so that the student could read through the text in its entirety as part of an introductory course in respiratory pathophysiology. Over time and subsequent editions, additional material has been added, with the intent of keeping pace with new diseases, advances in our understanding of basic disease mechanisms, evolving diagnostic tools, and new forms of treatment. I have also tried to incorporate sufficient clinical information to make the book useful to an audience broader than preclinical medical students, without sacrificing the readability and the pathophysiologic approach that are so important for an introductory textbook.

Since the Third Edition, the text and the references have been updated throughout, but the overall structure of the book is unchanged. New figures have been added, especially new radiographs, and the popular margin notes and appendices (covering quantitative aspects of pulmonary physiology, interpretation of pulmonary function tests, and interpretation of arterial blood gases) have been continued.

In the course of preparing the Fourth Edition, I remain most grateful to my administrative assistant, Ms. Carol Murree, whose superb support has been invaluable to me, now spanning the last three editions of the book. Ms. Catherine Carroll, my editor at Elsevier, and two editorial assistants who have worked with her, Sabrina Martin and Dana Lamparello, have been a true pleasure to work with during all phases of this project. I remain most grateful to the many students, house staff, and colleagues who have used the book—at Harvard Medical School and at many other medical schools and settings in North America and around the world—and have provided valuable feedback and encouragement. Finally, I cannot sufficiently thank my wonderful family—my wife, Janet, and my two sons, Eric and Mark—for their continued patience, support, and inspiration.

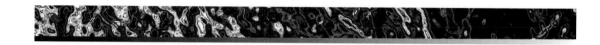

Contents

Pulmonary Anatomy and Physiology—The Basics

ANATOMY
PHYSIOLOGY
  Mechanical Aspects of the Lungs
    and Chest Wall
  Ventilation
  Circulation
  Diffusion
  Oxygen Transport

Carbon Dioxide Transport
Ventilation-Perfusion
  Relationships
**ABNORMALITIES IN
GAS EXCHANGE**
  Hypoxemia
  Hypercapnia

To be effective at gas-exchange, the lungs cannot act in isolation; they must interact with the central nervous system (which provides the rhythmic drive to breathe), the diaphragm and muscular apparatus of the chest wall (which respond to signals from the central nervous system and act as a bellows for movement of air), and the circulatory system (which provides blood flow and, therefore, gas transport between the tissues and the lungs). The processes of oxygen uptake and carbon dioxide elimination by the lungs depend on the functioning of all these systems, and a disturbance in any of them can result in clinically important abnormalities in gas transport and thus arterial blood gases. In this chapter, an initial overview of pulmonary anatomy is followed by a discussion of mechanical properties of the lungs and chest wall and a consideration of some aspects of the contribution of the lungs and the circulatory system to gas-exchange. Additional discussion about pulmonary and circulatory physiology is presented in Chapters 4, 8, and 12, and neurologic, muscular, and chest wall interactions with the lungs are discussed further in Chapter 17.

ANATOMY

It is appropriate when discussing the anatomy of the respiratory system to include the entire pathway for airflow from the mouth or nose down to the alveolar sacs. En route to the alveoli, gas flows through the oropharynx or nasopharynx, the larynx, the trachea, and finally a progressively arborizing system of bronchi and bronchioles (Fig. 1-1). The trachea divides at the carina into right and left mainstem bronchi, which branch into lobar bronchi (three on the right, two on the left), segmental bronchi, and an extensive system of subsegmental and smaller bronchi. These conducting airways divide approximately 15 to 20 times down to the level of terminal bronchioles, which are the smallest units that do not actually participate in gas-exchange.

Conducting airways include all airways down to the level of the terminal bronchioles.

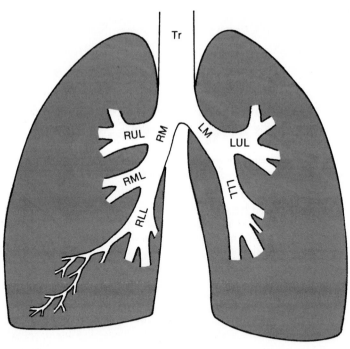

Figure 1-1 ▬▬ Schematic diagram of airway branching. Tr = trachea; RM = right mainstem bronchus; LM = left mainstem bronchus; RUL = right upper lobe bronchus; RML = right middle lobe bronchus; RLL = right lower lobe bronchus; LUL = left upper lobe bronchus; LLL = left lower lobe bronchus.

The acinus includes structures distal to a terminal bronchiole: respiratory bronchioles, alveolar ducts, and alveoli (alveolar sacs).

Beyond the terminal bronchioles, further divisions include the respiratory bronchioles, the alveolar ducts, and the alveoli. From the respiratory bronchioles on, these divisions form the portion of the lung involved in gas-exchange and constitute the terminal respiratory unit or *acinus*. At this level, inhaled gas comes into contact with alveolar walls (septa), and pulmonary capillary blood loads O_2 and unloads CO_2 as it courses through the septa.

The surface area for gas-exchange provided by the alveoli is enormous. It is estimated that the adult human lung has on the order of 300 million alveoli, with a total surface area approximately the size of a tennis court. This vast surface area of gas in contact with alveolar walls is a highly efficient mechanism for O_2 and CO_2 transfer between alveolar spaces and pulmonary capillary blood.

The pulmonary capillary network and the blood within provide the other crucial requirement for gas-exchange: a transportation system for O_2 and CO_2 to and from other body tissues and organs. After blood arrives at the lungs via the pulmonary artery, it courses through a widely branching system of smaller pulmonary arteries and arterioles to the major locale for gas-exchange, the pulmonary capillary network. The capillaries generally allow red blood cells to flow through in single file only, so that gas-exchange between each cell and alveolar gas is facilitated. On completion of gas-exchange and travel through the pulmonary capillary bed, the oxygenated blood flows through pulmonary venules and veins and arrives at the left side of the heart for pumping to the systemic circulation and distribution to the tissues.

Further details about the anatomy of airways, alveoli, and the pulmonary vasculature, particularly with regard to structure-function relationships and cellular anatomy, are in Chapters 4, 8, and 12.

PHYSIOLOGY

Mechanical Aspects of the Lungs and Chest Wall

This discussion of pulmonary physiology begins with an introduction to a few concepts about the mechanical properties of the respiratory system, which have important implications for assessment of pulmonary function and its derangement in disease states.

The lungs and the chest wall have elastic properties—they have a particular resting size (or volume) that they would assume if no internal or external pressure were exerted on them, and any deviation from this volume requires some additional influencing force. If the lungs were removed from the chest and no longer had the external influences of the chest wall and the pleural space acting on them, they would be almost airless; they would have a much lower volume than they have within the thoracic cage. To expand these lungs, positive pressure would have to be exerted on the air spaces, as could be done by putting positive pressure through the airway. (Similarly, a balloon is essentially airless unless positive pressure is exerted on the opening to distend the elastic wall and fill it with air.)

Alternatively, instead of positive pressure exerted on alveoli through the airways, negative pressure could be applied outside the lungs to cause their expansion. Thus, what increases the volume of the isolated lungs from the resting, essentially airless, state is the application of a positive *transpulmonary pressure*—the pressure inside the lungs relative to the pressure outside. Internal pressure can be made positive, or external pressure can be made negative; the net effect is the same. With the lungs inside the chest wall, the internal pressure is alveolar pressure, whereas external pressure is the pressure within the pleural space (Fig. 1-2). Therefore, transpulmonary pressure is defined as alveolar pressure (P_{alv}) minus pleural pressure (P_{pl}), and the presence of air in the lungs requires that pleural pressure be relatively negative compared with alveolar pressure.

The relationship between transpulmonary pressure and lung volume can be described for a range of transpulmonary pressures. The plot of this relationship, shown in Figure 1-3*A*, is the *compliance curve* of the lung. As transpulmonary pressure increases, lung volume naturally increases. The relationship, however, is not linear, but curvilinear; at relatively high volumes, the lungs reach their limit of distensibility, and even rather large increases in transpulmonary pressure do not result in significant increases in lung volume.

Switching from the lungs to the chest wall, if the lungs were removed from the chest, the chest wall would expand to a larger size when no external or internal pressures were exerted on it. Thus, the chest wall has a spring-like character; the resting volume is relatively high, and distortion to either a smaller or larger volume requires an alteration of either the external or internal pressures acting on it. The pressure across the chest wall is akin to the transpulmonary pressure. Again, with the lungs back inside the chest wall, the pressure across the chest wall is the pleural pressure (internal pressure) minus the external pressure surrounding the chest wall (atmospheric pressure).

The compliance curve of the chest wall in Figure 1-3*B* relates the volume enclosed by the chest wall to the pressure across the chest wall. The curve becomes relatively flat at low lung volumes, at which the chest wall becomes quite stiff; further changes in the pressure across the chest wall cause little further decrement in volume.

Transpulmonary pressure = $P_{alv} - P_{pl}$.

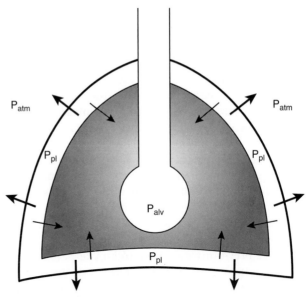

Figure 1-2 ■— Simplified diagram showing the pressures on both sides of the chest wall (heavy line) and the lung (shaded area). P_{pl} = pleural pressure; P_{alv} = alveolar pressure; P_{atm} = atmospheric pressure. Thin arrows show the direction of elastic recoil of the lung (at the resting end-expiratory position); thick arrows show the direction of elastic recoil of the chest wall.

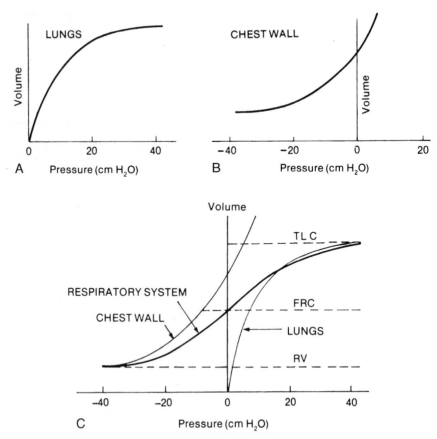

Figure 1-3 ■— *A*, Relationship between lung volume and distending (transpulmonary) pressure, i.e., compliance curve of the lung. *B*, Relationship between volume enclosed by the chest wall and distending (trans–chest wall) pressure, i.e., compliance curve of the chest wall. *C*, Combined compliance curves of the lung and chest wall, showing relationship between respiratory system volume and distending (trans–respiratory system) pressure. RV = residual volume; FRC = functional residual capacity; TLC = total lung capacity.

In order to examine how the lungs and chest wall behave in situ, remember that the elastic properties of each are acting in opposite directions. At the normal resting end-expiratory position of the respiratory system (*functional residual capacity* [FRC]), the lung is expanded to a volume greater than the resting volume it would have in isolation, whereas the chest wall is contracted to a volume smaller than it would have in isolation. However, at FRC the tendency of the lung to become smaller (the inward or elastic recoil of the lung) is exactly balanced by the tendency of the chest wall to expand (the outward recoil of the chest wall). As Figure 1-3*C* shows, the transpulmonary pressure at FRC is equal in magnitude to the pressure across the chest wall but acts in an opposite direction. Pleural pressure is therefore negative, a consequence of the inward recoil of the lungs and the outward recoil of the chest wall.

> At FRC, the inward elastic recoil of the lung is balanced by the outward elastic recoil of the chest wall.

The chest wall and the lungs can be considered as a unit, the *respiratory system*. The respiratory system has its own compliance curve, which is essentially a combination of the individual compliance curves of the lungs and chest wall (see Fig. 1-3*C*). The transrespiratory system pressure, again defined as internal minus external pressure, is therefore airway pressure minus atmospheric pressure. At a transrespiratory system pressure of 0, the respiratory system is at its normal resting end-expiratory position, and the volume within the lungs is FRC.

Two additional lung volumes can be defined as well as the factors that determine each of them. The first, *total lung capacity* (TLC), is the volume of gas within the lungs at the end of a maximal inhalation. At this point the lungs are stretched well above their resting position, and even the chest wall is stretched beyond its resting position. We are able to distort both the lungs and the chest wall so far from FRC by using our inspiratory muscles, which exert an outward force to counterbalance the inward elastic recoil of the lung and, at TLC, the chest wall. However, at TLC it is primarily the extreme stiffness of the lungs that prevents even further expansion by inspiratory muscle action. Therefore, the primary determinants of TLC are the expanding action of the inspiratory musculature balanced by the inward elastic recoil of the lung.

> At TLC, the expanding action of the inspiratory musculature is limited primarily by the inward elastic recoil of the lung.

At the other extreme, when we exhale as much as possible, we reach *residual volume* (RV). At this point, there is still a significant amount of gas within the lungs; that is, we can never exhale enough to empty the lungs entirely of gas. Again, the reason can be seen by looking at the compliance curves in Figure 1-3*C*. The chest wall becomes so stiff at low volumes that additional effort by the expiratory muscles is unable to decrease the volume any further. Therefore, RV is determined primarily by the balance of the outward recoil of the chest wall and the contracting action of the expiratory musculature. However, this simple model for RV applies only to the young individual with normal lungs and airways. With age or with disease of the airways, further expulsion of gas during expiration is limited not by the outward recoil of the chest wall but rather by the tendency for airways to close during expiration and for gas to be trapped behind the closed airways.

> At RV, either outward recoil of the chest wall or closure of airways prevents further expiration.

Ventilation

To maintain normal gas-exchange to the tissues, an adequate volume of air must pass through the lungs for provision of O_2 to and removal of CO_2 from the blood. A normal person at rest typically breathes approximately 500 mL of air per breath at a frequency of 12 to 16 times per minute, resulting in a

> The volume of each breath (tidal volume [V_T]) is divided into dead space volume (V_D) and alveolar volume (V_A).

ventilation of 6 to 8 L/min (the *minute ventilation*, abbreviated $\dot{V}_E$).* The volume of each breath (*tidal volume* [V_T]) is not used entirely for gas-exchange; a portion stays in the conducting airways and does not reach the distal part of the lung capable of gas-exchange. The portion of the tidal volume that is "wasted" (in the sense of gas-exchange) is termed *dead space* (V_D), and the volume that reaches the gas-exchanging portion of the lung is the *alveolar volume* (V_A). The *anatomic dead space,* which includes the larynx, trachea, and bronchi down to the level of the terminal bronchioles, is approximately 150 mL in a normal person; thus, 30 percent of a tidal volume of 500 mL is wasted.

As for CO_2 elimination by the lung, the alveolar ventilation ($\dot{V}_A$), which is equal to the breathing frequency (f) multiplied by V_A, bears a direct relationship to the amount of CO_2 removed from the body. In fact, the partial pressure of CO_2 in arterial blood (Pa_{CO_2}) is inversely proportional to $\dot{V}_A$; as $\dot{V}_A$ increases, Pa_{CO_2} decreases. Additionally, Pa_{CO_2} is affected by the body's rate of CO_2 production ($\dot{V}_{CO_2}$); if $\dot{V}_{CO_2}$ increases without any change in $\dot{V}_A$, Pa_{CO_2} shows a proportional increase as well. Thus, it is easy to understand the relationship in Equation 1-1:

$$Pa_{CO_2} \propto \dot{V}_{CO_2}/\dot{V}_A \qquad (1\text{-}1)$$

> Arterial P_{CO_2} (Pa_{CO_2}) is inversely proportional to alveolar ventilation ($\dot{V}_A$) and directly proportional to CO_2 production ($\dot{V}_{CO_2}$).

This defines the major factors determining Pa_{CO_2}. When a normal individual exercises, $\dot{V}_{CO_2}$ increases, but $\dot{V}_A$ increases proportionately so that Pa_{CO_2} remains relatively constant.

As mentioned already, the dead space comprises that amount of each breath going to parts of the tracheobronchial tree not involved in gas-exchange. The anatomic dead space consists of the conducting airways. In disease states, however, areas of lung that normally participate in gas-exchange (parts of the terminal respiratory unit) may not receive normal blood flow, even though they continue to be ventilated. In these areas, some of the ventilation is thus wasted; such regions contribute additional volume to the dead space.

Hence, a more useful clinical concept than anatomic dead space is *physiologic dead space,* which takes into account the volume of each breath not involved in gas-exchange, whether at the level of the conducting airways or the terminal respiratory units. Primarily in certain disease states, in which there may be areas with normal ventilation but decreased or no perfusion, the physiologic dead space is larger than the anatomic dead space.

Quantitation of the physiologic dead space, or, more precisely, the fraction of the tidal volume that is represented by the dead space (V_D/V_T), can be made by measuring P_{CO_2} in arterial blood (Pa_{CO_2}) and expired gas (Pe_{CO_2}) and by using Equation 1-2, known as the *Bohr equation* for physiologic dead space:

> The Bohr equation can be used to quantitate the fraction of each breath that is wasted, the dead space to tidal volume ratio (V_D/V_T).

$$V_D/V_T = (Pa_{CO_2} - Pe_{CO_2})/Pa_{CO_2} \qquad (1\text{-}2)$$

For gas coming directly from alveoli that have participated in gas-exchange, the P_{CO_2} approximates that of arterial blood. For gas coming from the dead space, the P_{CO_2} is 0, because the gas never came into contact with pulmonary capillary blood.

---

*By convention, a dot over a letter adds a time dimension. Hence, $\dot{V}_E$ stands for volume of expired gas per minute, i.e., minute ventilation. Other similar abbreviations that are used in this chapter include $\dot{V}_{CO_2}$ (volume of CO_2 produced per minute) and $\dot{Q}$ (blood flow per minute).

Consider the two extremes. If the expired gas came entirely from perfused alveoli, P_{ECO_2} would equal Pa_{CO_2}, and, according to the equation, V_D/V_T would equal 0. On the other hand, if expired gas came totally from the dead space, it would contain no CO_2, P_{ECO_2} would equal 0, and V_D/V_T would equal 1. In practice, this equation is used in situations between these two extremes, and it quantitates the proportion of expired gas coming from alveolar gas ($P_{CO_2} = Pa_{CO_2}$) versus dead space gas ($P_{CO_2} = 0$).

In summary, each normal or tidal volume breath can be divided into alveolar volume and dead space, just as the total minute ventilation can be divided into alveolar ventilation and wasted (or dead space) ventilation. Elimination of CO_2 by the lungs is proportional to alveolar ventilation, and therefore Pa_{CO_2} is inversely proportional to alveolar ventilation, not to minute ventilation. The wasted ventilation can be quantitated by the Bohr equation, with use of the principle that increasing amounts of dead space ventilation augment the difference between P_{CO_2} in arterial blood and expired gas.

Circulation

Because the entire cardiac output flows from the right ventricle to the lungs and back to the left side of the heart, the pulmonary circulation handles a blood flow of approximately 5 L/min. If the pulmonary vasculature were similar in structure to the systemic vasculature, large pressures would need to be generated because of the thick walls and high resistance offered by systemic-type arteries. Pulmonary arteries, however, are quite different in structure from systemic arteries, with thin walls that provide much less resistance to flow. Thus, despite equal right and left ventricular outputs, the normal mean pulmonary artery pressure of 15 mm Hg is much lower than the normal mean aortic pressure of approximately 95 mm Hg.

One important feature of blood flow in the pulmonary capillary bed is the distribution of flow in different areas of the lung. The pattern of flow is explained by gravity and the need for blood to be pumped "uphill" to reach the apices of the lungs. In the upright person, the apex of each lung is approximately 25 cm higher than the base, so that the pressure in pulmonary vessels at the apex is 25 cm H_2O (19 mm Hg) lower than in pulmonary vessels at the bases. Because flow through these vessels depends on the perfusion pressure, the capillary network at the bases receives much more flow than do capillaries at the apices. In fact, flow at the lung apices falls to 0 during the part of the cardiac cycle when pulmonary artery pressure is insufficient to pump blood up to the apices.

As a result of gravity, there is more blood flow to dependent regions of the lung.

West developed a model of pulmonary blood flow that divides the lung into zones, based on the relationships among pulmonary arterial, venous, and alveolar pressures (Fig. 1-4). As stated before, the vascular pressures—that is, pulmonary arterial and venous—depend in part on the vertical location of the vessels in the lung because of the hydrostatic effect. Apical vessels have much lower pressure than do basilar vessels, the difference being the vertical distance between them (divided by a correction factor of 1.3 to convert from cm H_2O to mm Hg).

At the apex of the lung (zone 1 in Fig. 1-4), alveolar pressure exceeds arterial and venous pressures, and no flow results. Normally, such a condition does not arise, unless pulmonary arterial pressure is decreased or alveolar pressure is increased (by exogenous pressure applied to the airways and alveoli). In zone 2, arterial but not venous pressure exceeds alveolar pressure, and the driving force for flow is determined by the difference between arterial and

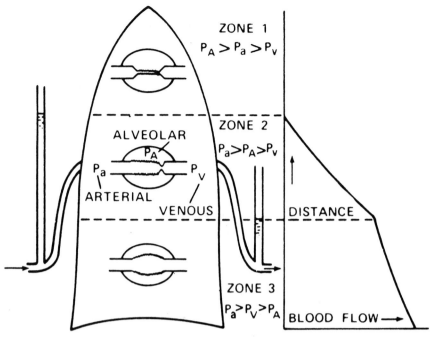

Figure 1-4 ■— Three-zone model of pulmonary blood flow, showing relationships among alveolar pressure (P_A), arterial pressure (P_a), and venous pressure (P_v) in each zone. On right side of figure, blood flow (per unit volume of lung) is shown as function of vertical distance. (From West JB, Dollery CT, and Naimark A: J Appl Physiol 19:713–724, 1964.)

alveolar pressures. In zone 3, arterial and venous pressures exceed alveolar pressure, and the driving force is the difference between arterial and venous pressures, as is the case in the systemic vasculature.

When cardiac output is increased (e.g., on exercise) the normal pulmonary vasculature is able to handle the increase in flow by recruiting previously unperfused vessels and by distending previously perfused vessels. The ability to expand the pulmonary vascular bed and thus decrease vascular resistance allows major increases in cardiac output with exercise to be accompanied by only small increments in mean pulmonary artery pressure. In disease states that affect the pulmonary vascular bed, however, the ability to recruit additional vessels with increased flow may not exist, and significant increases in pulmonary artery pressure may result.

Diffusion

Normally, equilibration of O_2 and CO_2 between alveolar gas and pulmonary capillary blood is complete in one-third the time spent by blood in the pulmonary capillary bed.

For O_2 and CO_2 to be transferred between the alveolar space and blood in the pulmonary capillary, diffusion through several compartments must take place—alveolar gas, alveolar and capillary walls, plasma, and membrane and cytoplasm of the red blood cell. In normal circumstances, the process of diffusion of both gases is relatively rapid, and full equilibration occurs during the transit time of blood flowing through the pulmonary capillary bed. In fact, the Po_2 in capillary blood rises from the mixed venous level of 40 torr* to the end-capillary level of 100 torr in approximately 0.25 second, or one-third the total

*The terms torr and mm Hg are used interchangeably throughout the text: 1 torr = 1 mm Hg.

transit time (0.75 second) that an erythrocyte spends within the pulmonary capillaries. Similarly, CO_2 transfer is complete within approximately the same amount of time.

Although diffusion of O_2 is normally a rapid process, it is not instantaneous. Resistance to diffusion is provided primarily by the alveolar-capillary membrane and by the reaction that forms oxygenated hemoglobin within the erythrocyte. Each factor provides approximately equal resistance to the transfer of O_2, and each can be disturbed in various disease states. However, as discussed later in this chapter, even when diffusion is measurably impaired, it rarely is a cause of impaired gas-exchange. Generally sufficient time still exists for full equilibration of O_2 or CO_2 to occur, unless transit time is significantly shortened, as with exercise.

Even though diffusion limitation rarely contributes to hypoxemia, an abnormality in diffusion may be a useful marker for diseases of the pulmonary parenchyma that affect the alveolar-capillary membrane or the volume of blood in the pulmonary capillaries, or both. Rather than using O_2 to measure diffusion within the lung, clinicians generally use carbon monoxide, which also combines with hemoglobin and provides a technically easier test to perform and interpret. The usefulness and meaning of the measurement of diffusing capacity are discussed in Chapter 3.

Oxygen Transport

Because the eventual goal of tissue oxygenation requires transport of O_2 from the lungs to the peripheral tissues and organs, any discussion of oxygenation is incomplete without consideration of these transport mechanisms.

In preparation for this discussion, an understanding of the concepts of *partial pressure, gas content,* and *percent saturation* is essential. The partial pressure of any gas is the product of the ambient total gas pressure and the proportion of total gas composition made up by the specific gas of interest. For example, air is composed of approximately 21 percent O_2; assuming a total pressure of 760 mm Hg (760 torr) at sea level and no water vapor pressure, the partial pressure of O_2 (Po_2) is 0.21×760, or 160 torr. If the gas is saturated with water vapor at body temperature (37° C), the water vapor has a partial pressure of 47 torr; the partial pressure of O_2 is then calculated on the basis of the remaining pressure, or $760 - 47 = 713$ torr. Therefore, when room air is saturated at body temperature, the Po_2 is $0.21 \times 713 = 150$ torr. Because inspired gas is normally humidified by the upper airway, it becomes fully saturated by the time it reaches the trachea and bronchi, where inspired Po_2 is approximately 150 torr.

In clinical situations, we must also consider the concept of partial pressure of a gas within a body fluid, primarily blood. When a liquid is in contact with a gas mixture, the partial pressure of a particular gas in the liquid is the same as its partial pressure in the gas mixture, assuming full equilibration has taken place. Therefore, the partial pressure of the gas acts as the "driving force" for the gas to be carried by the liquid phase.

However, the quantity of a gas that can be carried by the liquid medium depends on the "capacity" of the liquid for that particular gas. If a specific gas is quite soluble within a liquid, more of that gas is carried for a given partial pressure than is a less soluble gas. In addition, if a component of the liquid is able to bind the gas, more of the gas is transported at a particular partial pressure. This is true, for example, of the interaction of hemoglobin and O_2, as more detailed discussion will show.

The content of a gas in a liquid, such as blood, is the actual amount of the gas contained within the liquid. For O_2 in blood, the content is expressed as milliliters of O_2 per 100 mL blood. The percent saturation of a gas is the ratio of the actual content of the gas to the maximum possible content if there is a limit or plateau in the amount that can be carried.

Oxygen is transported in blood in two ways, either dissolved in the blood or bound to the heme portion of hemoglobin. Oxygen is not very soluble in plasma, and only a small amount of O_2 is carried this way under normal conditions. The amount dissolved is proportional to the partial pressure of O_2, with 0.0031 mL dissolved for each torr of partial pressure. The amount bound to hemoglobin is a function of the *oxyhemoglobin dissociation curve,* which relates the driving pressure (P_{O_2}) to the quantity of O_2 bound. As can be seen in Figure 1-5, this curve reaches a plateau, indicating that hemoglobin can hold only so much O_2 before it becomes fully saturated. At a P_{O_2} of 60 torr, hemoglobin is approximately 90 percent saturated, so that only relatively small amounts of additional O_2 are transported at a P_{O_2} above this level.

This curve can shift to the right or left, depending on a variety of conditions. Thus, the relationships between arterial P_{O_2} and saturation are not fixed. For instance, a decrease in pH or an increase in P_{CO_2} (largely by means of a pH effect), temperature, or 2,3-diphosphoglycerate (2,3-DPG) levels shifts the oxyhemoglobin dissociation curve to the right, making it easier to unload (or harder to bind) O_2 for any given P_{O_2} (see Fig. 1-5). The opposite changes in pH, P_{CO_2}, temperature, or 2,3-DPG shift the curve to the left and make it harder to unload (or easier to bind) O_2 for any given P_{O_2}.

Perhaps the easiest way to understand O_2 transport is to follow O_2 and hemoglobin as they course through the circulation in a normal person. When blood leaves the pulmonary capillaries, it has already been oxygenated by equilibration with alveolar gas, and the P_{O_2} should be identical to that in the alveoli. Because of O_2 uptake at the level of the alveolar-capillary interface, alveolar

---

Almost all O_2 transported in the blood is bound to hemoglobin; a small fraction is dissolved in plasma.

Hemoglobin is 90 percent saturated with O_2 at an arterial P_{O_2} of 60 torr.

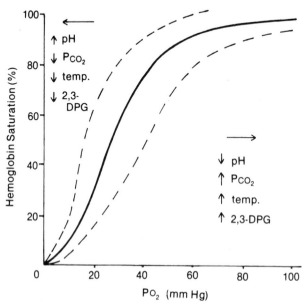

Figure 1-5 ·— Oxyhemoglobin dissociation curve, relating percent hemoglobin saturation and P_{O_2}. Oxygen content can be determined on the basis of hemoglobin concentration and percent hemoglobin saturation (see text). Normal curve is depicted with solid line; curves shifted to right or left (along with conditions leading to them) are shown with broken lines.

P_{O_2} is less than the 150 torr that was calculated for inspired gas within the airways. Alveolar P_{O_2} in a normal individual (breathing air at sea level) is approximately 100 torr. However, the P_{O_2} measured in arterial blood is actually slightly lower than this value for alveolar P_{O_2}, partly because of the presence of small amounts of "shunted" blood that do not participate in gas-exchange at the alveolar level—e.g., (1) desaturated blood from the bronchial circulation draining into pulmonary veins and (2) venous blood from the coronary circulation draining into the left ventricle via thebesian veins.

Assuming a P_{O_2} of 95 torr in arterial blood, the total O_2 content is the sum of the quantity of O_2 bound to hemoglobin plus the amount dissolved. To calculate the quantity bound to hemoglobin, the patient's hemoglobin level and the percent saturation of the hemoglobin with O_2 need to be known. Because each gram of hemoglobin can carry 1.34 mL O_2 when fully saturated, the O_2 content is calculated by Equation 1-3:

$$O_2 \text{ content bound to hemoglobin } = 1.34 \times \text{Hemoglobin} \times \text{Saturation} \tag{1-3}$$

Assume that hemoglobin is 97 percent saturated at $P_{O_2} = 95$ torr and that the individual has a hemoglobin level of 15 g/100 mL blood. Thus (Equation 1-4):

$$
\begin{aligned}
O_2 \text{ content bound to hemoglobin } &= 1.34 \times 15 \times 0.97 \\
&= 19.5 \text{ mL } O_2/100 \text{ mL blood} \tag{1-4}
\end{aligned}
$$

In contrast, the amount of dissolved O_2 is much smaller and is proportional to the P_{O_2}, with 0.0031 mL O_2 dissolved per 100 mL blood per torr P_{O_2}. Therefore, at an arterial P_{O_2} of 95 torr (Equation 1-5):

$$\text{Dissolved } O_2 \text{ content } = 0.0031 \times 95 = 0.3 \text{ mL } O_2/100 \text{ mL blood} \tag{1-5}$$

The total O_2 content is the sum of the hemoglobin-bound O_2 plus the dissolved O_2, or $19.5 + 0.3 = 19.8$ mL $O_2/100$ mL blood.

Arterial P_{O_2} is not the sole determinant of O_2 content; the hemoglobin level is also crucial. With anemia (a reduced hemoglobin level), there are fewer binding sites available for O_2, and the O_2 content falls even though P_{O_2} remains unchanged. In addition, the O_2 content of blood is a static measurement of the quantity of $O_2/100$ mL blood. The actual delivery of oxygen to tissues is dynamic and depends on blood flow (cardiac output) as well as O_2 content. Thus, three factors determine tissue O_2 delivery: arterial P_{O_2}, hemoglobin level, and cardiac output. Disturbances in any one of these can result in decreased or insufficient O_2 delivery.

> Oxygen content in arterial blood depends on arterial P_{O_2} and the hemoglobin level; tissue oxygen delivery depends on these two factors and cardiac output.

When blood reaches the systemic capillaries, O_2 is unloaded to the tissues, and P_{O_2} falls. The extent to which P_{O_2} falls depends on the balance of O_2 supply and demand: The local venous P_{O_2} of blood leaving a tissue falls to a greater degree if more O_2 is extracted per volume of blood because of increased tissue requirements or decreased supply (e.g., as a result of decreased cardiac output).

On average, in a resting individual, the P_{O_2} falls to approximately 40 torr after O_2 extraction occurs at the tissue-capillary level. Because a P_{O_2} of 40 torr is associated with 75 percent saturation of hemoglobin, the total O_2 content in venous blood is calculated by Equation 1-6:

$$
\begin{aligned}
\text{Venous } O_2 \text{ content } &= (1.34 \times 15 \times 0.75) + (0.0031 \times 40) \tag{1-6} \\
&= 15.2 \text{ mL } O_2/100 \text{ mL blood}
\end{aligned}
$$

The quantity of O_2 consumed at the tissue level is the difference between the arterial and venous O_2 contents, or $19.8 - 15.2 = 4.6$ mL $O_2/100$ mL blood.

The total O_2 consumption ($\dot{V}O_2$) is the product of cardiac output and the difference noted previously in arterial-venous O_2 content. Because (1) normal resting cardiac output for a young man is about 5 to 6 L/min and (2) 46 mL O_2 is extracted per liter of blood flow (note difference in units), the resting O_2 consumption is approximately 250 mL/min.

When venous blood returns to the lungs, oxygenation of this desaturated blood occurs at the level of the pulmonary capillaries, and the entire cycle can then repeat.

Carbon Dioxide Transport

Carbon dioxide is carried in blood as (1) bicarbonate, (2) dissolved CO_2, and (3) carbaminohemoglobin.

Carbon dioxide is transported through the circulation in three different forms: (1) as bicarbonate (HCO_3^-), quantitatively the largest component, (2) as CO_2 dissolved in plasma, and (3) as carbaminohemoglobin, bound to terminal amino groups on hemoglobin. The first of these, bicarbonate, results from the combination of CO_2 with H_2O to form carbonic acid (H_2CO_3), catalyzed by the enzyme carbonic anhydrase, and the subsequent dissociation to H^+ and HCO_3^-. This reaction takes place primarily within the red blood cell, but HCO_3^- then diffuses out into the plasma in exchange for Cl^-.

Although dissolved CO_2, the second transport mechanism, constitutes only a small portion of the total CO_2 transported, it is quantitatively more important for CO_2 transport than dissolved O_2 is for O_2 transport, because CO_2 is approximately 20 times more soluble in plasma than is O_2. Carbaminohemoglobin, formed by the combination of CO_2 with hemoglobin, is the third transport mechanism. The oxygenation status of hemoglobin is important in determining the quantity of CO_2 that can be bound, deoxygenated hemoglobin having a greater affinity for CO_2 than oxygenated hemoglobin (known as the Haldane effect). Therefore, oxygenation of hemoglobin in the pulmonary capillaries decreases its ability to bind CO_2 and facilitates the elimination of CO_2 by the lungs.

In the same way that the oxyhemoglobin dissociation curve depicts the relationship between the PO_2 and O_2 content of blood, a curve can be constructed relating the total CO_2 content to the PCO_2 of blood. However, within the range of gas tensions encountered under physiologic circumstances, the PCO_2–CO_2 content relationship is almost linear, compared with the curvilinear relationship of PO_2 and O_2 content (Fig. 1-6).

The PCO_2 in mixed venous blood is approximately 46 torr, whereas normal arterial PCO_2 is approximately 40 torr. This decrease of 6 torr in going from mixed venous to arterial blood, combined with the effect of oxygenation of hemoglobin on release of CO_2, corresponds to a change in CO_2 content of approximately 3.6 mL/100 mL blood. Assuming a cardiac output of 5 to 6 L/min, CO_2 production can be calculated as the product of the cardiac output and the arteriovenous CO_2 content difference, or approximately 200 mL/min.

Ventilation-Perfusion Relationships

Ventilation, blood flow, and diffusion and their relationship to gas-exchange (O_2 uptake and CO_2 elimination) are more complicated than initially presented, because the distribution of ventilation and blood flow within the lung was not considered. Effective gas-exchange depends critically on the relationship between ventilation and perfusion in individual gas-exchanging units; a disturbance in this relationship, even if the total amounts of ventilation and

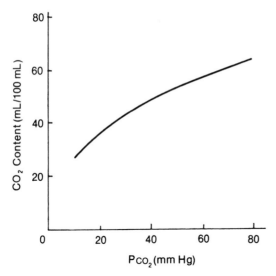

Figure 1-6 ── Relationship between P_{CO_2} and CO_2 content. Curve shifts slightly to left as O_2 saturation of blood decreases; curve shown is for blood completely saturated with O_2.

blood flow are normal, is frequently responsible for markedly abnormal gas-exchange in disease states.

The optimal efficiency for gas-exchange would be provided by an even distribution of ventilation and perfusion throughout the lung, so that a matching of ventilation and perfusion is always present. In reality, such a circumstance does not exist, even in normal lungs. Because blood flow is determined to a large extent by hydrostatic forces, the dependent regions of the lung receive a disproportionately large share of the perfusion, whereas the uppermost regions are relatively underperfused. Similarly, there is a gradient of ventilation throughout the lung, with greater amounts going to the dependent areas. However, even though ventilation and perfusion are both greater in the gravity-dependent regions of the lung, this gradient is more marked for perfusion than for ventilation. Consequently, the ratio of ventilation ($\dot{V}$) to perfusion ($\dot{Q}$) is higher in apical regions of the lung than in basal regions. As a result, gas-exchange throughout the lung is not uniform, but varies depending on the $\dot{V}/\dot{Q}$ ratio of each region.

From top to bottom of the lung, the gradient is more marked for perfusion ($\dot{Q}$) than for ventilation ($\dot{V}$); thus, the $\dot{V}/\dot{Q}$ ratio is lower in the dependent regions of the lung.

To understand the effects on gas-exchange of altering the $\dot{V}/\dot{Q}$ ratio, first consider the individual alveolus and then the more complex model with multiple alveoli and variable $\dot{V}/\dot{Q}$ ratios. In a single alveolus, a continuous spectrum exists for the possible relationships between $\dot{V}$ and $\dot{Q}$ (Fig. 1-7). At one extreme, where $\dot{V}$ is maintained and $\dot{Q}$ approaches 0, the $\dot{V}/\dot{Q}$ ratio approaches infinity. When there is actually no perfusion ($\dot{Q} = 0$), the ventilation is wasted insofar as gas exchange is concerned, and the alveolus is part of the dead space. At the other extreme, $\dot{V}$ approaches 0 while $\dot{Q}$ is preserved, and the $\dot{V}/\dot{Q}$ ratio approaches 0. When there is no ventilation ($\dot{V} = 0$), a "shunt" exists, oxygenation does not occur during transit through the pulmonary circulation, and the hemoglobin is still desaturated when it leaves the pulmonary capillary.

Ventilation-perfusion ratios within each alveolar-capillary unit range from $\dot{V}/\dot{Q} = \infty$ (dead space) to $\dot{V}/\dot{Q} = 0$ (shunt).

Again dealing with the extremes, for an alveolar-capillary unit acting as dead space ($\dot{V}/\dot{Q} = \infty$), P_{O_2} in the alveolus is equal to that in air, i.e., 150 torr (taking into account the fact that air in the alveolus is saturated with water vapor), whereas P_{CO_2} is 0, because no blood and therefore no CO_2 is in contact with alveolar gas. With a region of true dead space, there is no blood flow, so there are no gas tensions in blood leaving the alveolus. If there were a minute

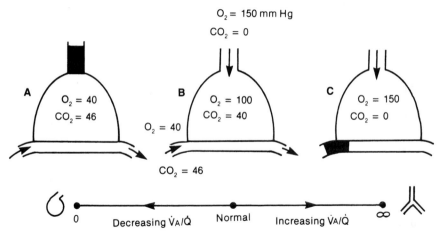

Figure 1-7 ■— Spectrum of ventilation-perfusion ratios within single alveolar-capillary unit. In B, ventilation and perfusion are well matched. In A, ventilation is obstructed, but perfusion is preserved, and alveolar-capillary unit is behaving as a shunt. In C, no blood flow is reaching the alveolus; thus, ventilation is wasted, serving as dead space ventilation. (Adapted from West JB: Ventilation/Blood Flow and Gas Exchange, 3rd ed. Oxford, Blackwell Scientific Publications, 1977, p 36.)

amount of blood flow, that is, if the $\dot{V}/\dot{Q}$ ratio approached but did not reach ∞, then the blood also would have a P_{O_2} approaching (but slightly less than) 150 torr and a P_{CO_2} approaching (but slightly more than) 0 torr. At the other extreme, for an alveolar-capillary unit acting as a shunt ($\dot{V}/\dot{Q} = 0$), blood leaving the capillary has gas tensions identical to those in mixed venous blood, i.e., $P_{O_2} = 40$ torr and $P_{CO_2} = 46$ torr, assuming the rest of the lung functioned well enough to maintain normal arterial and mixed venous gas tensions.

In reality, alveolar-capillary units may fall anywhere along this continuum of $\dot{V}/\dot{Q}$ ratios. The higher the $\dot{V}/\dot{Q}$ ratio in an alveolar-capillary unit, the closer the unit comes to behaving like an area of dead space and the more the P_{O_2} approaches 150 torr and the P_{CO_2} approaches 0 torr. The lower the $\dot{V}/\dot{Q}$ ratio, the closer the unit comes to behaving like a shunt, and the more the P_{O_2} and P_{CO_2} of blood leaving the capillary approach the gas tensions in mixed venous blood (40 and 46 torr, respectively). This continuum is depicted in Figure 1-8, in which moving to the left signifies decreasing the $\dot{V}/\dot{Q}$ ratio and moving to the right means increasing the $\dot{V}/\dot{Q}$ ratio. The ideal circumstance lies between these extremes, in which $P_{O_2} = 100$ torr and $P_{CO_2} = 40$ torr.

When multiple alveolar-capillary units are considered, the net P_{O_2} and P_{CO_2} of the resulting pulmonary venous blood depend on the total O_2 or CO_2 content and the total volume of blood collected from each of the contributing units. Considering P_{CO_2} first, areas with relatively high $\dot{V}/\dot{Q}$ ratios contribute blood with a lower P_{CO_2} than do areas with low $\dot{V}/\dot{Q}$ ratios. However, inasmuch as the relationship between CO_2 content and P_{CO_2} is nearly linear over the range of concern, if blood having a higher P_{CO_2} and CO_2 content mixes with an equal volume of blood having a lower P_{CO_2} and CO_2 content, an intermediate P_{CO_2} and CO_2 content (approximately halfway between) results.

In contrast, a high P_{O_2} in blood coming from a region with a high $\dot{V}/\dot{Q}$ ratio cannot compensate for blood with a low P_{O_2} from a region with a low $\dot{V}/\dot{Q}$ ratio. The difference stems from the shape of the oxyhemoglobin dissociation curve; once hemoglobin is nearly saturated with O_2, increasing the P_{O_2} does not boost the O_2 content. Therefore, blood with a higher than normal

Regions of the lung with a high $\dot{V}/\dot{Q}$ ratio and a high P_{O_2} cannot compensate for regions with a low $\dot{V}/\dot{Q}$ ratio and low P_{O_2}.

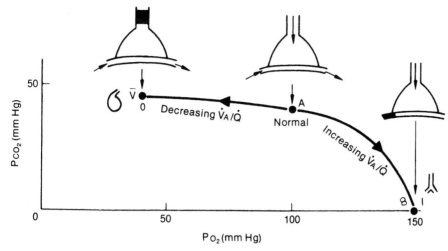

Figure 1-8 ▪— Continuum of alveolar gas composition at different ventilation-perfusion ratios within single alveolar-capillary unit. Line is called "ventilation-perfusion ratio line"; at extreme left side of line, $\dot{V}/\dot{Q} = 0$ (shunt), at extreme right side of line, $\dot{V}/\dot{Q} = \infty$ (dead space). (Adapted from West JB: Ventilation/Blood Flow and Gas Exchange, 3rd ed. Oxford, Blackwell Scientific Publications, 1977, p 37.)

PO_2 does not have a correspondingly higher O_2 content and cannot compensate for blood with a low PO_2 and low O_2 content.

In the normal lung, regional differences in the $\dot{V}/\dot{Q}$ ratio affect gas tensions in blood coming from specific regions as well as gas tensions in the resulting arterial blood. At the apices, where the $\dot{V}/\dot{Q}$ ratio is approximately 3.3, $PO_2 = 132$ torr and $PCO_2 = 28$ torr; at the bases, where the $\dot{V}/\dot{Q}$ ratio is approximately 0.63, $PO_2 = 89$ torr and $PCO_2 = 42$ torr. As discussed, the net PO_2 and PCO_2 of the combined blood coming from the apices, the bases, and the areas in between are a function of the relative amounts of blood from each of these areas and the gas contents of each.

In disease states, ventilation-perfusion mismatch frequently is much more extreme, resulting in clinically significant gas-exchange abnormalities. When an area of lung behaves as a shunt or even as a region of very low $\dot{V}/\dot{Q}$ ratio, blood coming from this area has a low O_2 content and saturation, which cannot be compensated for by blood from relatively preserved regions of lung. If $\dot{V}/\dot{Q}$ mismatch is severe, particularly with areas of a high $\dot{V}/\dot{Q}$ ratio, this can effectively produce dead space and therefore decrease the alveolar ventilation to other areas of the lung carrying a disproportionate share of the perfusion. Because CO_2 excretion depends on alveolar ventilation, PCO_2 may rise unless there is an overall increase in the minute ventilation to restore the effective alveolar ventilation.

ABNORMALITIES IN GAS EXCHANGE

The net effect of disturbances in the normal pattern of gas-exchange can be assessed by measurement of the gas tensions (PO_2 and PCO_2) in arterial blood. Although the information that can be obtained from arterial blood gas measurement is discussed further in Chapter 3, the mechanisms of hypoxemia (decreased arterial PO_2) and hypercapnia (increased PCO_2) are considered here because they relate to the physiologic principles just discussed.

Hypoxemia

Blood that has traversed pulmonary capillaries leaves with a P_{O_2} that should be in equilibrium with and almost identical to the P_{O_2} in companion alveoli. Although it is difficult to measure the O_2 tension in alveolar gas, it can be conveniently calculated by a formula known as the *alveolar gas equation*. A simplified version of this formula is relatively easy to use and can be extremely useful in the clinical setting, particularly when trying to deduce why a patient is hypoxemic. The alveolar O_2 tension $(P_{A_{O_2}})$* can be calculated by Equation 1-7:

$$P_{A_{O_2}} = F_{I_{O_2}}(P_B - P_{H_2O}) - P_{A_{CO_2}}/R \qquad (1\text{-}7)$$

$F_{I_{O_2}}$ is the fractional content of inspired O_2 ($F_{I_{O_2}}$ of air = 0.21); P_B is barometric pressure (approximately 760 torr at sea level); P_{H_2O} is the vapor pressure of water in the alveoli (at full saturation at 37° C, P_{H_2O} = 47 torr); $P_{A_{CO_2}}$ is alveolar CO_2 tension (which can be assumed to be identical to arterial CO_2 tension, $P_{a_{CO_2}}$); and R is the respiratory quotient (CO_2 production divided by O_2 consumption, usually about 0.8). In practice, for the patient breathing room air ($F_{I_{O_2}}$ = 0.21), the equation is often simplified. When numbers are substituted for $F_{I_{O_2}}$, P_B, and P_{H_2O}, and when $P_{a_{CO_2}}$ is used instead of $P_{A_{CO_2}}$, the resulting equation (at sea level) is the following (Equation 1-8):

$$P_{A_{O_2}} = 150 - 1.25 \times P_{a_{CO_2}} \qquad (1\text{-}8)$$

By calculating the $P_{A_{O_2}}$, the expected $P_{a_{O_2}}$ can be determined. Even in a normal person, $P_{A_{O_2}}$ is greater than $P_{a_{O_2}}$ by an amount that is called the *alveolar-arterial oxygen difference* or *gradient* (commonly abbreviated $A_aD_{O_2}$). There are two main reasons why a gradient exists even in normal individuals: (1) A small amount of the cardiac output behaves as a shunt, without ever going through the pulmonary capillary bed. This includes venous blood from the bronchial circulation, a portion of which drains into the pulmonary veins, and coronary venous blood draining via thebesian veins directly into the left ventricle. Desaturated blood from these sources lowers the O_2 tension in the resulting arterial blood. (2) Ventilation-perfusion gradients from the top to the bottom of the lung result in somewhat less oxygenated blood from the bases combining with better oxygenated blood from the apices.

The $A_aD_{O_2}$ normally is less than approximately 15 torr, although it increases with age. There are several reasons why it may be elevated in disease. First, a shunt may be present, so that some desaturated blood combines with fully saturated blood and lowers the P_{O_2} in the resulting arterial blood. The following are common causes of a shunt:

1. Intracardiac lesions, with a right-to-left shunt at the atrial or ventricular level—for example, in an atrial or ventricular septal defect. Note that a left-to-right shunt does not affect either the $A_aD_{O_2}$ or the arterial P_{O_2}, because its net effect is to recycle already oxygenated blood through the pulmonary vasculature, not to dilute oxygenated blood with desaturated blood.
2. Structural abnormalities of the pulmonary vasculature that result in direct communication between pulmonary arterial and venous systems—for example, pulmonary arteriovenous malformations.
3. Pulmonary diseases that result in filling of the alveolar spaces with fluid (e.g., pulmonary edema) or complete alveolar collapse. Either

*By convention, "A" refers to alveolar, "a" to arterial.

process can result in complete loss of ventilation to the affected alveoli, while some perfusion through the associated capillaries may continue.

Another cause of an elevated $AaDo_2$ is ventilation-perfusion mismatch. Even when total ventilation and total perfusion to both lungs are normal, if some areas receive less ventilation and more perfusion (low $\dot{V}/\dot{Q}$ ratio) while others receive more ventilation and less perfusion (high $\dot{V}/\dot{Q}$ ratio), then the $AaDo_2$ increases, and hypoxemia results. As just mentioned, the reason for this phenomenon is that areas having a low $\dot{V}/\dot{Q}$ ratio provide relatively desaturated blood with a low O_2 content. Blood coming from regions with a high $\dot{V}/\dot{Q}$ ratio cannot compensate for this problem, inasmuch as the hemoglobin is already fully saturated and cannot increase its O_2 content further by the increased ventilation (Fig. 1-9).

In practice, true shunt ($\dot{V}/\dot{Q} = 0$) and $\dot{V}/\dot{Q}$ mismatch (with areas of $\dot{V}/\dot{Q}$ that are low but not 0) can be distinguished by having the patient inhale 100

Ventilation-perfusion mismatch and shunting are the two important mechanisms for elevation of the alveolar-arterial O_2 difference ($AaDo_2$).

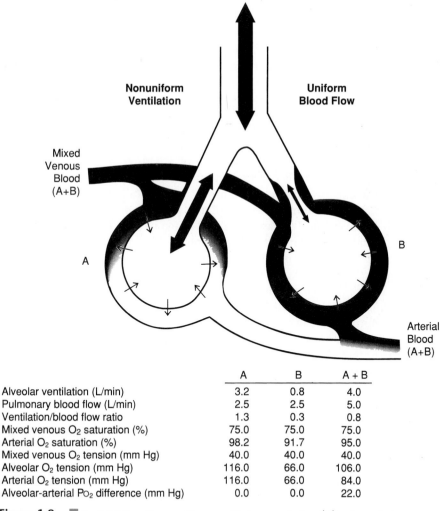

	A	B	A + B
Alveolar ventilation (L/min)	3.2	0.8	4.0
Pulmonary blood flow (L/min)	2.5	2.5	5.0
Ventilation/blood flow ratio	1.3	0.3	0.8
Mixed venous O_2 saturation (%)	75.0	75.0	75.0
Arterial O_2 saturation (%)	98.2	91.7	95.0
Mixed venous O_2 tension (mm Hg)	40.0	40.0	40.0
Alveolar O_2 tension (mm Hg)	116.0	66.0	106.0
Arterial O_2 tension (mm Hg)	116.0	66.0	84.0
Alveolar-arterial Po_2 difference (mm Hg)	0.0	0.0	22.0

Figure 1-9 ▬— Example of nonuniform ventilation producing $\dot{V}/\dot{Q}$ mismatch in two-alveolus model. In this instance, perfusion is equally distributed between the two alveoli. The calculations demonstrate how $\dot{V}/\dot{Q}$ mismatch lowers arterial PO_2 and causes elevated alveolar-arterial oxygen difference. (Adapted from Comroe JH: The Lung, 2nd ed. Chicago, Year Book Medical Publishers, 1962, p 94.)

percent O_2. In the former case, increasing the inspired PO_2 does not add further O_2 to the shunted blood, and O_2 content does not increase significantly. In the latter case, the alveolar and capillary PO_2 rise considerably with additional O_2, fully saturating blood coming even from regions with a low $\dot{V}/\dot{Q}$ ratio, and arterial PO_2 rises substantially.

A third cause for an elevated $AaDO_2$ can be postulated theoretically, although in reality it rarely occurs. This cause is a "diffusion block" in which the PO_2 in pulmonary capillary blood does not reach equilibrium with alveolar gas. If the interface (i.e., the tissue within the alveolar wall) between the capillary and the alveolar lumen were thickened, one could hypothesize that O_2 would not diffuse as readily and that the PO_2 in pulmonary capillary blood would never reach the PO_2 of alveolar gas. Even with a thickened alveolar wall, however, there is still sufficient time for this equilibrium; unless the transit time of erythrocytes also is significantly shortened, failure to equilibrate does not appear to be a problem. One of the rare times this occurs may be during exercise in a patient with interstitial lung disease, as will be discussed later. For most practical purposes, a diffusion block should be considered only a hypothetical rather than a realistic mechanism for increasing the $AaDO_2$ and causing hypoxemia.

Increasing the difference between alveolar and arterial PO_2 is not the only mechanism that results in hypoxemia. The alveolar PO_2 can be decreased, which must necessarily lower arterial PO_2 if the $AaDO_2$ remains constant. Referring back to the alveolar gas equation, it is relatively easy to see that alveolar PO_2 drops if barometric pressure falls (e.g., with altitude) or if alveolar PCO_2 rises (e.g., with hypoventilation). In the latter circumstance, when total alveolar ventilation falls, PCO_2 in alveolar gas rises at the same time that alveolar PO_2 falls. Hypoventilation is relatively common in lung disease and can easily be identified by the presence of a high PCO_2 accompanying the hypoxemia. If the PCO_2 is elevated and the $AaDO_2$ is normal, then hypoventilation is the exclusive cause of the low PO_2. If $AaDO_2$ is elevated, then either $\dot{V}/\dot{Q}$ mismatch or shunting also contributes to the hypoxemia.

In summary, lung disease can result in hypoxemia for multiple reasons. Shunting and ventilation-perfusion mismatch are associated with an elevated $AaDO_2$; they can often be distinguished, if necessary, by inhalation of 100 percent O_2, which markedly increases PaO_2 with $\dot{V}/\dot{Q}$ mismatch but not with true shunting. In contrast, hypoventilation (identified by a high $PaCO_2$) and a low inspired PO_2 lower alveolar PO_2 and cause hypoxemia, although $AaDO_2$ remains normal. Because many of the disease processes examined in this text cause several pathophysiologic abnormalities, it is not at all uncommon to see more than one of the aforementioned mechanisms producing hypoxemia in a particular patient.

Hypercapnia

As discussed earlier in the section on Ventilation, alveolar ventilation is the prime determinant of arterial PCO_2, assuming that CO_2 production remains constant. It is clear that alveolar ventilation is compromised either by decreasing the total minute ventilation (without changing the relative proportion of dead space and alveolar ventilation) or by keeping the total minute ventilation constant and increasing the relative proportion of dead space to alveolar ventilation. A simple way to produce the latter circumstance is to change the pattern of breathing, that is, by decreasing the tidal volume and increasing the frequency of breathing. With a lower tidal volume, a larger proportion

---

When hypoventilation is the sole cause of hypoxemia, $AaDO_2$ is normal.

Mechanisms of hypoxemia:

1. Shunt
2. $\dot{V}/\dot{Q}$ mismatch
3. Hypoventilation
4. Low inspired PO_2

of each breath ventilates the anatomic dead space, and the proportion of alveolar ventilation to total ventilation must decrease.

In addition, if significant ventilation-perfusion mismatching is present, well-perfused areas may be underventilated, whereas underperfused areas receive a disproportionate amount of ventilation. The net effect of having a large proportion of ventilation go to poorly perfused areas is similar to that of increasing the dead space. By wasting this ventilation, the remainder of the lung with the large share of the perfusion is underventilated, and the net effect is to decrease the effective alveolar ventilation. In many disease conditions, when such significant $\dot{V}/\dot{Q}$ mismatch exists, any increase in the P_{CO_2} stimulates breathing, increases the total minute ventilation, and compensates for the effectively wasted ventilation.

Therefore, several causes of hypercapnia can be defined, all of which have in common a decrease in the effective alveolar ventilation. These include a decrease in the minute ventilation, an increase in the proportion of wasted ventilation, and significant ventilation-perfusion mismatch. By increasing the total minute ventilation, however, a patient is often capable of compensating for the latter two situations so that CO_2 retention does not result.

Increasing CO_2 production necessitates an increase in alveolar ventilation to avoid CO_2 retention. Thus, if alveolar ventilation does not rise to compensate for additional CO_2 production, hypercapnia also will result.

As is the case with hypoxemia, pathophysiologic explanations for hypercapnia do not necessarily follow such simple rules in which each case can be fully explained by one mechanism. In reality, several of these mechanisms may be operative, even in a particular patient.

A decrease in alveolar ventilation is the primary mechanism that causes hypercapnia.

References

Crystal RG, West JB, Weibel ER, and Barnes PJ (eds): The Lung: Scientific Foundations, 2nd ed. Philadelphia, Lippincott-Raven, 1997.

Hughes JMB and Pride NB (eds): Lung Function Tests: Physiological Principles and Clinical Applications. London, WB Saunders Co., 2000.

Leff AR and Schumacker PT: Respiratory Physiology: Basics and Applications. Philadelphia, WB Saunders Co., 1993.

Weibel ER: The Pathway for Oxygen: Structure and Function in the Mammalian Respiratory System. Cambridge, Harvard University Press, 1984.

Weinberger SE, Schwartzstein RM, and Weiss JW: Hypercapnia. N Engl J Med 321:1223–1231, 1989.

West JB: Respiratory Physiology—The Essentials, 6th ed. Baltimore, Lippincott Williams & Wilkins, 2000.

West JB: Ventilation/Blood Flow and Gas-Exchange, 5th ed. Oxford, Blackwell Scientific Publications, 1990.

chapter 2

Presentation of the Patient with Pulmonary Disease

DYSPNEA
COUGH
HEMOPTYSIS
CHEST PAIN

The patient with a pulmonary problem generally comes to the attention of the clinician for one of two reasons: (1) a complaint of a symptom that can be traced to a respiratory cause, or (2) an incidental finding of an abnormality on a chest radiograph. Although the former presentation is more common, the latter is not uncommon when a radiograph is obtained either as part of a routine examination or for evaluation of a seemingly unrelated problem. In this chapter the focus is on the first case, the patient who comes to the physician with a respiratory-related complaint. In the next and in subsequent chapters, there is frequent reference to abnormal radiographic findings as the clue to the presence of a pulmonary disorder.

Four particularly common (as well as a number of less common) symptoms bring the patient with lung disease to the physician: dyspnea (and its variants), cough (with or without sputum production), hemoptysis, and chest pain. Each of these symptoms, however, to a greater or lesser extent, may result from a nonpulmonary disorder, especially primary cardiac disease. For each symptom, a discussion of some of the important clinical features is followed by the pathophysiologic features and the differential diagnosis.

DYSPNEA

Dyspnea, or shortness of breath, is frequently a difficult symptom for the physician to evaluate because it is such a subjective feeling experienced by the patient. It is perhaps best defined as an uncomfortable sensation (or awareness) of one's own breathing, to which, normally, little attention is paid. However, the term dyspnea probably subsumes several sensations that are qualitatively distinct. As a result, when patients are asked to describe in more detail their sensation of breathlessness, their descriptions tend to fall into three primary categories: (1) air hunger or suffocation, (2) increased effort or work of breathing, and (3) chest tightness.

Not only is the symptom of dyspnea highly subjective and describable in different ways, but the patient's appreciation of it and its importance to the physician depend heavily on the stimulus or amount of activity required to precipitate it. The physician also must take into account how the stimulus, when quantified, compares with the patient's usual level of activity. For example, a patient who is limited in exertion by a nonpulmonary problem may not experience any shortness of breath even in the presence of additional and significant lung disease; if the person were more active, however, dyspnea would become readily apparent. A marathon runner who experiences a new symptom of shortness of breath after 5 miles of running may warrant more concern than would an elderly man who for many years has had a stable symptom of shortness of breath after walking 3 blocks.

Dyspnea should be distinguished from several other signs or symptoms that may have an entirely different significance. *Tachypnea* is a rapid respiratory rate (greater than the usual value of 12 to 20/min). Tachypnea may be present with or without dyspnea, just as dyspnea does not necessarily entail the finding of tachypnea on physical examination. *Hyperventilation* is ventilation that is greater than the amount required to maintain normal CO_2 elimination. Hence, a decrease in PCO_2 in arterial blood is the hallmark of hyperventilation. Finally, the symptom of exertional fatigue must be distinguished from dyspnea. Fatigue may be due to cardiovascular, neuromuscular, or other nonpulmonary diseases, and the implication of this symptom is quite different from that of true shortness of breath.

> Dyspnea is distinct from tachypnea, hyperventilation, and exertional fatigue.

There are also some variations on the theme of dyspnea. *Orthopnea*, or shortness of breath on assuming the recumbent position, is often quantitated by the number of pillows or angle of elevation necessary to relieve or prevent the sensation. One of the main causes of orthopnea is an increase in venous return and central intravascular volume on assuming the recumbent position. In patients with cardiac decompensation and either overt or subclinical congestive heart failure, the increment in left atrial and left ventricular filling may result in pulmonary vascular congestion and pulmonary interstitial or alveolar edema. Thus, orthopnea frequently suggests cardiac disease and some element of congestive heart failure. However, some patients with primary pulmonary disease experience orthopnea, such as those with a significant amount of secretions who have more difficulty handling their secretions when they are recumbent.

> Orthopnea, often associated with left ventricular failure, may also accompany primary pulmonary disease.

Paroxysmal nocturnal dyspnea is waking from sleep with dyspnea. As with orthopnea the recumbent position is important, but this symptom differs from orthopnea in that it does not occur soon after lying down. Although the implication with regard to underlying cardiac decompensation still applies, the increase in central intravascular volume is due more to a slow mobilization of tissue fluid, such as peripheral edema, than to a rapid redistribution of intravascular volume from peripheral to central vessels.

Variants that are much more uncommon will only be mentioned. *Platypnea* is shortness of breath when in the upright position; it is the opposite of orthopnea. *Trepopnea* is shortness of breath when lying on one's side. Patients with this symptom report dyspnea on either the right or the left side; it can be relieved by moving to the opposite lateral position.

Returning to the more general symptom of dyspnea, there are a number of proposed sources or mechanisms rather than a single common thread linking the diverse responsible conditions. In particular, neural output reflecting central nervous system respiratory drive appears to be integrated with input from a variety of mechanical receptors in the chest wall, respiratory muscles, airways, and pulmonary vasculature. Presumably, the relative contributions of each source differ from disease to disease and from patient to

The sensation of dyspnea probably has a number of underlying pathophysiologic mechanisms.

patient, and are responsible for the qualitatively different sensations all subsumed under the term dyspnea.

In an attempt to link dyspnea with underlying pathophysiologic mechanisms, we can return to the three qualitatively distinct sensations of breathlessness mentioned at the beginning of this section. Patients who describe their breathlessness as a sense of air hunger or suffocation often have increased respiratory drive, which can in part be related to either a high PCO_2 or a low PO_2, but can also occur even in the absence of respiratory system or gas-exchange abnormalities. The sensation of increased effort or work of breathing is commonly experienced by patients who have increased resistance to airflow or abnormally stiff lungs. The sensation of chest tightness, frequently noted by patients with asthma, probably arises from intrathoracic receptors that are stimulated by bronchoconstriction. Because some disorders may produce breathlessness by more than one mechanism (e.g., asthma may have components of all three of the above mechanisms), there may often be overlap or a mixture of these different sensations.

There is a broad differential diagnosis of the disorders that result in dyspnea (Table 2-1), and it is perhaps best to separate them into the major categories of respiratory and cardiovascular disease. In addition, dyspnea may be present in conditions associated with increased respiratory drive, even in the absence of underlying respiratory or cardiovascular disease, or it may have an anxiety-related or psychosomatic origin.

The first major category consists of disorders at many levels of the respiratory system—airways, pulmonary parenchyma, pulmonary vasculature, pleura, and bellows—that can cause dyspnea. Airway diseases that cause dyspnea result primarily from obstruction to airflow, occurring anywhere from the upper airway to the large, medium, and small intrathoracic bronchi and bronchioles. Upper airway obstruction, which is defined here as obstruction above or including the level of the vocal cords, is caused primarily by foreign bodies, tumors, edema (e.g., with anaphylaxis), and stenosis. A clue to upper airway obstruction may be the presence of disproportionate difficulty during inspiration and an audible, prolonged gasping sound called *inspiratory stridor*. The reason for the inspiratory problem is considered in Chapter 7, in which the pathophysiology of upper airway obstruction is discussed.

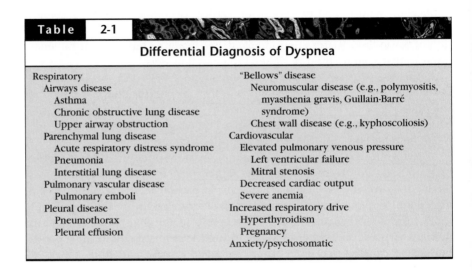

Table 2-1

Differential Diagnosis of Dyspnea

Respiratory
  Airways disease
    Asthma
    Chronic obstructive lung disease
    Upper airway obstruction
  Parenchymal lung disease
    Acute respiratory distress syndrome
    Pneumonia
    Interstitial lung disease
  Pulmonary vascular disease
    Pulmonary emboli
  Pleural disease
    Pneumothorax
    Pleural effusion
"Bellows" disease
  Neuromuscular disease (e.g., polymyositis, myasthenia gravis, Guillain-Barré syndrome)
  Chest wall disease (e.g., kyphoscoliosis)
Cardiovascular
  Elevated pulmonary venous pressure
    Left ventricular failure
    Mitral stenosis
  Decreased cardiac output
  Severe anemia
Increased respiratory drive
  Hyperthyroidism
  Pregnancy
Anxiety/psychosomatic

Airways below the level of the vocal cords, from the trachea down to the small bronchioles, are the ones more commonly involved with disorders that produce dyspnea. An isolated problem, such as an airway tumor, usually does not by itself cause dyspnea unless it occurs in the trachea or in a major bronchus. In contrast, diseases such as asthma and chronic obstructive pulmonary disease have widespread effects throughout the tracheobronchial tree, with airway narrowing resulting from spasm, edema, secretions, or loss of radial support (see Chapter 4). With this type of obstruction, difficulty with expiration generally predominates over that with inspiration, and the physical findings associated with obstruction (wheezing, prolongation of airflow) are more prominent on expiration.

The category of pulmonary parenchymal disease includes disorders causing inflammation, infiltration, fluid accumulation, or scarring of the alveolar structures. Such disorders may be diffuse in nature, as with the many causes of pulmonary fibrosis, or they may be more localized, as occurs with a bacterial pneumonia.

Pulmonary vascular disease results in blockage or loss of vessels in the lung. The most common acute type of this disease is pulmonary embolism, in which one or many pulmonary vessels are occluded by thrombi originating in systemic veins. Chronically, vessels may be blocked by recurrent pulmonary emboli or by inflammatory or scarring processes that result in thickening of vessel walls or obliteration of the vascular lumen.

Two major disorders affecting the pleura may result in dyspnea: pneumothorax (air in the pleural space) and pleural effusion (liquid in the pleural space). With pleural effusions, there generally must be a substantial amount of fluid in the pleural space to result in dyspnea, unless the patient also has significant underlying cardiopulmonary disease or there are additional complicating features.

The term *bellows* is used here for the final category of respiratory-related disorders causing dyspnea. It refers to the pump system that works under the control of a central nervous system generator to expand the lungs and allow airflow. This pump system includes a variety of muscles (primarily but not exclusively diaphragm and intercostal) and the chest wall. Primary disease affecting the muscles, their nerve supply, or neuromuscular interaction—including polymyositis, myasthenia gravis, and Guillain-Barré syndrome—may result in dyspnea. Deformity of the chest wall, particularly kyphoscoliosis, produces dyspnea by several pathophysiologic mechanisms, not the least of which is the increased work of breathing. These disorders of the respiratory bellows are covered in Chapter 19.

The second major category of disorders that produce dyspnea is cardiovascular. In the majority of cases, the feature that such patients have in common is an elevated pressure in the pulmonary veins and capillaries, which leads to a transudation or leakage of fluid into the pulmonary interstitium and the alveoli. Left ventricular failure, from either ischemic or valvular heart disease, is the most common example. In addition, mitral stenosis, with increased left atrial pressure, produces elevated pulmonary venous and capillary pressures even though left ventricular function and pressure are normal. A frequent accompaniment of the dyspnea associated with these forms of cardiac disease is orthopnea or paroxysmal nocturnal dyspnea, or both. Although a worsening of dyspnea in the supine position is not specific to pulmonary venous hypertension and can also be found in some patients with pulmonary disease, improvement of dyspnea in the supine position is a point against left ventricular failure as the causative factor.

The third category of conditions associated with dyspnea includes those characterized by increased respiratory drive but no underlying cardiopulmonary disease. Both thyroid hormone and progesterone augment respiratory drive, and patients with hyperthyroidism and women who are pregnant commonly complain of dyspnea. Dyspnea during pregnancy often starts before the abdomen is noticeably distended, indicating that diaphragmatic elevation from the enlarging uterus is not the primary explanation for the dyspnea.

Finally, dyspnea may be due to anxiety or to other psychosomatic problems. Because the sensation of dyspnea is such a subjective one, any awareness of one's breathing may start a self-perpetuating problem; the patient breathes faster, becomes more aware of breathing, and finally has a sensation of frank dyspnea. At the extreme, one can hyperventilate and lower the arterial P_{CO_2} sufficiently to cause additional symptoms of lightheadedness and tingling, particularly of the fingers and around the mouth. Of course, patients who may seem anxious or who have a history of psychologic problems can also have lung disease. Similarly, patients with lung or heart disease can also at times have dyspnea with a functional cause unrelated to their underlying disease process.

COUGH

Cough is a symptom that everyone has experienced at some point. It is a physiologic mechanism for clearing and protecting the airway and does not necessarily imply disease. Normally, cough is protective against food or other foreign material entering the airway, and it is also responsible for aiding in clearance of secretions produced within the tracheobronchial tree. Generally, mucociliary clearance is adequate to propel secretions upward through the trachea and into the larynx so that they can be removed from the airway and swallowed. If, however, the mucociliary clearance mechanism is temporarily damaged or not functioning well, or if it is overwhelmed by excessive production of secretions, then cough becomes an important additional mechanism for clearing the tracheobronchial tree.

Irritant receptors triggering cough are located primarily in larger airways.

Cough is usually initiated by stimulation of receptors (called irritant receptors) at any of a number of locations. These irritant receptor nerve endings are found primarily in the larynx, trachea, and major bronchi, particularly at points of bifurcation. However, there are also sensory receptors located in other parts of the upper airway as well as on the pleura, the diaphragm, and even the pericardium. Irritation of these nerve endings initiates an impulse that travels via afferent nerves (primarily the vagus but also trigeminal, glossopharyngeal, and phrenic) to a poorly defined cough center in the medulla. The efferent signal is then carried in the recurrent laryngeal nerve (a branch of the vagus), which controls closure of the glottis, and in phrenic and spinal nerves, which effect contraction of the diaphragm and the expiratory muscles of the chest and abdominal walls. The initial part of the cough sequence is a deep inspiration to a high lung volume, followed by closure of the glottis, contraction of the expiratory muscles, and opening of the glottis. When the glottis suddenly opens, contraction of the expiratory muscles and relaxation of the diaphragm produce an explosive rush of air at high velocity, which transports airway secretions or foreign material out of the tracheobronchial tree.

The major causes of cough are listed in Table 2-2. Cough commonly results from an airway irritant, regardless of whether the person has respira-

Table	2-2	
Differential Diagnosis of Cough		
Airway irritants	Bronchiectasis	
Inhaled smoke, dusts, fumes	Neoplasm	
Aspiration	External compression by a node or mass lesion	
Gastric contents	Reactive airways disease (asthma)	
Oral secretions	Parenchymal disease	
Foreign body	Pneumonia	
Postnasal drip	Lung abscess	
Airways disease	Interstitial lung disease	
Upper respiratory tract infection	Congestive heart failure	
Postinfectious cough	Miscellaneous	
Acute or chronic bronchitis	Drug-induced (angiotensin-converting enzyme	
Eosinophilic bronchitis	inhibitors)	

tory system disease. The most common inhaled irritant is cigarette smoke; noxious fumes, dusts, and chemicals also stimulate irritant receptors and result in cough. Secretions due to postnasal drip are a particularly common cause of cough, presumably triggering the symptom via stimulation of laryngeal cough receptors. Aspiration of gastric contents or upper airway secretions, which amounts to "inhalation" of liquid or solid material, can also result in cough, the cause of which may be unrecognized if the aspiration has not been clinically apparent. In the case of gastroesophageal reflux, in which gastric acid flows retrograde into the esophagus, cough is due not only to aspiration of gastric contents from the esophagus or pharynx into the tracheobronchial tree, but also to reflex mechanisms triggered by acid entry into the lower esophagus and mediated by the vagal nerve.

Cough caused by respiratory system disease comes mainly but not exclusively from disorders affecting the airway. Most commonly, viruses or other organisms (such as *Mycoplasma, Chlamydia,* and *Bordetella pertussis*) producing upper respiratory tract infections also affect parts of the tracheobronchial tree, and the airway inflammation results in a bothersome cough lasting sometimes from weeks to months. Bacterial infections of the lung, either acute (pneumonia, acute bronchitis) or chronic (bronchiectasis, chronic bronchitis, lung abscess), generally have an airway component and an impressive amount of associated coughing. Space-occupying lesions in the tracheobronchial tree (tumors, foreign bodies, granulomas) and external lesions compressing the airway (mediastinal masses, lymph nodes, other tumors) commonly manifest as cough secondary to airway irritation. Hyperirritable airways with airway constriction, as in asthma, are frequently associated with cough, even when a specific inhaled irritant is not identified. The more readily recognized manifestations of asthma—wheezing and dyspnea—may not be apparent, and cough may be the sole presenting symptom. Recently, an entity of unknown etiology called *eosinophilic bronchitis,* characterized by eosinophilic inflammation of the airway in the absence of asthma, has also been identified as a cause of chronic cough.

Patients with pulmonary interstitial disease may also have cough, probably owing more to secondary airway or pleural involvement, inasmuch as few irritant receptors are in the lung itself. In congestive heart failure, cough may be related to the same unclear mechanism operative in patients with interstitial lung disease, or it may be secondary to bronchial edema.

A variety of miscellaneous causes of cough, such as irritation of the tympanic membrane by wax or by a hair or of one of the afferent nerves by osteophytes or by neural tumors, have been identified but will not be discussed in further detail here. With the widespread use of angiotensin-converting enzyme inhibitors (e.g., captopril, enalapril) for treatment of hypertension and congestive heart failure, cough has been recognized as a relatively common side effect of these agents. Because angiotensin-converting enzyme breaks down bradykinin and other inflammatory peptides, accumulation of bradykinin or other peptides in patients taking these inhibitors may be responsible by stimulating receptors capable of initiating cough. Finally, coughing may be a nervous habit that can be especially prominent when the patient is anxious, although the physician must not neglect the possibility that an organic cause may also be present.

The symptom of cough is generally characterized by whether it is productive or nonproductive of sputum. Virtually any cause of cough may be productive at times of small amounts of clear or mucoid sputum. Thick yellow or green sputum, however, indicates the presence of numerous leukocytes in the sputum, either neutrophils or eosinophils. Neutrophils may be present with just an inflammatory process of the airways or parenchyma, but they also frequently reflect the presence of a bacterial infection. Specific examples include bacterial bronchitis, bronchiectasis, lung abscess, and pneumonia. Eosinophils, which can be seen after special preparation of the sputum, often occur with bronchial asthma, whether or not an allergic component plays a role, and in the much less common entity of eosinophilic bronchitis.

In clinical practice, cough is often divided into two categories, acute or chronic, depending upon the duration of the symptom. *Acute cough*, defined by a duration of less than three weeks, is most commonly due to an acute viral respiratory tract infection, such as the common cold. When cough following an upper respiratory tract infection lasts longer than three weeks, it is often called a *postinfectious cough* and is due to persistent airway inflammation, postnasal drip, or bronchial hyperresponsiveness (as one sees with asthma). The other major temporal category, *chronic cough,* is defined by a duration of three or more weeks. Whereas chronic bronchitis is a particularly common cause of cough in smokers, the three most common causes of chronic cough in nonsmokers are postnasal drip, gastroesophageal reflux, and asthma. In all cases, however, the clinician must keep in mind the broader differential diagnosis of cough that is outlined in Table 2-2, recognizing that cough may sometimes be a marker and the initial presenting symptom of a more serious disease, such as carcinoma of the lung.

Yellow or green sputum reflects the presence of numerous leukocytes, either neutrophils or eosinophils.

HEMOPTYSIS

Hemoptysis is coughing or spitting up blood derived from airways or the lung itself. When the patient complains of coughing or spitting up blood, it is not always apparent whether the blood has in fact originated from the respiratory system. Other sources of blood include the nasopharynx (particularly in the common nosebleed), the mouth (even lip or tongue biting can be mistaken for hemoptysis), and the upper gastrointestinal tract (esophagus, stomach, and duodenum). The patient is often able to distinguish some of these causes of pseudohemoptysis, but the physician also should search by examination for a mouth or nasopharyngeal source.

The major causes of hemoptysis can be divided into three categories by location: airways, pulmonary parenchyma, and vasculature (Table 2-3). Airways disease is the most common cause, with bronchitis, bronchiectasis, and bronchogenic carcinoma heading the list. Bronchial carcinoid tumor (bronchial adenoma), a less common neoplasm with variable malignant potential, also originates in the airway. In patients with acquired immunodeficiency syndrome, hemoptysis may be due to endobronchial (and/or pulmonary parenchymal) involvement with Kaposi's sarcoma.

Parenchymal causes of hemoptysis are frequently infectious in nature: tuberculosis, lung abscess, pneumonia, and a localized fungal infection (generally due to *Aspergillus* organisms) termed *mycetoma* ("fungus ball") or *aspergilloma.* Rarer causes of parenchymal hemorrhage are Goodpasture's syndrome, idiopathic pulmonary hemosiderosis, and Wegener's granulomatosis, some of which are discussed in Chapter 11.

Vascular lesions resulting in hemoptysis are generally related to problems with the pulmonary circulation. Pulmonary embolism, either with frank infarction or with reversible bleeding in the lung termed *congestive atelectasis,* is often a cause of hemoptysis. Elevated pressure in the pulmonary venous and capillary bed may also be associated with hemoptysis. Acutely elevated pressure, as in pulmonary edema, may have associated hemoptysis, commonly seen as pink- or red-tinged frothy sputum. Chronically elevated pulmonary venous pressure results from mitral stenosis, but this valvular lesion is relatively infrequent as a cause of significant hemoptysis. Vascular malformations, such as an arteriovenous malformation, may also be associated with the coughing of blood.

Finally, other miscellaneous etiologic factors in hemoptysis should be considered. Some of these fall into more than one of the aforementioned categories; others are included here because of their rarity. Cystic fibrosis affects both airways and pulmonary parenchyma. Although either component theoretically can cause hemoptysis, bronchiectasis (a common complication of cystic fibrosis) is most frequently responsible. Patients with impaired coagulation may rarely have pulmonary hemorrhage in the absence of other obvious causes of hemoptysis. An interesting but rare disorder is pulmonary endometriosis, in which implants of endometrial tissue in the lung can bleed coincident with the time of the menstrual cycle. Other causes are even more rare, and discussion of them is beyond the scope of this chapter.

> Diseases of the airways, e.g., bronchitis, are the most common causes of hemoptysis.

Table	2-3	
Differential Diagnosis of Hemoptysis		

Airways disease	Miscellaneous
Acute or chronic bronchitis	Goodpasture's syndrome
Bronchiectasis	Idiopathic pulmonary hemosiderosis
Bronchogenic carcinoma	Wegener's granulomatosis
Bronchial carcinoid tumor (bronchial	Vascular disease
adenoma)	Pulmonary embolism
Other endobronchial tumors (Kaposi's	Elevated pulmonary venous pressure
sarcoma, metastatic carcinoma)	Left ventricular failure
Parenchymal disease	Mitral stenosis
Tuberculosis	Vascular malformation
Lung abscess	Miscellaneous/rare causes
Pneumonia	Impaired coagulation
Mycetoma ("fungus ball")	Pulmonary endometriosis

CHEST PAIN

Chest pain can be associated with pleural, diaphragmatic, or mediastinal disease.

Chest pain as a reflection of respiratory system disease does not originate in the lung itself, which is free of sensory pain fibers. When chest pain does occur in this setting, its origin usually is either the parietal pleura (lining the inside of the chest wall), the diaphragm, or the mediastinum, each of which has extensive innervation by nerve fibers capable of pain sensation.

For the parietal pleura or the diaphragm, an inflammatory process of some sort generally produces the pain. When the diaphragm is involved, the pain commonly is referred to the shoulder. Pain from the parietal pleura, in contrast, is usually relatively well localized over the area of involvement. Pain involving the pleura or the diaphragm is often worsened on inspiration; in fact, chest pain that is particularly pronounced on inspiration is described as "pleuritic."

Inflammation of the parietal pleura producing pain is often secondary to pulmonary embolism or to pneumonia extending to the pleural surface. A pneumothorax may result in the acute onset of pleuritic pain, although the mechanism is not clear inasmuch as an acute inflammatory process is unlikely to be involved. Finally, some viruses, such as coxsackievirus, affect the pleura to produce pain; some diseases, particularly connective tissue disorders such as lupus, may result in episodes of pleuritic chest pain from a primary inflammatory process.

A variety of disorders originating in the mediastinum may result in pain; they may or may not be associated with additional problems in the lung itself. These disorders of the mediastinum are discussed in Chapter 16.

References

Dyspnea

American Thoracic Society: Dyspnea. Mechanisms, assessment, and management: a consensus statement. Am J Respir Crit Care Med 159:321-340, 1999.

Harver A, Mahler DA, Schwartzstein RM, and Baird JC: Descriptors of breathlessness in healthy individuals: distinct and separable constructs. Chest 118:679-690, 2000.

Luce JM and Luce JA: Management of dyspnea in patients with far-advanced lung disease. JAMA 285:1331-1337, 2001.

Manning HL and Schwartzstein RM: Pathophysiology of dyspnea. N Engl J Med 333:1547-1553, 1995.

Tobin MJ: Dyspnea: pathophysiologic basis, clinical presentation, and management. Arch Intern Med 150:1604-1613, 1990.

Wasserman K: Dyspnea on exertion: is it the heart or the lungs? JAMA 248:2039-2043, 1982.

Wasserman K and Casaburi R: Dyspnea: physiological and pathophysiological mechanisms. Annu Rev Med 39:503-515, 1988.

Cough

Carney IK et al: A systematic evaluation of mechanisms in chronic cough. Am J Respir Crit Care Med 156:211-216, 1997.

Gibson PG, Fujimara M, and Niimi A: Eosinophilic bronchitis: clinical manifestations and implications for treatment. Thorax 57:178-182, 2002.

Irwin RS, Curley FJ, and French CL: Chronic cough: the spectrum and frequency of causes, key components of the diagnostic evaluation, and outcome of specific therapy. Am Rev Respir Dis 141:640-647, 1990.

Irwin RS et al: Managing cough as a defense mechanism and as a symptom. A consensus panel report of the American College of Chest Physicians. Chest 114 (Suppl):133S-181S, 1998.

Irwin RS and Madison JM: The diagnosis and treatment of cough. N Engl J Med 343:1715-1721, 2000.

Irwin RS and Madison JM: Anatomical diagnostic protocol in evaluating chronic cough with specific reference to gastroesophageal reflux disease. Am J Med 108 (Suppl 4a):126S-130S, 2000.

Irwin RS and Madison JM: Symptom research on chronic cough: a historical perspective. Ann Intern Med 134:809-814, 2001.

Irwin RS and Madison JM: The persistently troublesome cough. Am J Respir Crit Care Med 165:1469-1474, 2002.
Israili ZH and Hall WD: Cough and angioneurotic edema associated with angiotensin-converting enzyme inhibitor therapy. Ann Intern Med 117:234-242, 1992.

Hemoptysis

Cahill BC and Ingbar DH: Massive hemoptysis: assessment and management. Clin Chest Med 15:147-168, 1994.
Israel RH and Poe RH: Hemoptysis. Clin Chest Med 8:197-205, 1987.
Jean-Baptiste E: Clinical assessment and management of massive hemoptysis. Crit Care Med 28:1642-1647, 2000.
Santiago S, Tobias J, and Williams AJ: A reappraisal of the causes of hemoptysis. Arch Intern Med 151:2449-2451, 1991.

Chest Pain

Branch WT Jr and McNeil BJ: Analysis of the differential diagnosis and assessment of pleuritic chest pain in young adults. Am J Med 75:671-679, 1983.
Donat WE: Chest pain: cardiac and noncardiac causes. Clin Chest Med 8:241-252, 1987.
Lee TH and Goldman L: Evaluation of the patient with acute chest pain. N Engl J Med 342:1187-1195, 2000.

chapter 3

Evaluation of the Patient with Pulmonary Disease

EVALUATION ON A MACRO-
SCOPIC LEVEL
   Physical Examination
   Chest Radiography
   Computed Tomography
   Magnetic Resonance Imaging
   Lung Scanning
   Pulmonary Angiography and CT
     Angiography
   Ultrasonography
   Bronchoscopy

EVALUATION ON A MICRO-
SCOPIC LEVEL
   Obtaining Specimens
   Processing Specimens
ASSESSMENT ON A FUNCTIONAL
LEVEL
   Pulmonary Function Tests
   Arterial Blood Gases
   Exercise Testing

In evaluating the patient with pulmonary disease, the physician is concerned with three levels of evaluation: the macroscopic level, the microscopic level, and the functional level. The methods for assessing each of these range from simple and readily available studies to highly sophisticated and elaborate techniques requiring state-of-the-art technology.

Each level is considered here, with an emphasis on the basic principles and utility of the studies. Subsequent chapters repeatedly refer to these methods, because they form the backbone of the physician's approach to the patient.

EVALUATION ON A MACROSCOPIC LEVEL

Physical Examination

The most accessible method for evaluating the patient with respiratory disease is the physical examination, which requires only a stethoscope; the eyes, ears, and hands of the examiner; and the examiner's skill in eliciting and recognizing abnormal findings. Because the purpose of this discussion is not to elaborate the details of a chest examination but rather to examine a few of the basic principles, the primary focus is on selected aspects of the examination and what is known about mechanisms that produce abnormalities.

Apart from general observation of the patient, the patient's respiratory rate, and the patient's pattern of and difficulty with breathing, the examiner relies primarily on palpation and percussion of the chest and auscultation with a stethoscope. Palpation is useful for comparing the expansion of the two sides of the chest; the examiner can determine if the two lungs are expanding symmetrically or if some process is affecting aeration much more on one side than on the other. Palpation of the chest wall is also useful for feeling the vibrations created by spoken sounds. When the examiner places a hand over an area of lung, vibration normally should be felt as the sound is transmitted to the chest wall. This vibration is called *vocal* or *tactile fremitus*. Some disease processes improve transmission of sound, and they augment the intensity of the vibration. Other conditions diminish transmission of sound and reduce the intensity of the vibration or eliminate it altogether. Elaboration of this concept of sound transmission and its relation to specific conditions is provided in the discussion of chest auscultation.

When percussing the chest, the examiner notes the quality of sound produced by tapping a finger of one hand against a finger of the opposite hand pressed closely to the patient's chest wall. The principle is similar to that of tapping a surface and judging whether what is underneath is solid or hollow. Normally, percussion of the chest wall overlying air-containing lung gives a resonant sound, whereas percussion over a solid organ such as the liver produces a dull sound. This contrast allows the examiner to detect areas with something other than air-containing lung beneath the chest wall, such as fluid in the pleural space (pleural effusion) or airless (consolidated) lung, each of which sounds dull to percussion. At the other extreme, air in the pleural space (pneumothorax) or a hyperinflated lung (as in emphysema) may produce a hyperresonant or more "hollow" sound, approaching what one hears when percussing over a hollow viscus, such as the stomach. Additionally, the examiner can locate the approximate position of the diaphragm by a change in the quality of the percussed note, from resonant to dull, toward the bottom of the lung. A convenient aspect of the whole-chest examination is the basically symmetric nature of the two sides of the chest; a difference in the findings between the two sides suggests a localized abnormality.

When auscultating the lungs with a stethoscope, the examiner listens for two major features: the quality of the breath sounds and the presence of any abnormal (commonly called *adventitious*) sounds. As the patient takes a deep breath, the sound of airflow can be heard through the stethoscope. When the stethoscope is placed over normal lung tissue, sound is heard primarily during inspiration, and the quality of the sound is relatively smooth and soft. These normal breath sounds heard over lung tissue are called *vesicular breath sounds.* There is no general agreement about where these sounds originate, but the source is presumably somewhere distal to the trachea and proximal to the alveoli.

Goals of auscultation:
1. Assessment of breath sounds
2. Detection of adventitious sounds

When the examiner listens over consolidated lung—that is, lung that is airless and filled with liquid or inflammatory cells—the findings are different. The sound is louder and harsher, more hollow or tubular in quality, and expiration is at least as loud and as long as inspiration. Such breath sounds are called *bronchial breath sounds,* as opposed to the normal vesicular sounds. This difference in quality of the sound is due to the ability of consolidated lung to transmit sound better than normally aerated lung. As a result, sounds generated by turbulent airflow in the central airways (trachea and major bronchi) are transmitted to the periphery of the lung and can be heard through the stethoscope. Normally, these sounds are not heard in the lung periphery; they can be demonstrated only by listening near their site of origin—for example, over the upper part of the sternum or the suprasternal notch. When the stethoscope is placed over large airways that are not quite so central or over an area of partially consolidated lung, the breath sounds are intermediate in quality between bronchial and vesicular and are therefore termed *bronchovesicular.*

Consolidated lung does not filter sound in the same way as does air-containing lung.

Better transmission of sound through consolidated rather than normal lung can also be demonstrated when the patient whispers or speaks. The enhanced transmission of whispered sound results in more distinctly heard syllables and is termed *whispered pectoriloquy.* Spoken words can be heard more distinctly through the stethoscope placed over the involved area, a phenomenon commonly called *bronchophony.* When the patient says the vowel "E," the resulting sound through consolidated lung has a nasal "A" quality; this E-to-A change is termed *egophony.* All these findings are variations on the same theme—an altered transmission of sound through airless lung—and basically have the same significance.

Two qualifications are important in interpreting the quality of breath sounds. First, normal transmission of sound depends on patency of the airway. If a relatively large bronchus is occluded, such as by tumor, secretions, or a foreign body, airflow into that region of lung is diminished or absent, and the examiner hears decreased or absent breath sounds over the affected area. A blocked airway proximal to consolidated or airless lung also eliminates the increased transmission of sound described previously. Second, either air or fluid in the pleural space acts as a barrier to sound, so that either a pneumothorax or a pleural effusion causes a diminution of breath sounds.

The second major feature the examiner listens for is adventitious sounds. Unfortunately, the terminology for these adventitious sounds varies considerably from examiner to examiner; therefore, only the most commonly used terms are considered here: crackles, wheezes, and friction rubs. A fourth category, rhonchi, is used inconsistently by different examiners, thus decreasing its clinical usefulness for communicating abnormal findings.

Crackles, also called *rales,* are a series of individual clicking or popping noises heard with the stethoscope over an involved area of lung. Their quality can range from the sound produced by rubbing hairs together to that generated by opening a Velcro™ fastener or crumpling a piece of cellophane. These

---

Crackles, heard during inspiration, are "opening" sounds of small airways and alveoli.

---

sounds are "opening" sounds of small airways or alveoli that have been collapsed or decreased in volume during expiration because of fluid, inflammatory exudate, or poor aeration. On each subsequent inspiration, opening of these distal lung units creates the series of clicking or popping sounds heard either throughout or at the latter part of inspiration. The most common disorders producing rales are pulmonary edema, pneumonia, interstitial lung disease, and atelectasis. Although some clinicians believe the quality of the crackles helps to distinguish the different disorders, others think that such distinctions in quality are of little clinical value.

Wheezes are high-pitched, continuous sounds that are generated by airflow through narrowed airways. The causes of such narrowing include airway smooth muscle constriction, edema, secretions, and collapse because of poorly supported walls. These individual pathophysiologic features are discussed in Chapters 4 to 7. For reasons that are also described later, the diameter of intrathoracic airways is less during expiration than inspiration, and wheezing generally is more pronounced or exclusively heard in expiration. However, at least some airflow is necessary to generate wheezing; wheezing may no longer be heard if airway narrowing is severe.

Wheezes reflect airflow through narrowed airways.

Although clinicians commonly use the term *rhonchi* in referring to sounds generated by secretions in airways, different examiners use the term in somewhat different ways. The term is used to describe low-pitched continuous sounds that are somewhat coarser than high-pitched wheezing; it is also used to describe the very coarse crackles that often result from airway secretions. The result is that the term is frequently used to describe the variety of noises and musical sounds that cannot be readily classified within the more generally accepted categories of crackles and wheezes but that all appear to have a common underlying cause: airway secretions.

A *friction rub* is the term for the sounds generated by inflamed or roughened pleural surfaces rubbing against each other during respiration. A rub is a series of creaky or rasping sounds heard during both inspiration and expiration. The most common causes are primary inflammatory diseases of the pleura or parenchymal processes that extend out to the pleural surface, such as pneumonia and pulmonary infarction.

Table 3-1 provides a summary of some of the pulmonary findings commonly seen in selected disorders affecting the respiratory system. Many of these are mentioned again in subsequent chapters when the specific disorders are discussed in more detail.

Although the focus here is on the chest examination itself as an indicator of pulmonary disease, other nonthoracic manifestations of primary pulmonary disease may be detected on physical examination. Briefly discussed here are clubbing (with or without hypertrophic osteoarthropathy) and cyanosis.

Clubbing is a change in the normal configuration of the nails and the distal phalanx of the fingers or toes (Fig. 3-1). Several features may be seen: (1) loss of the normal angle between the nail and the skin, (2) increased curvature of the nail, (3) increased sponginess of the tissue below the proximal part of the nail, and (4) flaring or widening of the terminal phalanx. Although several nonpulmonary disorders can result in clubbing (such as congenital heart disease with right-to-left shunting, endocarditis, chronic liver disease, and inflammatory bowel disease), the most common causes are clearly pulmonary. Occasionally, clubbing is familial and of no clinical significance. Carcinoma of the lung (or mesothelioma of the pleura) is the single leading etiologic factor; other pulmonary causes include chronic pulmonary infection with suppuration (such as bronchiectasis or lung abscess) and interstitial lung disease. Uncomplicated chronic obstructive lung disease is not associated with clubbing, and the presence of clubbing in this setting should suggest coexisting malignancy or suppurative disease.

Respiratory diseases associated with clubbing:
1. Carcinoma of the lung (or mesothelioma of the pleura)
2. Chronic pulmonary infection
3. Interstitial lung disease

Table	3-1

Typical Chest Examination Findings in Selected Clinical Conditions

Condition	Percussion	Fremitus	Breath Sounds	Voice Transmission	Crackles
Normal	Resonant	Normal	Vesicular (at lung bases)	Normal	Absent
Consolidation or atelectasis (with patent airway)	Dull	Increased	Bronchial	Bronchophony, whispered pectoriloquy, egophony	Present
Consolidation or atelectasis (with blocked airway)	Dull	Decreased	Decreased	Decreased	Absent
Emphysema	Hyperresonant	Decreased	Decreased	Decreased	Absent
Pneumothorax	Hyperresonant	Decreased	Decreased	Decreased	Absent
Pleural effusion	Dull	Decreased	Decreased*	Decreased*	Absent

*May be altered by collapse of underlying lung, which will increase transmission of sound.

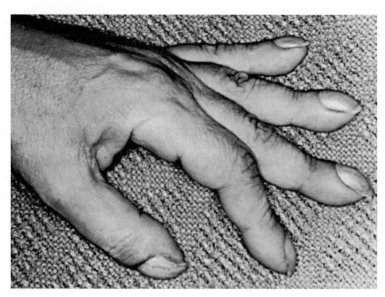

Figure 3-1   ■— Clubbing in patient with carcinoma of lung. Curvature of nail and loss of angle between nail and adjacent skin can be seen.

Clubbing may also be accompanied by *hypertrophic osteoarthropathy,* characterized by periosteal new bone formation, particularly in the long bones, and arthralgias and arthritis of any of several joints. When there is coexistent hypertrophic osteoarthropathy, either pulmonary or pleural tumor is the likely cause of the clubbing, because hypertrophic osteoarthropathy is relatively rare with the other causes of clubbing.

The mechanism of clubbing and hypertrophic osteoarthropathy is not at all clear. It has been observed that clubbing is associated with an increase in digital blood flow, whereas the osteoarthropathy is characterized by an overgrowth of highly vascular connective tissue. Why these changes occur, however, is a mystery. One interesting theory suggests an important role for nerve stimuli coming through the vagus nerve, because vagotomy frequently ameliorates some of the bone and nail changes. Another theory proposes that megakaryocytes and platelet clumps, bypassing the pulmonary vascular bed and impacting in the peripheral systemic circulation, release growth factors responsible for the soft-tissue changes of clubbing.

Cyanosis, the second extrapulmonary physical finding arising from lung disease, is a bluish discoloration of the skin (particularly under the nails) and mucous membranes. Whereas saturated hemoglobin gives the skin its usual pink color, a sufficient amount of unsaturated hemoglobin produces cyanosis. Cyanosis may be either generalized, owing to a low Po_2 or low systemic blood flow resulting in increased extraction of oxygen from the blood, or localized, owing to low blood flow and increased O_2 extraction within the localized area. With lung disease the common factor causing cyanosis is a low Po_2, and several different types of lung disease may be responsible. The total amount of hemoglobin affects the likelihood of detecting cyanosis. In the anemic patient, if the total quantity of desaturated hemoglobin is less than the amount needed to produce the bluish discoloration, even a very low Po_2 may not be associated with cyanosis. In the patient with polycythemia, in contrast, much less depression of the Po_2 is necessary before sufficient unsaturated hemoglobin exists to produce cyanosis.

Chest Radiography

The chest radiograph, which is largely taken for granted in the practice of medicine, is used not only in evaluating patients with suspected respiratory disease but also frequently in the routine evaluation of asymptomatic patients. Of all the viscera, the lungs are the best suited for radiographic examination. The reason is straightforward: air in the lungs provides an excellent background against which abnormalities can stand out. Additionally, the presence of two lungs allows each to serve as a control for the other, so that unilateral abnormalities can be more easily recognized.

A detailed description of interpretation of the chest radiograph is beyond the scope of this text. A few principles, however, can aid the reader in viewing films presented in this and subsequent chapters.

First, the appearance of any structure on a radiograph depends on the structure's density; the denser it is, the whiter it appears on the film. At one extreme is air, which is radiolucent and appears black on the film. At the other extreme are metallic densities, which appear white. In between, there is a spectrum of increasing density from fat to water to bone. The viscera and muscles fall within the realm of water density tissues and cannot be distinguished in their radiographic density from water or blood.

Second, in order for a line or an interface to appear between two adjacent structures on a radiograph, the two structures must differ in density. For example, within the cardiac shadow the heart muscle cannot be distinguished from the blood coursing within the chambers because both are of water density. In contrast, the borders of the heart are visible against the lungs, because the water density of the heart contrasts with the density of the lungs, which is closer to that of air. However, if the lung adjacent to a normally denser structure (such as the heart or diaphragm) is airless, either because of collapse or consolidation, the neighboring structures are now both of the same density, and no visible interface or boundary separates them. This principle is the basis of the useful *silhouette sign*; if an expected border with an area of lung is not visualized or is not distinct, the adjacent lung is abnormal and lacks full aeration.

Chest radiographs are usually taken in two standard views—posteroanterior (PA) and lateral (Fig. 3-2). For a PA film, the roentgen beam goes from the back to the front of the patient, and the patient's chest is adjacent to the film. The lateral view is taken with the patient's side against the film, and the beam is directed through the patient to the film. If a film cannot be taken with the patient standing and the chest adjacent to the film, as in the case of a bedridden patient, then an anteroposterior view is taken. For this view, which is generally used with portable chest radiographs in a patient's hospital room, the film is placed behind the patient (generally between the patient's back and the bed), and the beam is directed through the patient from front to back. Lateral decubitus views, either right or left, are obtained with the patient in a side-lying position, with the beam directed horizontally. Decubitus views are particularly useful for detecting free-flowing fluid within the pleural space and therefore are often used when a pleural effusion is suspected.

Knowledge of radiographic anatomy is fundamental for the interpretation of consolidation or collapse (atelectasis) and for localization of other abnormalities on the chest film. Lobar anatomy and the locations of fissures separating the lobes are shown in Figure 3-3. Localization of an abnormality often requires information from both the PA and lateral views, both of which should be taken when an abnormality is being evaluated. As can be seen in

Posteroanterior and lateral radiographs are often both necessary for localization of an abnormality.

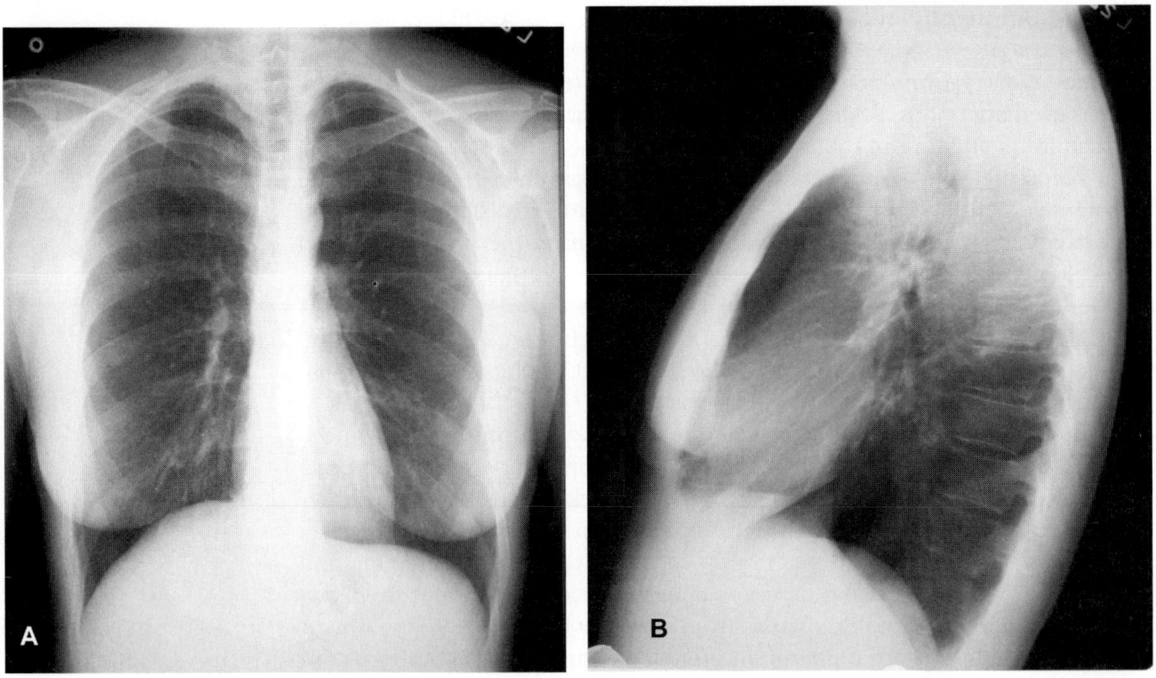

Figure 3-2 ■— Normal chest radiograph. *A,* PA view. *B,* Lateral view. Compare with Figure 3-3 for position of each lobe.

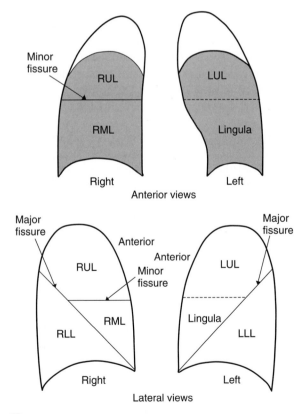

Figure 3-3 ■— Lobar anatomy as seen from anterior *(A)* and lateral *(B)* views. RUL = right upper lobe; RML = right middle lobe; RLL = right lower lobe; LUL = left upper lobe; LLL = left lower lobe. In anterior views, shaded regions represent lower lobes and are behind upper and middle lobes. Lingula is part of LUL, and dashed line between the two does not represent a fissure.

Figure 3-3, the major fissure separating the upper (and middle) lobes from the lower lobe runs obliquely through the chest. Thus it is easy to be misled about location on the PA film alone; a lower lobe lesion may appear in the upper part of the chest, whereas an upper lobe lesion may appear much lower in position.

When a lobe becomes filled with fluid or inflammatory exudate, as in pneumonia, it contains water rather than air density and therefore is easily delineated on the chest radiograph. With pure consolidation the lobe does not lose volume, and it therefore occupies its usual position and retains its usual size. An example of lobar consolidation on PA and lateral radiographs is shown in Figure 3-4.

In contrast, when a lobe has airless alveoli and collapses, it not only becomes more dense but also has features of volume loss characteristic for each individual lobe. Such features of volume loss include change in position of a fissure or the indirect signs of displacement of the hilum, diaphragm, trachea, or mediastinum in the direction of the volume loss (Fig. 3-5). A common mechanism of atelectasis is occlusion of the airway leading to the collapsed region of lung, caused, for example, by a tumor, an aspirated foreign body, or a mucous plug. All the aforementioned examples reflect either pure consolidation or pure collapse. In practice, however, a combination of these processes often occurs, leading to consolidation accompanied by partial volume loss.

When the chest film shows a diffuse or widespread pattern of increased density within the lung parenchyma, it is often useful to characterize the process further, based on the pattern of the radiographic findings. The two primary patterns are *interstitial* and *alveolar.* Although the naming of these patterns suggests a correlation with the type of pathologic involvement (i.e., interstitial, affecting the alveolar walls and the interstitial tissue; alveolar, involving filling of the alveolar spaces), such correlations are often lacking. Nevertheless, many diffuse lung diseases are characterized by one of these radiographic patterns, and the particular pattern may provide clues about the underlying type or cause of disease.

An interstitial pattern is generally described as *reticular* or *reticulo-nodular*, consisting of an interlacing network of linear and small nodular densities. In contrast, an alveolar pattern appears more fluffy, and the outlines of air-filled bronchi coursing through the alveolar densities are often seen. This latter finding is called an *air bronchogram* and is due to air in the bronchi being surrounded and outlined by alveoli that are filled with fluid. This finding does not occur with a purely interstitial pattern. Examples of chest radiographs that show diffuse abnormality as a result of interstitial disease and alveolar filling are presented in Figures 3-6 and 3-7, respectively.

Two additional terms used to describe patterns of increased density are worth mentioning. A *nodular* pattern refers to the presence of multiple discrete, typically spherical, nodules. A uniform pattern of relatively small nodules, several millimeters or less in diameter, is often called a *miliary* pattern, as can be seen with hematogenous (blood-borne) dissemination of tuberculosis throughout the lungs. Alternatively, the nodules can be larger (e.g., greater than 1 cm in diameter), as seen with hematogenous metastasis of carcinoma to the lungs. Another common term is *ground glass,* which is used to describe a hazy, translucent appearance to the region of increased density. Although the term can be used to describe a region or a pattern of increased density on a plain chest radiograph, it is more commonly used when describing abnormalities seen on computed tomography of the chest.

Diffuse increase in density on the radiograph often can be categorized as either alveolar or interstitial.

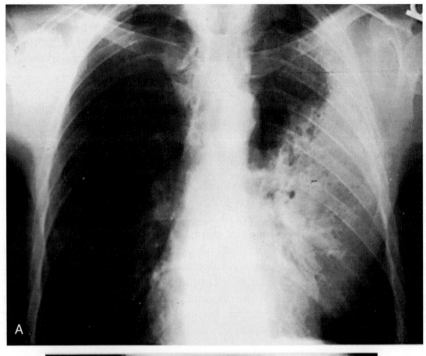

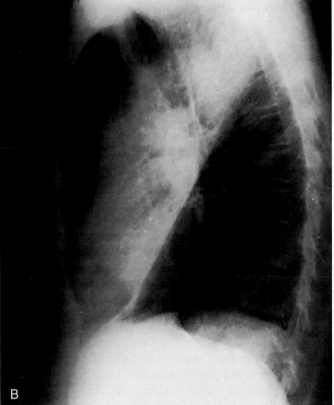

Figure 3-4 ▪— PA *(A)* and lateral *(B)* chest radiographs in patient with LUL consolidation due to pneumonia. The anatomic boundary is best appreciated on lateral view, where it is easily seen that the normally positioned major fissure defines lower border of consolidation (compare with Fig. 3-3). Part of LUL is spared. (Courtesy Dr. T. Scott Johnson.)

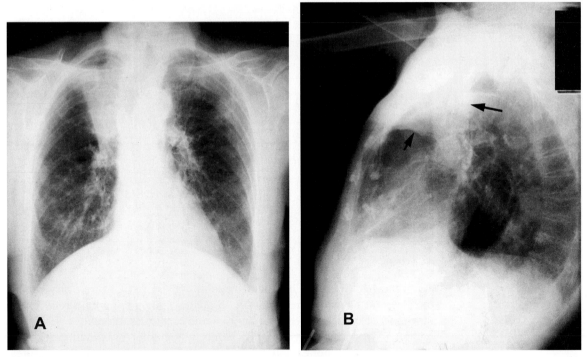

Figure 3-5 ▬ PA *(A)* and lateral *(B)* chest radiographs demonstrating RUL collapse. In *A*, displaced minor fissure outlines airless (dense) RUL. In *B*, RUL is outlined by elevated minor fissure *(short arrow)* and anteriorly displaced major fissure *(long arrow)*.

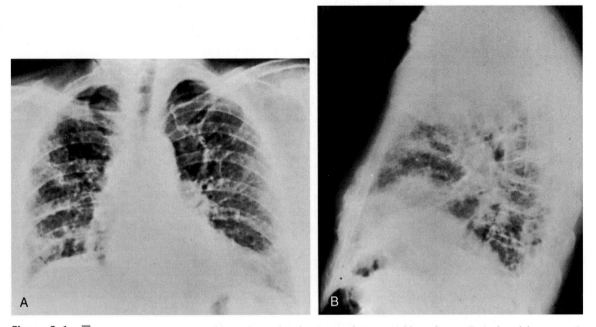

Figure 3-6 ▬ PA *(A)* and lateral *(B)* chest radiographs of patient with interstitial lung disease. Reticulonodular pattern is present throughout but is most prominent in right lung and at base of left lung.

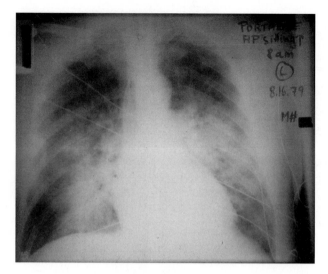

Figure 3-7 ■—
Chest radiograph show-ing a diffuse alveolar filling pattern, most prominent in the middle and lower lung fields.

Though the preceding focus on some typical abnormalities provides an introduction to pattern recognition on a chest radiograph, the careful exam-iner must also use a systematic approach in analyzing the film. A chest radi-ograph shows not merely the lungs alone; radiographic examination also may detect changes in bones, soft tissues, the heart, other mediastinal structures, and the pleural space.

Computed Tomography

Within a relatively short time, computed tomography (CT) has revolutionized the field of diagnostic radiology. With this technique a narrow beam of x-rays is passed through the patient and sensed by a rotating detector on the other side of the patient. The beam is partially absorbed within the patient, depend-ing on the density of the intervening tissues. Computerized analysis of the information received by the detector allows a series of cross-sectional images to be constructed (Fig. 3-8). Use of different "windows" allows the collected data to be displayed in different ways, depending on the densities of the struc-tures of interest. With the technique of helical (spiral) CT scanning, the entire chest is scanned continuously (typically during a single breathhold) as the patient's body is moved through the CT apparatus (the gantry). If radiographic contrast is injected intravenously, images of the pulmonary arterial system obtained during helical scanning (CT angiography) can be used for detection of pulmonary emboli, as described in Chapter 13.

CT provides cross-sectional views of the chest and detects subtle differences in tissue density.

CT is particularly useful in detecting subtle differences in tissue density that cannot be distinguished by conventional radiography. In addition, the cross-sectional views obtained from the slices provide very different informa-tion from that provided by the vertical orientation of plain films. Chest CT has been used extensively in evaluating pulmonary nodules and the medi-astinum. It has also been quite valuable in characterizing chest wall and pleural disease, and it is increasingly being used for detection of pulmonary emboli through the technique of CT angiography. As the technology has advanced, CT has become progressively more useful in the diagnostic evaluation of various diseases affecting the pulmonary parenchyma and the airways. With high-resolution CT, the thickness of individual cross-sectional images is reduced to 1 to 2 mm instead of the traditional 5 to 10 mm. As a result, excep-tionally fine detail can be seen, allowing earlier recognition of subtle disease and better characterization of specific disease patterns (Fig. 3-9).

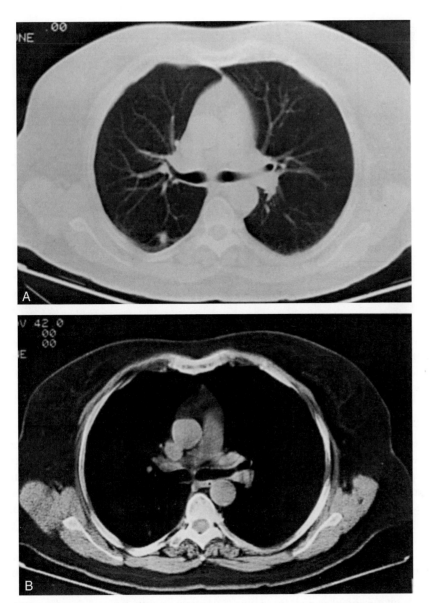

Figure 3-8 ▬▬ Cross-sectional slice from a CT scan performed for evaluation of solitary peripheral pulmonary nodule. Nodule can be seen in posterior portion of right lung. The two images were taken using different "windows" at the same cross-sectional level. In *A*, settings were chosen to optimize visualization of the lung parenchyma. In *B*, settings were chosen to distinguish different densities of soft tissues, such as structures within the mediastinum.

Sophisticated software protocols now allow images obtained by CT scanning to be reconstructed and presented in any plane that best displays the abnormalities of interest. Additionally, it is now possible to produce three-dimensional images from the data acquired by CT scanning. For example, one can display a three-dimensional view of the airways in a manner resembling what is seen inside the airway lumen during bronchoscopy (which is described later in this chapter). This methodology creates an imaging tool that has been dubbed *virtual bronchoscopy.*

Magnetic Resonance Imaging

Another radiologic technique available for evaluation of intrathoracic disease is magnetic resonance imaging (MRI). The physical principles of MRI, which

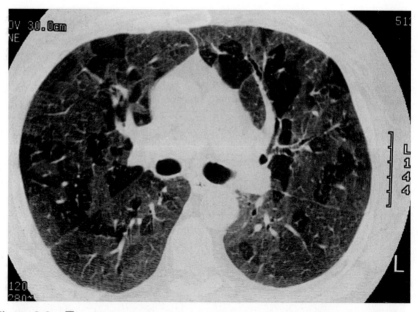

Figure 3-9 ▬— High-resolution CT scan of a patient with dyspnea and a normal chest radiograph. There are well-demarcated areas of lower density (normal lung) interspersed between hazy areas of increased ("ground-glass") density. Biopsy specimen showed findings of hypersensitivity pneumonitis.

are complicated and beyond the training of most physicians and students, are cited here only briefly. The interested reader should refer to other sources for an in-depth discussion of the principles of MRI. In brief, the technique depends on the way that nuclei within a stationary magnetic field change their orientation and release energy delivered to them by a radio frequency pulse. The time required to return to the baseline energy state can be analyzed by a complex computer algorithm, and a visual image can be created.

In the evaluation of intrathoracic disease, MRI provides several important features. First, flowing blood produces a "signal void" and appears black, so that blood vessels can be readily distinguished from nonvascular structures, without the need to use intravenous contrast agents. Second, images can be constructed in any plane, so that the information obtained can be displayed as sagittal, coronal, or transverse (cross-sectional) views. Third, differences can be seen between normal and diseased tissues that are adjacent to each other, even when they are of the same density and therefore could not be distinguished by routine radiography or CT. Some of these features are illustrated in Figure 3-10.

Because MRI scanning is expensive, it is generally used when it can provide information not otherwise obtainable by less expensive, equally noninvasive means. Although it is newer than CT, it does not replace CT but rather often provides complementary diagnostic information. It can be a valuable tool in evaluating hilar and mediastinal disease as well as in defining intrathoracic disease that extends to the neck or the abdomen. It appears to be less useful than CT in the evaluation of pulmonary parenchymal disease. However, knowledge about the power and the limitations of this technique continues to grow, and applications are likely to expand with further refinements in technology.

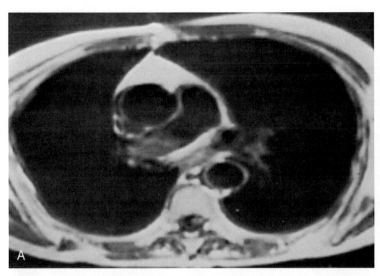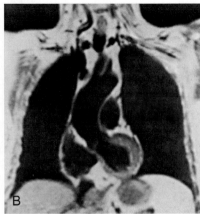

A   B

Figure 3-10 ■— Magnetic resonance images of normal chest: cross-sectional *(A)* and coronal *(B)* views. Lumen of structures that contain blood appears black because flowing blood produces signal void.

Lung Scanning

Injected or inhaled radioisotopes readily provide information about pulmonary blood flow and ventilation. Imaging of the gamma radiation from these isotopes produces a picture showing the distribution of blood flow and ventilation throughout both lungs (Fig. 3-11). Other isotopes have been used for detecting and evaluating infectious, inflammatory, and neoplastic processes affecting the lungs.

Perfusion and Ventilation Scanning

For lung perfusion scanning, the most common technique involves injecting aggregates or microspheres of human albumin labeled with a radionuclide, usually technetium 99 m, into a peripheral vein. These particles, which are approximately 10 to 60 μm in diameter, travel through the right side of the heart, enter the pulmonary vasculature, and become lodged in small pulmonary vessels. Only areas of the lung receiving perfusion from the pulmonary arterial system demonstrate uptake of the tracer, whereas nonperfused regions show no uptake of the labeled albumin.

For ventilation scanning, a gaseous radioisotope, usually xenon 133, is inhaled, and sequential pictures are obtained that show how the gas distributes within the lung. Pictures at different times after inhalation reveal information about gas distribution after the first breath (wash-in phase), after a longer time of breathing the gas (equilibrium phase), and after the patient again breathes air to eliminate the radioisotope (wash-out phase). Ventilation scanning shows which regions of the lungs are being ventilated and whether there are significant localized problems with expiratory airflow and "gas trapping" of the radioisotope during the wash-out phase.

Perfusion and ventilation scans are performed chiefly for two reasons: detection of pulmonary emboli and assessment of regional lung function. When a pulmonary embolus occludes a pulmonary artery, blood flow ceases to the lung region normally supplied by that vessel, and a corresponding perfusion defect results. Generally, ventilation is preserved, and a ventilation scan does not show a corresponding ventilation defect. In practice, many

Perfusion and ventilation lung scans are useful for detection of pulmonary emboli and evaluation of regional lung function.

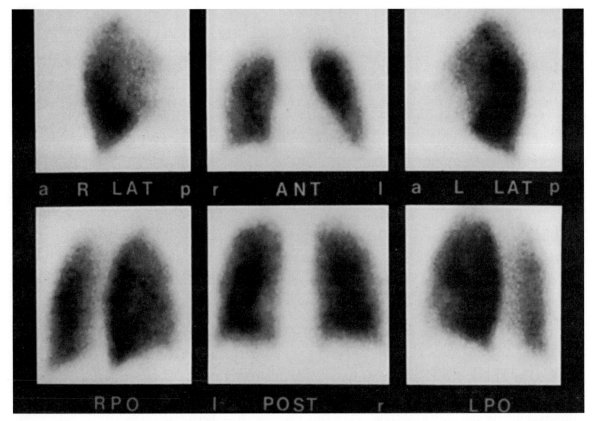

Figure 3-11 ■— Normal perfusion lung scan. Six views are shown. LAT = lateral; ANT = anterior; RPO = right posterior oblique; POST = posterior; LPO = left posterior oblique; a = anterior; p = posterior; r = right; l = left. (Courtesy Dr. Henry Royal.)

pieces of information are considered in the interpretation of the scan, including the appearance of the chest radiograph and the size and distribution of the defects on the perfusion scan. These issues are discussed in more detail in Chapter 13.

Scans to assess regional lung function are sometimes performed before surgery involving resection of a part of the lung, usually one or more lobes. By visualizing which areas of lung receive ventilation and perfusion, the physician can determine how much the area to be resected is contributing to overall lung function. When the scanning techniques are used in conjunction with pulmonary function testing, the physician can predict postoperative pulmonary function, which is a guide to postoperative respiratory problems and impairment.

Gallium Scanning

The most commonly used radioisotope for detection and evaluation of infectious and inflammatory disorders affecting the lungs is gallium 67, in the form of gallium citrate. Gallium scanning has been used for detection of *Pneumocystis carinii* in patients with acquired immunodeficiency syndrome, although uptake of gallium can also be seen in a variety of other opportunistic infections. Gallium scanning has additionally been used as a marker of inflammation and disease activity in patients with a variety of noninfectious inflammatory disorders affecting the lungs. However, its use in this setting is controversial.

Fluorodeoxyglucose Scanning

Based on the principle that malignant tumors typically exhibit increased metabolic activity, scanning following injection of a radiolabeled glucose analog, 18-fluorodeoxyglucose (FDG), has been used as a way of identifying malignant lesions in the lungs and the mediastinum. Malignant cells, as a consequence of their increased uptake and utilization of glucose, take up the FDG but cannot metabolize it beyond the initial phosphorylation step, and the FDG is trapped within the cell. The radiolabeled FDG emits positrons, which are detected by positron emission tomography (PET) using a specialized imaging system or by adapting a gamma camera for imaging of positron-emitting radionuclides. PET imaging with FDG, which remains a very expensive technique that is not universally available, has been used primarily for evaluation of solitary pulmonary nodules and for staging of lung cancer, particularly for mediastinal lymph node involvement. However, the distinction between benign and malignant disease is not perfect, and false-negative and false-positive results can be seen with hypometabolic malignant lesions and highly active inflammatory lesions, respectively. Because of concerns about the expense and the specificity of FDG-PET imaging in the identification of malignant disease, its overall role relative to other diagnostic modalities is not yet well established.

Pulmonary Angiography and CT Angiography

Although the perfusion lung scan provides useful information about pulmonary blood flow and is often the first procedure performed to diagnose pulmonary embolism, it has limitations, particularly in patients with other forms of underlying lung disease. For this reason the physician must frequently turn to additional diagnostic methods such as pulmonary angiography, a radiographic technique in which a catheter is guided from a peripheral vein, through the right atrium and ventricle, and into the main pulmonary artery or one of its branches. A radiopaque dye is then injected, and the pulmonary arterial tree is visualized on a series of rapidly exposed chest films (Fig. 3-12). A clot in a pulmonary vessel appears either as an abrupt termination ("cutoff") of the vessel or as a filling defect within its lumen.

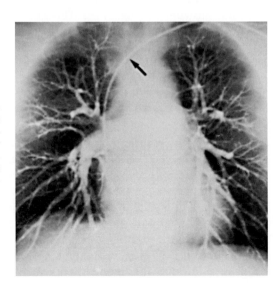

Figure 3-12 ▆— Normal pulmonary angiogram. Radiopaque dye was injected directly into pulmonary artery, and the pulmonary arterial tree is well visualized. Catheter used for injecting dye is indicated by arrow. (Courtesy Dr. Morris Simon.)

The pulmonary angiogram has other uses, including investigation of congenital vascular anomalies and invasion of a vessel by tumor. Use of the angiogram in these situations, however, is much less frequent than its use for diagnosis of pulmonary emboli.

Recently, CT angiography, in which the pulmonary arterial system is visualized by helical CT scanning following injection of radiographic contrast into a peripheral vein, has been increasingly used in place of traditional pulmonary angiography. Its attractiveness is based on its being less invasive than traditional pulmonary angiography, although it is not as sensitive as traditional angiography for detecting emboli in relatively small pulmonary arteries, i.e., peripheral pulmonary emboli.

Ultrasonography

The ability of different types of tissue to transmit sound and of tissue interfaces to reflect sound has made ultrasonography useful for evaluating a variety of body structures. A piezoelectric crystal generates sound waves, and the reflected echoes are detected and recorded by the same crystal. Images are displayed on a screen and can be photographed for a permanent record.

The heart is the intrathoracic structure most frequently studied by ultrasonography, but the technique is also useful in evaluating pleural disease. In particular, ultrasonography is capable of detecting small amounts of pleural fluid and is often used to guide placement of a needle for sampling a small amount of this fluid. Additionally, it can detect walled-off compartments (loculations) within pleural effusions and distinguish fluid from pleural thickening.

Ultrasonography is also capable of localizing the diaphragm and detecting disease immediately below the diaphragm, such as a subphrenic abscess. In contrast, ultrasonography is not useful for defining structures or lesions within the pulmonary parenchyma, because the ultrasound beam penetrates air poorly.

Bronchoscopy

Direct visualization of the airways is possible by bronchoscopy, performed originally with a hollow, rigid metal tube and now much more commonly with a flexible instrument (Fig. 3-13). The flexible instrument transmits images either via flexible fiberoptic bundles (a traditional fiberoptic bronchoscope) or via a digital chip at the tip of the bronchoscope, which then displays the images on a monitor screen. Because the bronchoscope is flexible, the bronchoscopist can bend the tip with a control lever and maneuver into airways at least down to the subsegmental level.

With the fiberoptic bronchoscope, airways are visualized and laboratory samples are obtained.

The bronchoscopist can obtain an excellent view of the airways (Fig. 3-14) and collect a variety of samples for cytologic, pathologic, and microbiologic examination. Sterile saline can be injected through the bronchoscope and suctioned back into a collection chamber. This technique, called *bronchial washing,* samples cells and, if present, microorganisms from the lower respiratory tract. When the bronchoscope is passed as far as possible and wedged into an airway before saline is injected, the washings are able to sample the contents of the alveolar spaces; this technique is called *bronchoalveolar lavage* (BAL).

A long, flexible wire instrument with a small brush at the tip can also be passed through the bronchoscope. The surface of a lesion within a

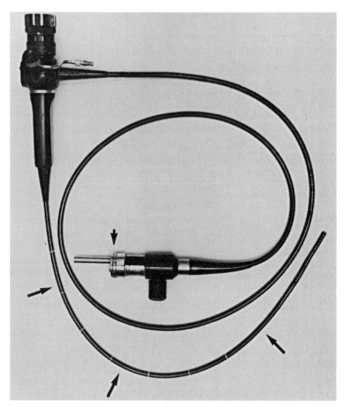

Figure 3-13 ■— Fiberoptic bronchoscope. Long arrows point to flexible part passed into patient's airways. Short arrow points to portion of bronchoscope connected to light source. Controls for clinician performing the procedure are shown at upper left.

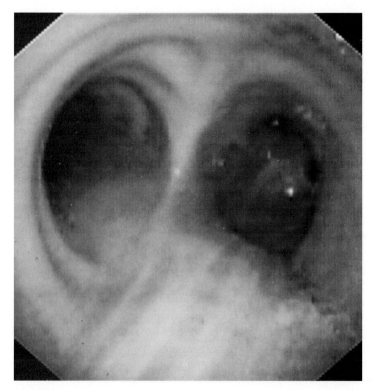

Figure 3-14 ■— Airways as seen through a fiberoptic bronchoscope. At this level, the carina can be seen separating the right and left mainstem bronchi. A large endobronchial mass (a squamous cell carcinoma of the lung) obstructs the right main-stem bronchus.

bronchus can be brushed and the cells collected or smeared onto a slide for cytologic examination. Brushes are also frequently passed into diseased areas of the lung parenchyma; the material collected by the bristles is then subjected to cytologic and microbiologic analysis.

A needle at the end of a long catheter passed through the bronchoscope can puncture an airway wall and sample cells from lymph nodes or lesions adjacent to the airway. This technique, called *transbronchial needle aspiration,* can be used as a way of trying to obtain malignant cells from mediastinal lymph nodes in the staging of known or suspected lung cancer.

With a small biopsy forceps passed through the bronchoscope, the clinician can extract a biopsy specimen from a lesion visualized on the bronchial wall (*endobronchial biopsy*). When a fluoroscope is used to aid in passage of the forceps, the lung parenchyma is quite accessible after the forceps puncture a small bronchus and move out into the distal parenchyma. This procedure, known as a *transbronchial biopsy,* yields pieces of tissue that are small but that have a sizable number of alveoli.

There are many indications for bronchoscopy, usually with a fiberoptic instrument, although there are occasional circumstances in which the rigid instrument is preferred. Some of the indications for bronchoscopy include the following: (1) evaluation of a suspected endobronchial malignancy, (2) sampling of an area of parenchymal disease by bronchoalveolar lavage, brushings, or biopsy, (3) evaluation of hemoptysis, and (4) removal of a foreign body (with special instruments that can be passed through the bronchoscope and are capable of snagging objects). A variety of newer therapeutic modalities are being delivered to the airways via either flexible or rigid bronchoscopic techniques. These include laser techniques for shrinkage of endobronchial tumors causing airway obstruction; placement of stents to maintain patency of airways whose lumen is compromised or obstructed; procedures for dilation of strictures; placement of radioactive seeds directly into malignant airway lesions (brachytherapy); and delivery of electric current (electrocautery), low temperature (cryotherapy), or certain wavelengths of light (phototherapy) to endobronchial masses.

Over the past 35 years or so, bronchoscopy has become a common, useful technique in evaluating and managing pulmonary disease. Even though the physician who first suggested placing a tube into the larynx and bronchi was censured in 1847 for proposing a technique that is "an anatomical impossibility and an unwarrantable innovation in practical medicine," bronchoscopy generally is well tolerated and complications are infrequent.

EVALUATION ON A MICROSCOPIC LEVEL

Microscopy often provides the definitive diagnosis of pulmonary disease suggested by the history, physical examination, or chest radiograph. Several types of disorders are particularly amenable to diagnosis by microscopy: lung tumors (by either histology or cytology), pulmonary infection (by microscopic identification of a specific organism), and a variety of miscellaneous pulmonary diseases, particularly those affecting the interstitium of the lung (by histology). Frequently, when a diagnosis is uncertain, the same techniques are utilized to obtain samples that are processed both for histologic (or cytologic) examination and for identification of microorganisms. This section first provides a discussion of how specimens are obtained and then considers how the specimens are processed.

Obtaining Specimens

The three main types of specimens the physician uses for microscopic analysis in diagnosing the patient with lung disease are (1) tracheobronchial secretions, (2) tissue from the lung parenchyma, and (3) fluid or tissue from the pleura. A number of methods are available for obtaining each of these types of specimens, and knowledge of the yield and the complications determines the most appropriate method.

The easiest way to obtain a specimen of tracheobronchial secretions is to collect sputum that is expectorated spontaneously by the patient. The sample can be used for identifying inflammatory or malignant cells and for staining (and culturing) microorganisms. Although collecting sputum sounds simple, it presents several potential problems. First, the patient may not have any spontaneous cough and sputum production. If this is the case, sputum frequently can be induced by having the patient inhale an irritating aerosol, such as hypertonic saline. Second, what is thought to be sputum originating from the tracheobronchial tree is frequently either nasal secretions or "spit" expectorated from the mouth or the back of the throat. Finally, as a result of passage through the mouth, even a good, deep sputum specimen is contaminated by microorganisms from the mouth. Because of this contamination, care is required in interpreting the results of sputum culture, particularly with regard to the normal flora of the upper respiratory tract. Despite these limitations, sputum remains a valuable resource when looking for malignancy and infectious processes such as bacterial pneumonia and tuberculosis.

Tracheobronchial secretions can also be obtained by two other routes: transtracheal aspiration and bronchoscopy. With transtracheal aspiration, a small plastic catheter is passed inside (or over) a needle inserted through the cricothyroid membrane and into the trachea. The catheter induces coughing, and secretions are collected either with or without the additional instillation of saline through the catheter. This technique avoids the problem of contamination by upper airway flora, and it also allows collection of a sample even when the patient has no spontaneous sputum production. However, it is not without risk; bleeding complications and, to a lesser extent, subcutaneous emphysema (air dissecting through tissues in the neck) are potentially serious sequelae. Because of these potential complications, the availability of alternative methods of sampling, and physicians' inexperience with the procedure, transtracheal aspiration is rarely performed at most institutions.

Bronchoscopy, generally with a flexible instrument, is also a suitable way to obtain tracheobronchial secretions. It has the additional benefit of allowing visualization of the airways. Bronchoscopy has distinct advantages in collecting material for cytologic analysis, because specimens can be collected from a localized area directly visualized with the bronchoscope. However, because the instrument passes through the upper respiratory tract, collection of specimens for culture is subject to contamination by upper airway flora. Specially designed systems with a protected brush can decrease contamination, and quantitating the bacteria recovered can be helpful in distinguishing upper airway contamination from true lower respiratory infection.

BAL has become an increasingly popular method for obtaining specimens from the lower respiratory tract. The fluid obtained by BAL has been used quite effectively for detecting *Pneumocystis carinii,* particularly in patients with acquired immunodeficiency syndrome (AIDS). In some of the interstitial lung diseases (see Chapters 9 and 11), analysis of the cellular and

Tracheobronchial secretions are provided by

1. Expectorated sputum
2. Transtracheal aspiration
3. Fiberoptic bronchoscopy

biochemical components of BAL may provide information that is useful diagnostically and for research about basic disease mechanisms.

As is true of tracheobronchial secretions, tissue specimens for microscopic examination can be collected in numerous ways. A brush or a biopsy forceps can be passed through a bronchoscope. The brush is often used to scrape cells from the surface of an airway lesion, but it also can be passed more distally into the lung parenchyma to obtain specimens directly from a diseased area. The biopsy forceps is used in a similar fashion to sample tissue either from a lesion in the airway (endobronchial biopsy) or from an area of disease in the parenchyma (transbronchial biopsy, so named because the forceps must puncture a small bronchus to sample the parenchyma). In the case of bronchial brushing, the specimen that adheres to the brush is smeared onto a slide for staining and microscopic examination. For both endobronchial and transbronchial biopsies, the tissue obtained can be fixed and sectioned, and slides can be made for subsequent microscopic examination.

In addition to its accessibility through an airway approach, a lesion or diseased area in the lung parenchyma can also be reached with a needle through the chest wall. Depending on the type of needle used, a small sample may be aspirated or taken by biopsy. Bleeding and pneumothorax are potential complications, just as they are for a transbronchial biopsy with a bronchoscope.

Lung tissue is also frequently obtained by a surgical procedure involving an approach through the chest wall. Traditionally, a surgeon made an incision in the chest wall, allowing direct visualization of the lung surface and removal of a small piece of lung tissue. This type of open lung biopsy has largely been supplanted by a less invasive procedure called thoracoscopy (or video-assisted thoracic surgery). Video-assisted thoracic surgery involves placement of a thoracoscope and biopsy instruments through small incisions in the chest wall, and a high-quality image obtained through the thoracoscope can be displayed on a monitor screen. The surgeon uses the video image as a guide for manipulating the instruments to obtain a biopsy sample of peripheral lung tissue or to remove a peripheral lung nodule.

Finally, fluid in the pleural space is frequently sampled in the evaluation of a patient with a pleural effusion. A small needle is inserted through the chest wall and into the pleural space, and fluid is withdrawn. The fluid can be examined for malignant cells and microorganisms; chemical analysis of the fluid (see Chapter 15) often provides additional useful diagnostic information. A biopsy specimen of the parietal pleural surface (the tissue layer lining the pleural space) may also be obtained either blindly, with a special needle passed through the chest wall, or under direct visualization using a thoracoscope. The tissue can be used for microscopic examination and microbiologic studies.

> Lung biopsy specimens can be obtained by
>
> 1. Flexible bronchoscopy
> 2. Percutaneous needle aspiration or biopsy
> 3. Video-assisted thoracic surgery
> 4. Open surgical procedure

Processing Specimens

Once the specimens are obtained, the techniques of processing and the types of examination performed are common to those used for many types of tissue and fluid specimens.

Diagnosis of pulmonary infections depends on smears and cultures of the material obtained, such as sputum, other samples of tracheobronchial secretions, or pleural fluid. The standard Gram's stain technique often allows initial identification of organisms, and inspection also may reveal inflammatory cells (particularly polymorphonuclear leukocytes) and upper airway (squamous epithelial) cells, the latter indicating contamination of sputum by upper

> Specimens can be processed for staining and culture of microorganisms and for cytologic and histopathologic examination.

airway secretions. Final culture results give definitive identification of an organism, but the results must always be interpreted with the knowledge that the specimen may be contaminated and that what is grown is not necessarily causally related to the clinical problem.

Identification of mycobacteria, the causative agent for tuberculosis, requires special staining and culturing techniques. Mycobacteria are stained by agents such as carbolfuchsin or auramine-rhodamine, and the organisms are almost unique in their ability to retain the stain after acid is added. Hence, the expression *acid-fast bacilli* is used commonly in referring to mycobacteria. Frequently used staining methods are the Ziehl-Neelsen stain or a modification called the Kinyoun stain. A more sensitive and faster way to detect mycobacteria involves use of a fluorescent dye such as auramine-rhodamine; mycobacteria take up the dye and fluoresce, and they can be detected relatively easily even when present in small numbers. Because mycobacteria grow slowly, they usually require about 6 weeks for growth and identification on culture media.

Organisms other than the common bacterial pathogens and mycobacteria often require other specialized staining and culture techniques. Fungi may be diagnosed by special stains, such as methenamine silver or periodic acid–Schiff stains, applied to tissue specimens. Fungi can also be cultured on special media favorable to the growth of fungi. *Pneumocystis carinii,* a pathogen of uncertain taxonomic status (see Chapter 25) that is most common in patients with impaired defense mechanisms, is stained in tissue and tracheobronchial secretions by methenamine silver, toluidine blue, or Giemsa stains. An immunofluorescent stain using monoclonal antibodies against *Pneumocystis* is particularly sensitive for detection of the organism in sputum and BAL fluid. The organism identified in 1976 as *Legionella pneumophila,* the causative agent of legionnaires' disease, can be diagnosed by silver impregnation or immunofluorescence staining; it can also be grown, with difficulty, on some special media.

Cytologic examination for malignant cells is available for expectorated sputum, specimens obtained by needle aspiration, bronchial washings or brushings obtained with a bronchoscope, and pleural fluid. A specimen can be smeared directly onto a slide (as with a bronchial brushing), subjected to concentration (bronchial washings, pleural fluid), or digested (sputum) prior to smearing on the slide. The slide is then stained by the Papanicolaou technique, and the cells are examined for findings suggestive or diagnostic of malignancy.

Pathologic examination of tissue sections obtained by biopsy is most useful for diagnosis of malignancy or infection, as well as for a variety of other processes affecting the lungs and the pleura. In many circumstances, examination of tissue obtained by biopsy is the gold standard for diagnosis, although even biopsy results can show false-negative findings or can give misleading information.

Tissue obtained by biopsy is routinely stained with hematoxylin and eosin for histologic examination. A wide assortment of other stains are available that more or less specifically stain collagen, elastin, and a variety of microorganisms. Further discussion of the specific techniques and stains can be found in standard pathology textbooks.

There has been great interest in applying state-of-the-art molecular biologic techniques to respiratory specimens to diagnose certain types of respiratory tract infection. For example, the polymerase chain reaction uses specific synthetic oligonucleotide "primer" sequences and DNA polymerase to amplify

DNA that is unique to a specific organism. If the particular target DNA sequence is present, even if only from a single organism, sequential amplification allows production of millions of copies, which can then be detected by gel electrophoresis. This technique can be applied to samples such as sputum and BAL, providing an exquisitely sensitive test for identifying organisms such as mycobacteria, *P. carinii,* and cytomegalovirus. These newer molecular techniques are becoming more readily available and are likely to see increasing clinical use over time.

ASSESSMENT ON A FUNCTIONAL LEVEL

Pulmonary evaluation on a macroscopic or microscopic level aims at a diagnosis of lung disease, but neither can determine the extent to which normal functions of the lung are impaired. This final aspect of evaluation adds an important dimension to overall assessment of the patient, because it reflects how much the disease may limit a patient's daily activities. The two most common methods for determining a patient's functional status are pulmonary function testing and measuring gas-exchange (using either arterial blood gases or pulse oximetry). In addition, a variety of measurements can be taken during exercise that help determine how much exercise a patient can perform and what factors contribute to any limitation of exercise. Many other types of functional studies are useful for clinical or research purposes, but they are not discussed in this chapter.

Pulmonary Function Tests

Pulmonary function testing provides an objective method for assessing functional changes in a patient with known or suspected lung disease. With the results of screening tests that are available at most hospitals, the physician is able to answer several questions, such as the following: (1) Does the patient have significant lung disease sufficient to cause respiratory impairment and to account for his or her symptoms? (2) What functional pattern of lung disease does the patient have—restrictive or obstructive disease?

In addition, serial evaluation of pulmonary function allows the physician to quantitate any improvement or deterioration in a patient's functional status. Information obtained from such objective evaluation may be essential in deciding when to treat a patient with lung disease and in assessing whether a patient has responded to therapy. Preoperative evaluation of patients can also be useful in predicting which patients are likely to have significant postoperative respiratory problems and which are likely to have adequate pulmonary function after lung resection.

Three main categories of information can be obtained with routine pulmonary function testing:

1. Lung volumes, which provide a measurement of the size of the various compartments within the lung
2. Flow rates, which measure maximal flow within the airways
3. Diffusing capacity, which indicates how readily gas transfer occurs from the alveolus to pulmonary capillary blood

Before examining how these tests indicate what type of functional lung disease a patient has, the tests and their performance within each category are discussed.

Lung Volumes. Although the lung can be subdivided into compartments in different ways, four volumes are particularly important (Fig. 3-15):

1. Total lung capacity (TLC): the total volume of gas within the lungs after a maximal inspiration
2. Residual volume (RV): the volume of gas remaining within the lungs after a maximal expiration
3. Vital capacity (VC): the volume of gas expired when going from TLC to RV
4. Functional residual capacity (FRC): the volume of gas within the lungs at the resting state, that is, at the end of expiration during the normal tidal breathing pattern

Vital capacity can be measured by having the patient breathe into a spirometer from TLC down to RV; by definition, the volume expired in this manner is the VC. However, because RV, FRC, and TLC all include the amount of gas left within the lungs even after a maximal expiration, these volumes cannot be determined simply by having the patient breathe into a spirometer. To quantitate these volumes, a variety of methods are available that can measure one of these three volumes, and the other two can then be calculated or derived from the spirometric tracing. Two methods are described here:

1. Dilution tests: A known volume of an inert gas (usually helium) at a known concentration is inhaled into the lungs. This gas is diluted by the volume of gas already present within the lungs, and the concentration of expired gas (relative to inspired) therefore reflects the initial volume of gas in the lungs.
2. Body plethysmography: The patient, sitting inside an airtight box, performs a maneuver that causes expansion and compression of gas within the thorax. By quantitating volume and pressure changes and by applying Boyle's law, the volume of gas in the thorax can be calculated.

In many circumstances, dilution methods are adequate for determining lung volumes. However, for those patients who have air spaces within the lung that do not communicate with the bronchial tree (e.g., bullae), the inhaled gas

> Lung volumes are determined by spirometry and either gas dilution or body plethysmography.

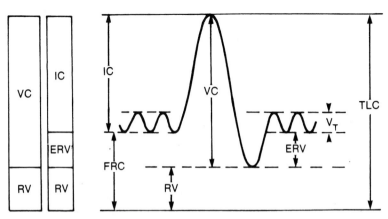

Figure 3-15 ■— Subcompartments of lung, i.e., lung volumes. On right side, lung volumes are labeled on spirographic tracing. On left side are block diagrams showing two ways that total lung capacity can be subdivided. VC = vital capacity; RV = residual volume; IC = inspiratory capacity; ERV = expiratory reserve volume; FRC = functional residual capacity; VT = tidal volume; TLC = total lung capacity.

is not diluted in these noncommunicating areas, and the measured lung volumes determined by dilution methods are falsely low. In such a situation, body plethysmography gives a more accurate reflection of intrathoracic gas volume inasmuch as it does not depend on ready communication of all peripheral air spaces with the bronchial tree.

Flow Rates. The measurement of flow rates on routine pulmonary function testing involves assessing airflow during maximal forced expiration, that is, with the patient breathing as hard and as fast as possible from TLC down to RV. The volume expired during this maneuver is the *forced vital capacity* (FVC), whereas the amount expired during the first second is the *forced expiratory volume in 1 second* (FEV_1) (Fig. 3-16). In interpreting flow rates, it is common to use the ratio between these two measurements (FEV_1/FVC) as an index of obstruction to airflow. Another parameter often calculated from the forced expiratory maneuver is the maximum midexpiratory flow rate (MMFR), which is the rate of airflow during the middle one-half of the expiration

> Maximal expiratory airflow is assessed by the FEV_1/FVC ratio and the MMFR ($FEF_{25\%-75\%}$).

(between 25 and 75 percent of the volume expired during the FVC). MMFR is frequently called the forced expiratory flow (FEF) between 25 and 75 percent of vital capacity, or the $FEF_{25\%-75\%}$. The MMFR or $FEF_{25\%-75\%}$ is a relatively sensitive index of airflow obstruction and may be abnormal when the FEV_1/FVC ratio is still preserved.

Diffusing Capacity. The diffusing capacity is a measurement of the rate of transfer of gas from the alveolus to the capillary measured in relation to the driving pressure of the gas across the alveolar-capillary membrane. Small concentrations of carbon monoxide are generally used for this purpose. Carbon monoxide combines readily with hemoglobin, and the rate of transfer of gas from the alveolus to the capillary depends on movement through the alveolar-capillary membrane and the amount of hemoglobin available for binding the carbon monoxide.

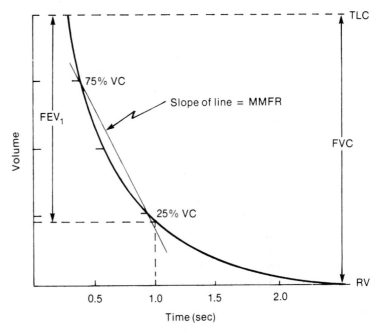

Figure 3-16 ■— Forced expiratory spirogram. Volume is plotted against time while patient breathes out as hard and fast as possible from TLC to RV. FEV_1 = forced expiratory volume in 1 second; TLC = total lung capacity; FVC = forced vital capacity; RV = residual volume; MMFR = maximal midexpiratory flow rate (also called forced expiratory flow from 25%-75% [$FEF_{25\%-75\%}$]).

Although the diffusing capacity may be influenced to some extent by the thickness of the alveolar-capillary membrane, it is most dependent on the number of functioning alveolar-capillary units, i.e., the surface area available for gas-exchange and the volume of blood (hemoglobin) in the pulmonary capillaries available to bind carbon monoxide. Because diffusing capacity may be depressed if a patient is anemic (owing to less available hemoglobin to bind carbon monoxide), the observed value is generally corrected for the patient's hemoglobin level. In practice, the diffusing capacity is commonly decreased in three categories of disease in which surface area for gas-exchange is lost or pulmonary capillary blood volume is decreased, or both: (1) emphysema, (2) interstitial lung disease, and (3) pulmonary vascular disease. In disorders that affect only the airways and not pulmonary parenchymal tissue (e.g., asthma, chronic bronchitis), diffusing capacity is generally preserved. On the other hand, the diffusing capacity may be elevated when there has been recent intrapulmonary hemorrhage, as a result of uptake of carbon monoxide by erythrocytes within the alveolar spaces.

> Diffusing capacity for carbon monoxide depends largely on the surface area for gas-exchange and the pulmonary capillary blood volume.

Interpretation of Normality in Pulmonary Function Testing

Interpretation of pulmonary function tests necessarily involves a qualitative judgment about normality or abnormality on the basis of the quantitative data obtained from these tests. To arrive at a relatively objective judgment, normal standards have been established for each test by using large numbers of normal, nonsmoking control subjects. Regression lines have been constructed to fit the data obtained from these normal control subjects. A "normal" or predicted value for a test in a given patient can then be found by putting the patient's age and height into the regression equation. The standards for determining what constitutes the "lower limits of normal" for a particular test may vary from laboratory to laboratory. Some laboratories utilize "95 percent confidence intervals," based on standard errors around the regression line, whereas others consider an observed value to be normal if it is greater than 80 percent of the predicted value. No matter which criteria are used, all the data must be considered to determine if certain patterns are consistently present. Interpretation of any test in isolation, with the assumption that a patient with a value of 79 percent has lung disease whereas one with a value of 81 percent is disease-free, is obviously dangerous.

Interpretation of the FEV_1/FVC ratio is the only exception to the general rule that a normal value is greater than 80 percent of the predicted value. If this ratio is compared with the predicted ratio (the latter often approximately 75 to 80 percent), this "ratio of the ratios" should be greater than about 95 percent. This 95 percent value does not refer to the actual FEV_1/FVC ratio but rather to the comparison of this observed ratio with the predicted ratio.

Patterns of Pulmonary Function Impairment

In the analysis of pulmonary function tests, abnormalities are usually categorized into one of two patterns (or a combination of the two): (1) an obstructive pattern, characterized mainly by obstruction to airflow, and (2) a restrictive pattern, with evidence of decreased lung volumes but no airflow obstruction.

An obstructive pattern, as seen in patients with asthma, chronic bronchitis, and emphysema, consists of a decrease in rates of expiratory airflow and usually manifests as a decrease in MMFR and the FEV_1/FVC ratio (Fig. 3-17). There is generally a high residual volume and an increased RV/TLC ratio, indicating air trapping due to closure of airways during forced

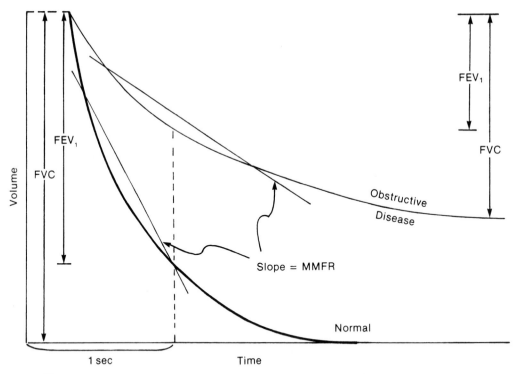

Figure 3-17 ■— Forced expiratory spirograms in normal individual and in patient with airflow obstruction. Note prolonged expiration and changes in FVC and FEV_1 in patient with obstructive disease.

Patterns of impairment:

1. Obstructive: diminished rates of expiratory airflow ($\downarrow FEV_1/FVC$, $\downarrow MMFR$)
2. Restrictive: diminished lung volumes (especially $\downarrow TLC$) and preserved expiratory airflow

expiration (Fig. 3-18). Hyperinflation, reflected by an increased total lung capacity, is often found, particularly in patients with either asthma or emphysema. Diffusing capacity tends to be decreased in those patients who have loss of alveolar-capillary bed (as seen in emphysema) but not in those without loss of available surface area for gas-exchange (as in chronic bronchitis and asthma).

The hallmark of restrictive disease is a reduction in lung volumes, whereas expiratory airflow is normal (see Fig. 3-18). Therefore, TLC, RV, VC, and FRC all tend to be reduced, whereas MMFR and FEV_1/FVC are preserved. In some patients with significant loss of volume from restrictive disease, the MMFR is decreased because of less volume available to generate a high flow rate. It is therefore difficult to interpret a low MMFR in the face of significant restrictive disease unless MMFR is clearly decreased out of proportion to the decrease in lung volumes.

A wide variety of parenchymal, pleural, neuromuscular, and chest wall diseases can demonstrate a restrictive pattern. Certain clues are often useful in distinguishing among these causes of restriction. For example, a decrease in the diffusing capacity for carbon monoxide suggests loss of alveolar-capillary units and points toward interstitial disease as the cause of the restrictive pattern. The finding of a relatively high RV can indicate either expiratory muscle weakness or a chest wall abnormality that makes the thoracic cage particularly stiff (noncompliant) at low volumes.

Although lung diseases often occur with one or the other of these patterns, a mixed picture of obstructive and restrictive disease can be present, making interpretation of the tests much more complex. These tests do not directly reflect a patient's overall capability for O_2 and CO_2 exchange, which is assessed by measurement of arterial blood gases.

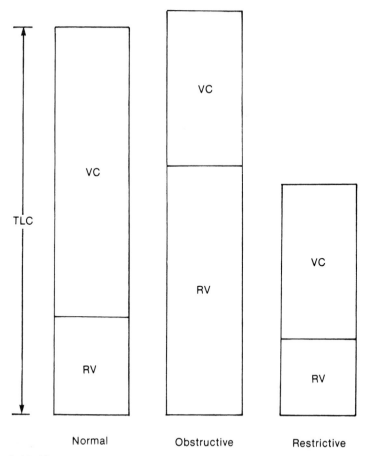

Figure 3-18 ■— Diagram of lung volumes (TLC and subcompartments VC and RV) in normal individual and in patients with obstructive and restrictive disease.

A simplified guide to the interpretation of pulmonary function tests is presented along with several sample problems in Appendix B.

Other Tests

A significant amount of work was done in the past to develop tests that detect early obstruction to airflow, particularly when due to small or peripheral airways obstruction. Such tests include maximal expiratory flow-volume loops, analysis of closing volume, and frequency-dependent dynamic compliance. Unfortunately, pathologic studies have shown that the correlation between tests of "small airways function" and the actual presence of disease in small airways (as demonstrated by histopathologic specimens) is inconsistent, making the value of these tests unclear. Despite this limitation, the maximal expiratory flow-volume loop is a test with sufficient routine clinical applicability to warrant a short discussion here.

The flow-volume loop is a graphic record of maximal inspiratory and maximal expiratory maneuvers. However, rather than the graph of volume versus time that is given with usual spirometric testing, the flow-volume loop has a plot of flow (on the Y axis) versus volume (on the X axis). Although the initial flows obtained during the early part of a forced expiratory maneuver are effort dependent, the flows during the latter part of the maneuver are effort independent and primarily reflect the mechanical properties of the lungs and the resistance to airflow.

In obstructive lung disease, the expiratory portion of the flow-volume curve has a "scooped out" or coved appearance.

In those patients with evidence of airflow obstruction, flow rates at a given volume are decreased, often giving the curve a "scooped out" or coved appearance. The flow data obtained from maximal expiratory flow-volume loops can be interpreted quantitatively (comparing observed flow rates at specified volumes with predicted values) or qualitatively (visually analyzing the shape and concavity of the expiratory portion of the curve). When routine spirometric parameters reflecting airflow obstruction (MMFR, FEV_1/FVC) are abnormal, the flow-volume loop is generally abnormal. In addition, however, in patients with early airflow obstruction, perhaps localized to small airways, the contour of the terminal part of the expiratory curve may be abnormal even when the FEV_1/FVC ratio is normal. Examples of flow-volume loops in a normal patient and in a patient with obstructive lung disease are shown in Figure 3-19.

Another important application of flow-volume loops is for diagnosing and localizing upper airway obstruction. By analyzing the contour of the inspiratory and expiratory portions of the curve, the obstruction can be categorized as *fixed* or *variable,* as well as *intrathoracic* or *extrathoracic.* In a fixed lesion, changes in pleural pressure do not affect the degree of obstruction, and a limitation in peak airflow (a plateau) is seen on both the inspiratory and the expiratory portions of the curve. In a variable lesion the amount of obstruction is determined by the location of the lesion and by the effect of alterations in pleural and airway pressure with inspiration and expiration (Fig. 3-20).

Upper airway obstruction is characterized by maximal inspiratory and expiratory flow-volume curves.

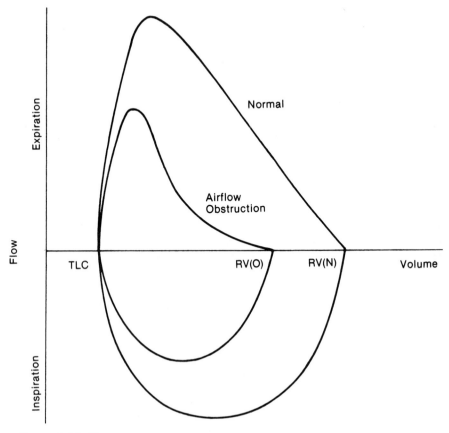

Figure 3-19 ■— Flow-volume loops in normal individual and in patient with airflow obstruction. Expiratory "coving" is apparent on tracing of patient with airflow obstruction. RV(O) = residual volume in patient with obstructive disease; RV(N) = residual volume in the normal individual.

expiration   inspiration   expiration   inspiration

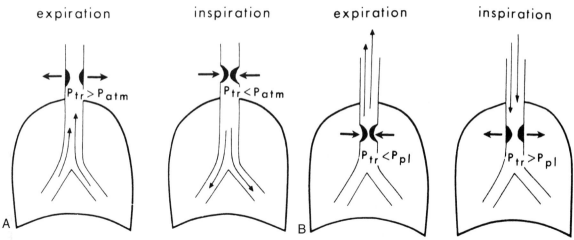

Figure 3-20 ■— Effect of phase of respiration on upper airway obstruction. *A,* Variable extrathoracic obstruction. During forced inspiration, airway or tracheal pressure (P_{tr}) becomes more negative than surrounding atmospheric pressure (P_{atm}), and airway diameter decreases. During forced expiration, more positive intratracheal pressure distends airway and decreases magnitude of obstruction. *B,* Variable intrathoracic obstruction. Pleural pressure surrounds and acts on large intrathoracic airways, affecting airway diameter. During forced expiration, pleural pressure is markedly positive, and airway diameter is decreased. During forced inspiration, negative pleural pressure causes intrathoracic airways to be increased in size, and obstruction is decreased. (Reprinted from Kryger M, Bode F, Antic R, and Anthonisen N: Diagnosis of obstruction of the upper and lower airways. Am J Med 61:85-93, 1976, with permission from Excerpta Medica Inc.)

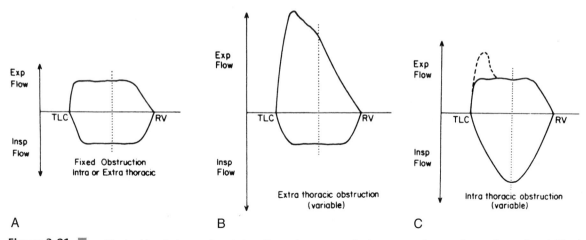

Figure 3-21 ■— Maximal inspiratory and expiratory flow-volume curves in three types of upper airway obstruction. *A,* Fixed obstruction, either intrathoracic or extrathoracic. Obstruction is equivalent during inspiration and expiration so that maximal inspiratory and expiratory flows are limited to the same extent. *B,* Variable extrathoracic obstruction. Obstruction is more marked during inspiration, and only inspiratory part of curve demonstrates plateau. *C,* Variable intrathoracic obstruction. Obstruction is more marked during expiration, and only expiratory part of curve demonstrates a plateau. Dashed line represents a higher initial flow that is occasionally observed before plateau in intrathoracic obstruction. (Reprinted from Kryger M, Bode F, Antic R, and Anthonisen N: Diagnosis of obstruction of the upper and lower airways. Am J Med 61:85-93, 1976, with permission from Excerpta Medica Inc.)

A variable intrathoracic lesion is characterized by expiratory limitation of airflow and a plateau on the expiratory portion of the flow-volume curve, whereas a variable extrathoracic lesion demonstrates inspiratory limitation of airflow and a plateau on the inspiratory portion of the flow-volume curve (Fig. 3-21).

Finally, a test of airflow that is commonly used in clinical practice, particularly in asthmatics as a method to follow severity of disease, is the *peak expiratory flow rate.* In performing this test, the patient blows out from TLC as hard as possible into a simple, readily available device that records the maximal (or peak) expiratory flow rate achieved. Patients with asthma frequently perform and record serial measurements of the test at home as a way of self-monitoring their disease. A significant drop in the peak flow rate from the usual baseline often indicates an exacerbation of the disease and the need for escalating or intensifying the therapeutic regimen.

Arterial Blood Gases

Despite the extensive information that pulmonary function tests provide, they do not show the net effect of lung disease on gas-exchange, which is easily assessed by studies performed on arterial blood. Arterial blood can be conveniently sampled by needle puncture of a radial artery or, less commonly and with more potential risk, of a brachial or femoral artery. The blood is collected into a heparinized syringe (to prevent clotting), and care is taken to expel air bubbles from the syringe and to analyze the sample quickly (or to keep it on ice until analyzed). Three measurements are routinely obtained: arterial Po_2, Pco_2, and pH.

Arterial Po_2 is normally between approximately 80 and 100 torr, but the expected value depends significantly on the patient's age and the simultaneous level of Pco_2 (reflecting alveolar ventilation, an important determinant of alveolar and, secondarily, arterial Po_2). From the arterial blood gases, the alveolar-arterial oxygen gradient ($AaDo_2$) can be calculated, as discussed in Chapter 1. Normally, the difference between alveolar and arterial Po_2 is less than 10 to 15 torr, but again this depends on the patient's age. As also shown in Chapter 1, the oxygen content of the blood does not begin to fall significantly until the arterial Po_2 drops below approximately 60 torr. Therefore, an abnormally low Po_2 generally does not affect O_2 transport to the tissues until it drops below this level and the saturation falls.

The range of normal arterial Pco_2 is approximately 36 to 44 torr, with a corresponding pH between 7.44 and 7.36. Respiratory and metabolic factors interact closely in determining these numbers and a patient's acid-base status. The Pco_2 and pH should be interpreted simultaneously, because both pieces of information are necessary to distinguish respiratory from metabolic abnormalities.

When the Pco_2 rises acutely, the concentration of H^+ also rises, and the pH therefore falls. As a general rule, the pH falls approximately 0.08 (or, rounded off, about 0.1) for each 10 torr increase in Pco_2. Such a rise in Pco_2 with an appropriate decrease in pH is an *acute respiratory acidosis*. Conversely, a drop in Pco_2 due to hyperventilation, with the attendant increase in pH, is an *acute respiratory alkalosis*. With time (hours to days), the kidneys attempt to compensate for a prolonged respiratory acidosis by retaining bicarbonate (HCO_3^-) or by excreting bicarbonate in the case of a prolonged respiratory alkalosis. In either case the compensation returns the pH value toward but not entirely to normal, and the disturbance is termed a *chronic* (i.e., compensated) *respiratory acidosis* or *alkalosis*.

On the other hand, a patient who is producing too much (or excreting too little) acid has a *primary metabolic acidosis*. Conversely, an excess of HCO_3^- (equivalent to a decrease in H^+) defines a *primary metabolic alkalosis*. In the same way that the kidneys attempt to compensate for a primary respiratory acid-base disturbance, respiratory elimination of CO_2 is adjusted to compensate for metabolic acid-base disturbances. Hence, metabolic acidosis stimulates ventilation, CO_2 elimination, and a rise in the pH toward the normal level, whereas metabolic alkalosis suppresses ventilation and CO_2 elimination, and the pH falls toward the normal range.

In practice, the clinician considers three fundamental questions in defining all acid-base disturbances: (1) Is there an acidosis or alkalosis? (2) Is the primary disorder of respiratory or metabolic origin? (3) Is there evidence for respiratory or metabolic compensation? Table 3-2 summarizes the findings in the major types of acid-base disturbances. Unfortunately, in clinical practice, matters are not always so simple, and it is quite common to see complex mixtures of acid-base disturbances in patients who have several diseases and are receiving a variety of medications.

A simplified guide to the interpretation of arterial blood gases is presented along with several sample problems in Appendix C.

Arterial P_{CO_2} and pH together determine the nature of an acid-base disorder and the presence or absence of compensation.

Pulse Oximetry

Although direct measurement of arterial blood gases provides the best method of assessing gas-exchange, it requires collection of blood by arterial puncture. Sampling of arterial blood is uncomfortable for patients, and there is a small but finite risk associated with arterial puncture. As a result, a noninvasive method of assessing arterial oxygenation—pulse oximetry—has come into widespread use, particularly for hospitalized patients. The pulse oximeter is clipped onto a patient's finger, and specific wavelengths of light are passed through the finger. Oxygenated and deoxygenated hemoglobin have different patterns of light absorption, and measurement of the pulsatile absorption of light by arteriolar blood passing through the finger allows quantitation of these two forms of hemoglobin. However, there are certain limitations inherent to pulse oximetry: (1) the oximeter measures O_2 saturation rather than P_{O_2}, and (2) no information is provided about CO_2 elimination and acid-base status.

Exercise Testing

Because limited exercise tolerance is frequently the most prominent symptom of patients with a variety of pulmonary problems, study of patients during exercise may provide valuable information about how much and why these patients are limited. Adding measurements of arterial blood gases during exercise provides an additional dimension and shows whether gas-exchange

Table 3-2			
Acid-Base Disturbances			
Condition	P_{CO_2}	pH	HCO_3^-
Normal	36–44 torr	7.36–7.44	23–30 mEq/L
Respiratory acidosis			
No metabolic compensation	↑	↓	Normal (or ↑)
With metabolic compensation	↑	↓	↑
Respiratory alkalosis			
No metabolic compensation	↓	↑	Normal (or ↓)
With metabolic compensation	↓	↑	↓
Metabolic acidosis			
No respiratory compensation	Normal	↓	↓
With respiratory compensation	↓	↓	↓
Metabolic alkalosis			
No respiratory compensation	Normal	↑	↑
With respiratory compensation	↑	↑	↑

↑ or ↓ indicates a greater change from normal than ↑ or ↓.

problems (either hypoxemia or hypercapnia) contribute to the impairment. Pulse oximetry is also commonly used during exercise, particularly because it is noninvasive; however, it provides less information than does direct measurement of arterial blood gases.

Although any form of exercise is theoretically possible for the testing procedure, the patient is usually studied while exercising on a treadmill or a stationary bicycle. Measurements that can be made at various points during exercise include work output, heart rate, ventilation, O_2 consumption, CO_2 production, expired gas tensions, and arterial blood gases. Analysis of these data can often distinguish whether ventilation, cardiac output, or problems with gas-exchange (particularly hypoxemia) provide the major limitation to exercise tolerance. The results may then guide the physician to specific therapy, based on the type of limitation found.

References

Physical Examination

Dickinson CJ: The aetiology of clubbing and hypertrophic osteoarthropathy. Eur J Clin Invest 23:330-338, 1993.

Hansen-Flaschen J and Nordberg J: Clubbing and hypertrophic osteoarthropathy. Clin Chest Med 8:287-298, 1987.

Loudon R and Murphy RLH Jr: Lung sounds. Am Rev Respir Dis 130:663-673, 1984.

Loudon RG and Murphy RLH. Lung sounds. *In* Crystal RG et al (eds): The Lung. Scientific Foundations. 2nd ed. Philadelphia, Lippincott-Raven, 1997, pp 1383-1391.

Maitre B, Similowski T, and Derenne J-P: Physical examination of the adult patient with respiratory diseases: inspection and palpation. Eur Respir J 8:1584-1593, 1995.

Martin L and Khalil H: How much reduced hemoglobin is necessary to generate central cyanosis? Chest 97:182-185, 1990.

Myers KA and Farquhar DRE: Does this patient have clubbing? JAMA 286:341-347, 2001.

Pasterkamp H, Kraman SS, and Wodicka GR: Respiratory sounds. Advances beyond the stethoscope. Am J Respir Crit Care Med 156:974-987, 1997.

Sridhar KS, Lobo CF, and Altman RD: Digital clubbing and lung cancer. Chest 114:1535-1537, 1998.

Chest Roentgenography

Chiles C: A radiographic approach to diffuse lung disease. Radiol Clin North Am 29:919-929, 1991.

Felson B: Chest Roentgenology. Philadelphia, WB Saunders Co., 1973.

Fraser RS et al (eds): Fraser and Paré's Diagnosis of Diseases of the Chest, vol. I, 4th ed. Philadelphia, WB Saunders Co., 1999.

Goodman LR: Felson's Principles of Chest Roentgenology: A Programmed Text. 2nd ed. Philadelphia, WB Saunders Co., 1999.

Computed Tomography

Ferretti GR, Bricault I, and Coulomb M: Virtual tools for imaging of the thorax. Eur Respir J 18:381-392, 2001.

Müller NL: Advances in imaging. Eur Respir J 18:867-871, 2001.

Müller NL: Computed tomography and magnetic resonance imaging: past, present and future. Eur Respir J 19(suppl 35):3s-12s, 2002.

Swensen SJ, Aughenbaugh GL, Douglas WW, and Myers JL: High resolution CT of the lungs: findings in various pulmonary diseases. AJR 158:971-979, 1992.

Touliopoulos P and Costello P: Helical (spiral) CT of the thorax. Radiol Clin North Am 33:843-861, 1995.

Webb WR, Müller NL, and Naidich DP: High-Resolution CT of the Lung, 3rd ed. Philadelphia, Lippincott Williams & Wilkins, 2001.

Magnetic Resonance Imaging

Bittner RC and Felix R: Magnetic resonance (MR) imaging of the chest: state-of-the-art. Eur Respir J 11:1392-1404, 1998.

Hatabu H et al: Magnetic resonance imaging of the thorax. Past, present, and future. Radiol Clin North Am 38:593-620, 2000.

Müller NL: Computed tomography and magnetic resonance imaging: past, present and future. Eur Respir J 19(suppl 35):3s-12s, 2002.

Naidich DP et al: Computed Tomography and Magnetic Resonance of the Thorax, 3rd ed. Philadelphia, Lippincott-Raven, 1999.

Lung Scanning

Gould MK et al: Accuracy of positron emission tomography for diagnosis of pulmonary nodules and mass lesions. A meta-analysis. JAMA 285:914-924, 2001.

Kramer EL and Divgi CR: Pulmonary applications of nuclear medicine. Clin Chest Med 12:55-75, 1991.

The PIOPED Investigators: Value of the ventilation/perfusion scan in acute pulmonary embolism. JAMA 263:2753-2759, 1990.

Vansteenkiste JF and Stroobants SG: The role of positron emission tomography with ^{18}F-fluoro-2-deoxy-D-glucose in respiratory oncology. Eur Respir J 17:802-820, 2001.

Pulmonary Angiography and CT Angiography

Greenspan RH: Pulmonary angiography and the diagnosis of pulmonary embolism. Prog Cardiovasc Dis 37:93-106, 1994.

Remy-Jardin M and Remy J: Spiral CT angiography of the pulmonary circulation. Radiology 212:615-636, 1999.

Ryu JH, Swensen SJ, Olson EJ, and Pellikka PA: Diagnosis of pulmonary embolism with use of computed tomographic angiography. Mayo Clin Proc 76:59-65, 2001.

Stein PD et al: Complications and validity of pulmonary angiography in acute pulmonary embolism. Circulation 85:462-468, 1992.

Ultrasonography

Beckh S, Bölcskei PL, and Lessnau K-D: Real-time chest ultrasonography. A comprehensive review for the pulmonologist. Chest 122:1759–1773, 2002.

Rosenberg ER: Ultrasound in the assessment of pleural densities. Chest 84:283-285, 1983.

Yang PC et al: Value of sonography in determining the nature of pleural effusion: analysis of 320 cases. AJR Am J Roentgenol 159:29-33, 1992.

Yu C-J, Yang P-C, Chang D-B, and Luh K-T: Diagnostic and therapeutic use of chest sonography: value in critically ill patients. AJR 159:695-701, 1992.

Bronchoscopy

Bolliger CT and Mathur PN: ERS/ATS statement on interventional pulmonology. Eur Respir J 19:356-373, 2002.

Mehta AC (ed): Flexible bronchoscopy in the 21st century. Clin Chest Med 20:1-217, 1999.

Mehta AC (ed): Flexible bronchoscopy update. Clin Chest Med 22:225-379, 2001.

Prakash UBS. Advances in bronchoscopic procedures. Chest 116:1403-1408, 1999.

Seijo LM and Sterman DH: Interventional pulmonology. N Engl J Med 344:740-749, 2001.

Wang K-P and Mehta AC (eds): Flexible Bronchoscopy. Cambridge, MA, Blackwell Science, 1995.

Obtaining and Processing Specimens

American Thoracic Society: Clinical role of bronchoalveolar lavage in adults with pulmonary disease. Am Rev Respir Dis 142:481-486, 1990.

American Thoracic Society Workshop: Rapid diagnostic tests for tuberculosis: what is the appropriate use? Am J Respir Crit Care Med 155:1804-1814, 1997.

Baughman RP and Conrado CE: Diagnosis of lower respiratory tract infections: what we have and what would be nice. Chest 113 (suppl 3):219S-223S, 1998.

Epstein RL: Constituents of sputum: a simple method. Ann Intern Med 77:259-265, 1972.

Ettinger NA: Invasive diagnostic approaches to pulmonary infiltrates. Semin Respir Infect 8:168-176, 1993.

Goldberg M and Unger M: Lung cancer. Diagnostic tools. Chest Surg Clin N Am 10:763-779, 2000.

Health and Public Policy Committee, American College of Physicians: Diagnostic thoracentesis and pleural biopsy in pleural effusions. Ann Intern Med 103:799-802, 1985.

Kaiser LR and Shrager JB: Video-assisted thoracic surgery: the current state of the art. AJR 165:1111-1117, 1995.

Larscheid RC, Thorpe PE, and Scott WJ: Percutaneous transthoracic needle aspiration biopsy: a comprehensive review of its current role in the diagnosis and treatment of lung tumors. Chest 114:704-709, 1998.

Leslie KO, Helmers RA, Lanza LA, and Colby TV: Processing and evaluation of lung biopsy specimens. Eur Respir Mon 5 (Monograph 14):55-62, 2000.

Loddenkemper R: Thoracoscopy: state of the art. Eur Respir J 11:213-221, 1998.

Mayaud C and Cadranel J: A persistent challenge: the diagnosis of respiratory disease in the non-AIDS immunocompromised host. Thorax 55:511-517, 2000.

Murray PR and Washington JA II: Microscopic and bacteriologic analysis of expectorated sputum. Mayo Clin Proc 50:339-344, 1975.

Perlmutt LM, Johnston WW, and Dunnick NR: Percutaneous transthoracic needle aspiration: a review. AJR 152:451-455, 1989.

Reynolds HY: Bronchoalveolar lavage. Am Rev Respir Dis 135:250-263, 1987.

Reynolds HY: Use of bronchoalveolar lavage in humans: past necessity and future imperative. Lung 178:271-293, 2000.

Salzman SH: Bronchoscopic techniques for the diagnosis of pulmonary complications of HIV infection. Semin Respir Infect 14:318-326, 1999.

Schluger NW and Rom WN: The polymerase chain reaction in the diagnosis and evaluation of pulmonary infections. Am J Respir Crit Care Med 152:11-16, 1995.

Shure D: Transbronchial biopsy and needle aspiration. Chest 95:1130-1138, 1989.

Soini H and Musser JM: Molecular diagnosis of mycobacteria. Clin Chem 47:809-814, 2001.

Assessment on a Functional Level

American Thoracic Society: Lung function testing: selection of reference values and interpretative strategies. Am Rev Respir Dis 144:1202-1218, 1991.

American Thoracic Society: Single-breath carbon monoxide diffusing capacity (transfer factor): recommendations for a standardized technique—1995 update. Am J Respir Crit Care Med 152:2185-2198, 1995.

American Thoracic Society: Standardization of spirometry—1994 update. Am J Respir Crit Care Med 152:1107-1136, 1995.

American Thoracic Society and American College of Chest Physicians: ATS/ACCP statement on cardiopulmonary exercise testing. Am J Respir Crit Care Med 167:211–277, 2003.

Bates DV: Respiratory Function in Disease, 3rd ed. Philadelphia, WB Saunders Co., 1989.

Chupp GL (ed): Pulmonary function testing. Clin Chest Med 22:599-859, 2001.

Crapo RO: Pulmonary-function testing. N Engl J Med 331:25-30, 1994.

European Respiratory Society. Clinical exercise testing with reference to lung disease: indications, standardization and interpretation strategies. Eur Respir J 10:2662-2689, 1997.

Hughes JMB and Pride NB: In defence of the carbon monoxide transfer coefficient K_{CO} (T_L/V_A). Eur Respir J 17:168-174, 2001.

Hughes JMB and Pride NB (eds): Lung Function Tests: Physiological Principles and Clinical Applications. London, WB Saunders Co., 2000.

Jain P, Kavuru MS, Emerman CL, and Ahmad M: Utility of peak expiratory flow monitoring. Chest 114:861-876, 1998.

Jones NL: Clinical Exercise Testing, 4th ed. Philadelphia, WB Saunders Co., 1997.

Jubran A: Pulse oximetry. In Tobin MJ (ed): Respiratory Monitoring: Contemporary Management in Critical Care. 1(4):79-100, 1991.

Narins RG and Emmett M: Simple and mixed acid-base disorders: a practical approach. Medicine 59:161-187, 1980.

Quanjer PH et al: Peak expiratory flow: conclusions and recommendations of a Working Party of the European Respiratory Society. Eur Respir J Suppl 24:2S-8S, 1997.

Raffin TA: Indications for arterial blood gas analysis. Ann Intern Med 105:390-398, 1986.

Shapiro BA, Peruzzi WT, and Kozelowski-Templin R: Clinical Application of Blood Gases, 5th ed. St. Louis, Mosby, 1994.

Wasserman K: Diagnosing cardiovascular and lung pathophysiology from exercise gas-exchange. Chest 112:1091–1101, 1997.

Wasserman K et al: Principles of Exercise Testing and Interpretation: Including Pathophysiology and Clinical Applications. 3rd ed. Philadelphia, Lippincott Williams & Wilkins, 1999.

Williams AJ: ABC of oxygen: assessing and interpreting arterial blood gases and acid-base balance. BMJ 317:1213-1216, 1998.

Anatomic and Physiologic Aspects of Airways

STRUCTURE
  Neural Control of Airways
FUNCTION
  Airway Resistance
  Maximal Expiratory Effort

In its transit from the nose or the mouth to the gas-exchanging region of the lung, air passes through the larynx and then along a series of progressively branching tubes, from the trachea down to the smallest bronchioles. In preparation for a discussion of diseases affecting the airways, this chapter describes the structure of these airways and then considers how they function.

STRUCTURE

The trachea, bronchi, and bronchioles down to the level of the terminal bronchioles constitute the *conducting airways;* their function is purely one of transport. Beyond the terminal bronchioles are the *respiratory bronchioles;* they mark the beginning of the *respiratory zone* of the lung, where gasexchange takes place. Respiratory bronchioles are considered part of the gasexchanging region of lung because alveoli are present along their walls. With successive generations of respiratory bronchioles, more alveoli appear along the walls up to the site of the alveolar ducts, which are entirely "alveolarized" (Fig. 4-1). The discussion in this chapter is limited to the conducting airways and to those aspects of the more distal airways that affect air movement but not gas-exchange. Alveolar structure is discussed further in Chapter 8.

The airways are composed of several layers of tissue (Fig. 4-2). Adjacent to the airway lumen is the mucosa, beneath which is a basement membrane separating the epithelial cells of the mucosa from the submucosa. Within the submucosa are mucous glands (the contents of which are extruded through the mucosa), smooth muscle, and loose connective tissue with some nerves and lymphatic vessels. Surrounding the submucosa is a fibrocartilaginous layer that contains the cartilage rings that support several generations of airways. Finally, a layer of peribronchial tissue, with fat, lymphatics, vessels, and nerves, encircles the rest of the airway wall. Each of these layers is considered here, with a description of the component cells and the way the structure changes in the distal progression through the tracheobronchial tree.

Conducting airways: trachea, bronchi, bronchioles down to the level of terminal bronchioles. Respiratory zone: respiratory bronchioles, alveolar ducts, and alveoli.

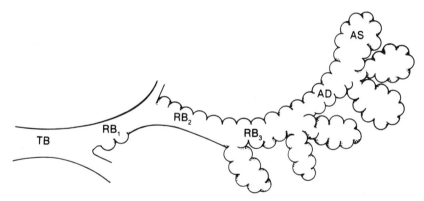

Figure 4-1 ■— Schematic diagram of the most distal portion of the respiratory tree. Each terminal bronchiole (TB) supplies several generations of respiratory bronchioles (RB_1 through RB_3), which have progressively more respiratory (alveolar) epithelium lining their walls. Alveolar ducts (AD) are entirely lined by alveolar epithelium, as are alveolar sacs (AS). Region of lung distal to and supplied by terminal bronchiole is termed *acinus*. (From Thurlbeck WM: Chronic obstructive lung disease. *In* Sommers SC (ed): Pathology Annual, vol 3. New York, Appleton-Century-Crofts, 1968.)

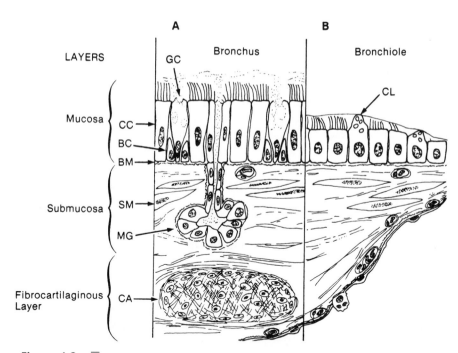

Figure 4-2 ■— Schematic diagram of components of airway wall. *A*, Level of large airways (trachea and bronchi); *B*, Level of small airways (bronchioles). CC = ciliated columnar epithelial cell; BC = basal cell; BM = basement membrane; SM = smooth muscle; MG = mucous gland; CA = cartilage; GC = goblet cell; CL = Clara cell. (Adapted from Weibel ER and Burri PH: Funktionelle Aspekte der Lungenmorphologie. *In* Fuchs WA and Voegeli E [eds]:Aktuelle Probleme der Roentgendiagnostik, vol 2. Bern, Huber, 1973.)

The mucosal layer of large airways consists of pseudo-stratified, ciliated columnar epithelial cells.

The surface layer (mucosa) consists of pseudostratified, columnar epithelial cells, which appear to be several cells thick in the trachea and large bronchi (see Fig. 4-2A). The ciliated cells, which are most superficial, are responsible for protecting the deeper airways by propelling tracheobronchial secretions (and inhaled particles) toward the pharynx. The cilia have the characteristic ultrastructure seen in other ciliated cells: a central pair of microtubules and an outer ring of nine double microtubules (see Fig. 22-1). Small side arms, called *dynein arms*, are on the outer double microtubules. Their presence appears to be important for normal functioning of the cilia; patients with cilia lacking the dynein side arms have impaired ciliary action and recurrent bronchopulmonary infections. Scattered between the ciliated epithelial cells are secretory cells called *goblet cells*, which produce and discharge mucus into the airway lumen. However, the goblet cells produce a relatively small proportion of total bronchial mucus, the largest portion of which is made by the bronchial mucous glands in the submucosa.

The surface epithelium appears to have other important functions that may be altered in certain clinical conditions. By virtue of tight junctions between epithelial cells at the luminal surface, the epithelium prevents access of inhaled foreign material to deeper levels of the airway wall. Whether a disturbance in this barrier function is important in asthma—perhaps by allowing inhaled foreign material to penetrate the epithelial surface—is not known with certainty. Another important function involves active transport of ions, particularly chloride, to maintain a favorable ionic environment in the mucous layer lining the airway wall. In cystic fibrosis, an abnormality in chloride transport by surface epithelial cells is believed to play a crucial role in the pathogenesis of the disease (see Chapter 7).

The deepest layer of epithelial cells, which abuts the basement membrane, includes cells called *basal cells*. The function of the basal cells is to differentiate into and replenish the more superficial cells of the mucosa, either the ciliated cells or the secretory goblet cells. Another important cell type found in the basal layer of the surface epithelium is the *Kulchitsky* or *K cell*, which is believed to have a neuroendocrine function. These cells are probably part of the amine precursor uptake and decarboxylation system and therefore may be capable of producing amine or polypeptide products, or both. In addition, K cells have cytoplasmic processes that extend to the luminal surface. As a result of these processes, K cells may be involved in sensing the composition of inspired gas, and it has been postulated that they play a role in the regional control of ventilation and perfusion. These different cell types are important not only because of their normal physiologic roles but also because of the way they respond to airway irritation and their potential for becoming neoplastic.

The submucosal layer has two major components: *bronchial mucous glands* and *bronchial smooth muscle*. The mucous glands are the main source of bronchial secretions; a duct transports the secretions through the mucosa and discharges them into the airway lumen. As mentioned earlier, superficial goblet cells also produce mucus, which qualitatively appears to be identical to mucus formed by the bronchial mucous glands. However, it is a mystery why both sources of mucus exist and whether both, in fact, are necessary. Airway smooth muscle is present from the trachea down to the level of the bronchioles and even appears in the alveolar ducts. Disturbances in the quantity and function of the smooth muscle are important in disease, particularly in the case of bronchial asthma.

Bronchial secretions are produced by submucosal glands and to a lesser extent by goblet cells in the mucosa.

Finally, the fibrocartilaginous layer is important because of the structural support that cartilage provides to the airways. The configuration of the cartilage varies significantly at different levels of the tracheobronchial tree, but the function at all levels is probably similar.

The preceding discussion describes the general structure of the airways. However, this structure varies considerably at different levels of the airway. Some of these differences are illustrated in Figure 4-2. In the progression

Airway structure changes considerably in the distal progression through the tracheobronchial tree.

distally through the tracheobronchial tree, the following changes are normally seen:

1. The epithelial layer of cells becomes progressively thinner until there is a single layer of cuboidal cells at the level of the terminal bronchioles.
2. Goblet cells decrease in number until they disappear approximately at the level of the terminal bronchiole. In their place are dome-shaped cells, called *Clara cells*, that project into the airway lumen. Although the function of the Clara cells is not known with certainty, it is believed that they may be involved in producing a liquid surface layer that coats the bronchiolar epithelium.
3. Mucous glands, which are present in the trachea and large bronchi, are most numerous in the medium-sized bronchi. They then become progressively fewer in number more distally and are absent from the bronchioles.
4. Smooth muscle changes in configuration at different levels of the tracheobronchial tree. In the trachea and large bronchi, the muscle is found either as bands or as a spiral network, whereas in the smaller bronchi and bronchioles a continuous layer of smooth muscle encircles the airway. As airway size decreases distally in the tracheobronchial tree, smooth muscle generally occupies a larger portion of the total thickness of the airway wall. This proportion of smooth muscle to airway wall thickness becomes maximal at the level of the terminal bronchiole.
5. Cartilage also changes in configuration. In the trachea, the cartilaginous rings are horseshoe-shaped, with the posterior aspect of the trachea being free of cartilage. In the bronchi, there are plates of cartilage, which become smaller and less numerous distally, until cartilage is absent in the bronchioles.

The preceding discussion describes many of the structural features of normal airways. However, with chronic exposure to an irritant, such as cigarette smoke, a variety of changes frequently occur. Some of these changes, particularly in the epithelial cells, are important because of the potential for eventual malignancy, as discussed in Chapter 20. Other changes are apparent in the mucus-secreting structures (bronchial mucous glands and goblet cells) and are important features of chronic bronchitis. With chronic irritation there is hypertrophy of the mucous glands; the goblet cells become more numerous and are found more distally than usual, even in the terminal bronchioles. The implications of these changes in disease states are discussed in Chapter 6.

Neural Control of Airways

The innervation (neural control) of airways is an important aspect of airway structure, with particular clinical relevance, as is discussed in Chapter 5. The neural control of airways affects not only the contraction and relaxation of bronchial smooth muscle but also the activity of bronchial mucous glands. An understanding of the innervation, receptors, and mediators involved in neural control of airway function is important both because of the potential role that neural control may have in the pathogenesis of asthma and because of the well-established role of pharmacotherapy in stimulating or blocking airway receptors. The following discussion focuses on three components of the neural control of airways: the parasympathetic (cholinergic) system, the sympathetic (adrenergic) system, and the nonadrenergic inhibitory system (Fig. 4-3).

The parasympathetic nervous system provides the primary bronchoconstrictor tone to the airways. This innervation comes from branches of the vagus nerve; stimulation of these branches causes contraction of smooth muscle in the airway wall. In addition, vagal fibers innervate bronchial mucous glands and goblet cells, resulting in increased secretions from both components of the mucus-secreting apparatus. The receptors on smooth muscle and on the mucus-secreting apparatus are muscarinic cholinergic receptors; the neurotransmitter is acetylcholine (ACh). These cholinergic receptors are more dense in central than in peripheral airways.

A role for the sympathetic (adrenergic) nervous system in controlling airway tone is much less clear, because there is sparse if any adrenergic innervation of human airways. However, despite the paucity of innervation by sympathetic nerves, there are adrenergic, primarily β_2-, receptors on bronchial smooth muscle. These receptors are stimulated by circulating catecholamines; when stimulated, the β_2-receptors activate adenylate cyclase, increasing the intracellular concentration of cyclic adenosine monophosphate and causing relaxation of bronchial smooth muscle. In contrast, stimulation of the less important α-adrenergic receptors results in bronchoconstriction. Receptor density for the β_2-adrenergic receptors is opposite that of the cholinergic

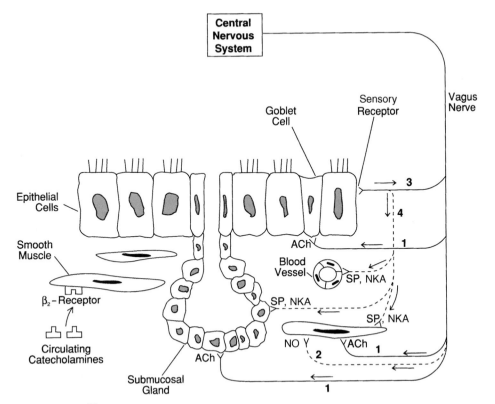

Figure 4-3 ■— Schematic diagram of neural control of airways. Parasympathetic fibers innervating airway smooth muscle cells, submucosal glands, and goblet cells are labeled 1; nonadrenergic, noncholinergic innervation of airway smooth muscle cells is labeled 2; afferent innervation of airway epithelial cells is labeled 3; neural traffic along pathway labeled 4 goes to vagus nerve but also has effects on airway smooth muscle cells, submucosal glands, and blood vessels via local reflexes. ACh = acetylcholine; SP = substance P; NKA = neurokinin A; NO = nitric oxide.

receptors; the β_2-adrenergic receptors are more dense in peripheral than in central airways.

A search for innervation of the airways with a smooth muscle relaxant (bronchodilating) effect has demonstrated a third component of neural control, often called the *nonadrenergic, noncholinergic inhibitory system*. These nerve fibers run in the vagal trunk, but when stimulated they cause bronchial smooth muscle to relax, not constrict. Evidence suggests that the bronchodilator transmitter for these nerves is nitric oxide.

Thus far only the neural output to—that is, the efferent control of—the airways has been discussed. In addition, there are airway receptors with sensory nerve innervation. These receptors, which are located in the airway epithelial layer and are responsive to various chemical and mechanical stimuli, include myelinated cough ("irritant") receptors and unmyelinated C fibers. Neural traffic is carried from these sensory endings in afferent fibers of the vagus nerve. This sensory information is not only communicated to the central nervous system via the afferent vagal fibers but also is responsible for activation of local reflexes causing release of mediators called *tachykinins* from nerve endings in the airway wall. The tachykinins, which include substance P and neurokinin A, can cause bronchoconstriction, increased submucosal gland secretion, and increased vascular permeability (see Fig. 4-3). However, the magnitude of their importance in disease states (e.g., asthma) is not yet known with certainty.

> Parasympathetic innervation provides bronchoconstrictor tone to the airways; nonadrenergic inhibitory innervation provides bronchodilator tone. Adrenergic receptors are present on bronchial smooth muscle despite the absence of significant sympathetic innervation.

FUNCTION

With each breath, air flows from the mouth, through the bronchial tree, to the regions of the lung responsible for gas-exchange. In order to generate this flow of air during inspiration, the pressure must be lower in the alveoli than at the mouth, because air flows from a region of higher to one of lower pressure. The diaphragm and inspiratory muscles of the chest wall cause expansion of the chest and lungs, producing negative pressure in the pleural space and in the alveoli, and thereby initiating airflow.

Flow in the airways can be considered analogous to the flow of current in an electrical system. However, rather than a voltage drop when electrons flow across a resistance, airways have a pressure difference between two points of airflow, and resistance to flow is provided by the airways themselves. The rate of airflow depends in part on this pressure difference between the two points and in part on the airway resistance. During inspiration, alveolar pressure is negative relative to mouth pressure (which is atmospheric), and air flows inward. In contrast, during expiration, alveolar pressure is positive relative to mouth pressure, and air flows outward from the alveoli toward the mouth.

Airway Resistance

The preceding description is comparatively simple; airflow is in fact a much more complex phenomenon. For instance, consider in more detail the problem of resistance. Normal airways resistance is approximately 0.5 to 2.0 cm $H_2O/L/s$; that is, a pressure difference of 0.5 to 2.0 cm H_2O between mouth and alveoli is required for air to flow at a rate of 1 L/s between these two points. Which airways provide most of the resistance? Although it is obvious that a single smaller airway provides more resistance to airflow than does a single larger airway, it does not follow that the aggregate of smaller airways provides the bulk of the resistance. In fact, the opposite is true. For example, even though the trachea is large, there is only one trachea, and the total cross-sectional area of the airways at this level is quite small. In contrast, at the level of small airways (e.g., <2 mm in diameter), the enormous number of these airways makes up for the small diameter of each one and results in a very large total cross-sectional area.

Table 4-1 shows the total cross-sectional area of the airways at different levels of the tracheobronchial tree. The major site of resistance (the smallest total cross-sectional area) is at the level of medium-sized bronchi. The small or peripheral airways, generally defined as airways less than 2 mm in diameter, contribute only about 10 to 20 percent of the total resistance. Hence, these airways are frequently called the "silent" zone, because disease in them can affect their size without significantly altering the total airways resistance. Unfortunately, despite a great deal of work by physiologists to develop methods capable of detecting increased resistance in small airways, the usefulness of such tests has not met original expectations. The correlation between these functional studies and histopathologic confirmation of disease in small airways has been inconsistent; consequently, these tests are used infrequently.

> Since resistance to airflow in the tracheobronchial tree depends on the total cross-sectional area of the airways, large and medium-sized airways provide greater resistance than do the more numerous small airways.

Maximal Expiratory Effort

The next important aspect of the physiology of airflow is the distinction between normal breathing and forced or maximal respiratory efforts. A great deal of information can be obtained by looking at flow during a forced expiration, that is, breathing out from total lung capacity down to residual volume as hard and as fast as possible. In a discussion of this concept, it is useful to consider the flow-volume curve, mentioned in Chapter 3 and shown again in Figure 4-4. In this figure, a series of expiratory curves shows the kind of flow rates generated by progressively greater expiratory efforts. Curve A shows expiratory flow with a relatively low effort, whereas curve D shows flow with a maximal expiratory effort.

During the first part of this curve, perhaps until approximately 30 percent of the vital capacity has been exhaled, the flow rate is quite dependent on the effort expended. That is, greater expiratory efforts cause a

Table	4-1		
Airway Numbers and Dimensions			
Name	Number	Diameter (mm)	Cross-Sectional Area (cm²)
Trachea	1	25	5
Main bronchi	2	11–19	3.2
Lobar bronchi	5	4.5–13.5	2.7
Segmental bronchi	19	4.5–6.5	3.2
Subsegmental bronchi	38	3–6	6.6
Terminal bronchi	1,000	1.0	7.9
Terminal bronchioles	35,000	0.65	116
Terminal respiratory bronchioles	630,000	0.45	1,000
Alveolar ducts and sacs	4×10^6	0.40	17,100
Alveoli	300×10^6	0.25–0.30	700,000 (surface area)

Adapted from Thurlbeck WM: Chronic obstructive lung disease. *In* Sommers SC (ed): Pathology Annual, vol. 3. New York, Appleton-Century-Crofts, 1968.

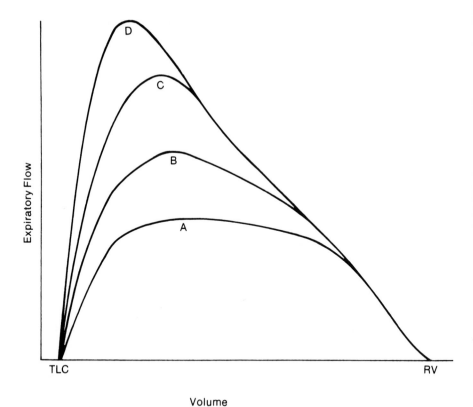

Figure 4-4 ▆— Expiratory flow-volume curves with progressively greater effort. Curve A represents the least effort; curve D represents maximal expiratory effort. On the downsloping part of the curve, beyond the point at which approximately 30 percent of the vital capacity has been exhaled, flow is limited by the mechanical properties of the airways and lungs, not by muscular effort. TLC = total lung capacity; RV = residual volume.

During most of a forced expiration, flow is limited by critical narrowing of the airway; further effort does not result in augmented flow.

continuing increase of expiratory flow rates, which results from increased pleural pressure and thus an increased driving force for expiratory airflow. This region of the vital capacity during maximal expiratory flow is often termed the *effort-dependent portion.*

Below 70 percent of vital capacity, there comes a point at which we can no longer increase the flow rate with increasing effort. In other words, something other than our muscular strength (hence, other than the pleural pressure we can generate) limits flow. In fact, the limiting factor is a critical narrowing of the airways. When we try harder, all we do is compress the airway further, without any increase in the flow rate. This part of the flow-volume curve is frequently termed the *effort-independent portion* at which, beyond a certain level of effort, further effort does not result in an augmented flow rate.

Two unanswered questions about maximal expiratory flow remain. First, why does critical narrowing of the airways occur, so that increasing effort proves fruitless in augmenting flow? Second, at what level in the airways does this critical narrowing occur? Answers to these questions that have been of great interest to pulmonary physiologists must be distilled from a large amount of theory and research.*

*This discussion uses a model based on the *equal pressure point* concept. A different model, based on *wave speed theory*, probably provides a more accurate conceptual framework for expiratory flow limitation, but it is more complicated and beyond the scope of this discussion.

During a forced expiration, there are several determinants of airway diameter. First and most obvious is the inherent size of the airway, which depends on its level in the tracheobronchial tree and the tone of the airway smooth muscle. In disease, smooth muscle tone may be increased (as in asthma), or secretions in the airway may narrow the lumen (as in asthma or chronic bronchitis). Second is the amount of radial traction exerted by surrounding lung tissue on the airway walls. Airways are not isolated structures but are surrounded by a supporting framework of alveolar walls that are constantly "pulling" or "tethering" the airways open. As will be discussed in Chapter 6, when lung parenchyma is destroyed, as in emphysema, the airways lose some of their normal support and are more likely to collapse. Third, and perhaps most difficult to understand, is the combination of pressures acting on the airway from without and from within. This balance of pressures is crucial in determining whether a particular airway remains open or closed during a forced expiration.

> Airway diameter depends on the level of the airway in the tracheobronchial tree, airway smooth muscle tone, traction on the airway from surrounding lung tissue, and internal and external pressures on the airway.

The external pressure acting on an airway is determined to a large extent by pleural pressure (Fig. 4-5). When pleural pressure is strongly positive, as with a forced expiration, the airway becomes compressed. It is only because of a counteracting pressure within the airways that they are able to remain open in the face of a strongly positive external pressure. Two factors contribute to this counteracting internal airway pressure: (1) the elastic recoil of the lungs and (2) pleural pressure transmitted to the alveoli and airways. Figure 4-5 shows that the alveolar wall is like a stretched balloon trying to expel its air. In the same way that a balloon, in trying to collapse, exerts pressure on the air inside, the alveolar wall has its elastic recoil that exerts pressure on the gas within. This pressure results in flow through the airways, but as mentioned earlier, flow through an airway must result in a pressure drop along the airway. At a certain point along the airway, the pressure falls enough so that pressure within the airway becomes equal to the pressure outside the airway (i.e., pleural pressure). This point is called the *equal pressure point.* If one increases the amount of effort, that is, the amount of pleural pressure, this pressure is exerted both on the alveolus and externally on the airway wall. The driving pressure—the difference between alveolar pressure and the pressure at the equal pressure point—remains the elastic recoil pressure of the lung. As Figure 4-5 shows, with additional effort the increased alveolar driving

> At the equal pressure point, internal and external pressures on the airway are equal. The net driving pressure from the alveolus to the equal pressure point is the elastic recoil pressure of the lung.

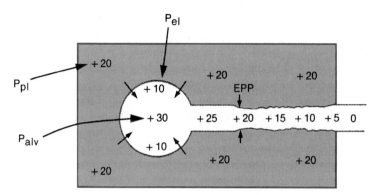

Figure 4-5 ■— Schematic diagram of equal pressure point (EPP) concept during a forced (maximal) expiration. Alveolus and its airway are shown inside box, which represents pleural space. Alveolar pressure (P_{alv}) has two contributing components—pleural pressure (P_{pl}) and elastic recoil pressure of lung (P_{el}). In this diagram, $P_{pl} = 20\,cm\,H_2O$, and $P_{el} = 10\,cm\,H_2O$. P_{alv}, the sum of P_{pl} and P_{el}, is therefore $30\,cm\,H_2O$.

pressure is exactly balanced by the increased external pressure on the airway. This increased external pressure promotes airway collapse. The net result is that the elastic recoil pressure is an important determinant of maximal expiratory flow, whereas pleural pressure produced by expiratory effort does not play a role, at least in the effort-independent or latter part of a forced expiration. Subsequent chapters show that in diseases with altered elastic recoil, maximal expiratory flow rates are affected by this change in the effective driving pressure for airflow.

The final question to be addressed here is the level at which this critical narrowing—that is, the equal pressure point—occurs. The answer depends on the lung volume; the equal pressure point does not remain at a constant position all along the flow-volume curve going toward residual volume. At higher lung volumes, the elastic recoil pressure is greater (the alveoli are stretched more), and a longer distance separates the alveoli from the equal pressure point. At lung volumes above functional residual capacity, this critical point of narrowing is within relatively large airways, segmental bronchi or larger. At lower lung volumes, the elastic recoil pressure is lower, the distance from alveoli to the equal pressure point is smaller, and critical narrowing occurs more peripherally. Because maximal airflow depends on elastic recoil and the resistance of the airways peripheral ("upstream") to the equal pressure point, the resistance of the small airways is a larger component of the upstream resistance at small lung volumes and is therefore a greater determinant of maximal expiratory flow at lower volumes along the flow-volume curve.

In summary, flow through the tracheobronchial tree reflects a combination of factors: airway size, support or radial traction exerted by the surrounding lung parenchyma, and driving pressure provided by the elastic recoil of the lung. Although pleural pressure contributes to the driving pressure for airflow, it also exerts a counterbalancing external pressure on the airway, promoting airway collapse. Later discussion of specific disorders will show how these different factors are interrelated as determinants of maximal expiratory airflow and how they can be altered in disease states.

> The equal pressure point moves peripherally (toward smaller airways) as lung volume decreases during a forced expiration; hence the resistance of small airways limits maximal expiratory flow more at low than at high lung volumes.

References

Barnes PJ: Neural control of airway smooth muscle. *In* Crystal RG, West JB, Weibel ER, and Barnes PJ (eds): The Lung: Scientific Foundations, 2nd ed. Philadelphia, Lippincott-Raven, 1997, pp 1269-1285.

Barnes PJ: Neurogenic inflammation in the airways. Respir Physiol 125:145-154, 2001.

Canning BJ and Fischer A: Neural regulation of airway smooth muscle tone. Respir Physiol 125:113-127, 2001.

Drazen JM, Gaston B, and Shore SA: Chemical regulation of pulmonary airway tone. Annu Rev Physiol 57:151-170, 1995.

Finkbeiner WE: Physiology and pathology of tracheobronchial glands. Respir Physiol 118:77-83, 1999.

Gail DB and Lenfant CJM: Cells of the lung: biology and clinical implications. Am Rev Respir Dis 127:366-387, 1983.

Hall IP: Second messengers, ion channels and pharmacology of airway smooth muscle. Eur Respir J 15:1120-1127, 2000.

Leff AR and Schumacker PT: Respiratory Physiology: Basics and Applications. Philadelphia, WB Saunders Co., 1993.

Wanner A, Matthias S, and O'Riordan TG: Mucociliary clearance in the airways. Am J Respir Crit Care Med 154:1868-1902, 1996.

Weibel ER: The Pathway for Oxygen. Cambridge, MA, Harvard University Press, 1984, pp 272-282.

West JB: Respiratory Physiology—The Essentials, 6th ed. Philadelphia, Lippincott Williams & Wilkins, 2000.

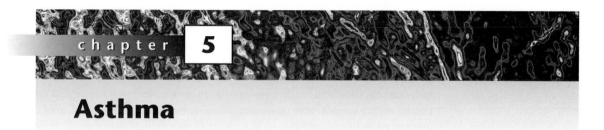

chapter 5

Asthma

ETIOLOGY AND PATHOGENESIS	PATHOPHYSIOLOGY
Predisposition to Asthma	CLINICAL FEATURES
Airway Inflammation and Bronchial Hyperresponsiveness	DIAGNOSTIC APPROACH
Common Provocative Stimuli	TREATMENT
PATHOLOGY	

Chapter 4 discussed the normal structure of airways and considered several aspects of airway function. The most common disorders disrupting the normal structure and function of the airways—asthma and chronic obstructive pulmonary disease—are discussed here and in Chapter 6, respectively, and several other miscellaneous diseases affecting airways are covered in Chapter 7.

Asthma is a condition characterized by episodes of reversible airway narrowing, associated with contraction of smooth muscle within the airway wall. It is a common disorder, affecting approximately 3 to 5 percent of the population. Although asthma can occur in any age group, it is particularly common in children and young adults and is probably the most common chronic disease found in these age groups.

The primary feature that patients with asthma appear to have in common is *hyperresponsiveness* of the airways, that is, an exaggerated response of airway smooth muscle to a wide variety of stimuli. This hyperresponsiveness is likely due to underlying airway inflammation with a variety of types of inflammatory cells, especially eosinophils. The particular constellation of stimuli triggering the attacks often varies from patient to patient, but the net effect (bronchoconstriction) is qualitatively similar. Because asthma is by definition a disease with at least some reversibility, the patient experiences exacerbations (attacks) interspersed between intervals of diminished symptoms or symptom-free periods. During an attack, the diagnosis is usually straightforward; during a symptom-free period, the diagnosis may be more difficult to make and may require provocation or challenge tests to induce airway constriction.

> Asthma is characterized by hyperreactivity of the airways and reversible episodes of bronchoconstriction.

ETIOLOGY AND PATHOGENESIS

Despite the prevalence of asthma in the general population and the many advances that have been made in treating the manifestations of the disease, a great deal about its etiology and pathogenesis remains speculative. This section focuses on two major questions: (1) What causes certain people to have airways that hyperreact to various stimuli? (2) What is the sequence of events from the time of exposure to the stimulus until the time of clinical response?

Predisposition to Asthma

Potential factors that may predispose an individual to developing asthma can be either inherited or acquired. There has been significant interest in and investigation of genetic and environmental factors that may contribute to the development of asthma, but the roles of these factors and their possible interactions have not been fully elucidated.

Genetics. A substantial proportion of patients with asthma have an underlying history of allergies (allergic rhinitis and eczema) along with accompanying markers for allergic disease, such as positive skin tests and elevated immunoglobulin E (IgE) levels. In addition, these patients' asthma is frequently exacerbated by exposure to various allergens to which they have been previously sensitized. In patients with an allergic component to their asthma, there is often also a strong family history of asthma or other allergies, suggesting that genetic factors may play a role in the development of asthma as well as the underlying allergic diathesis (often called *atopy*). However, no simple pattern of Mendelian inheritance has been identified to suggest a single responsible gene for either atopy or asthma.

Epidemiologic studies have confirmed an increased frequency of asthma and atopy in first-degree relatives of asthmatic subjects compared with control subjects, and studies in twins indicate a much higher concordance for asthma in monozygotic than in dizygotic twins. Attempts to identify chromosomal regions carrying genes associated with asthma have found a number of such regions, particularly on the long arm of chromosomes 5, 11, and 12 (5q, 11q, and 12q, respectively) and on the short arm of chromosome 6 (6p). Examples of candidate genes proposed to be involved in the predisposition to asthma include the β subunit gene of the high-affinity receptor for IgE (on chromosome 11q), a gene cluster for production of various cytokines (on chromosome 5q), and the gene encoding the β_2-adrenergic receptor (on chromosome 5q). Despite these intriguing associations, there is general agreement that the genetic influences in asthma are complex, and multiple genes and gene products are likely to interact in the pathogenesis of the disease.

Acquired (Environmental) Factors. A variety of environmental factors have been proposed that might predispose an individual to develop asthma, perhaps interacting with one or more genetic factors. Exposure to allergens, possibly at a critical time during childhood, may be an important environmental factor. Some of these allergens are common environmental allergens, such as those derived from house dust mites, domestic animals, and cockroaches. These allergens are found indoors, often concentrated in bedding and carpets, and are present throughout the year.

Another potential environmental factor is maternal cigarette smoking. This has been suggested as a predisposing factor for development of childhood asthma, possibly related to increasing the immune responsiveness of the child. Finally, viral respiratory tract infections are known to precipitate airway inflammation and trigger acute exacerbations of asthma, but their potential role as an inducer or cause of asthma in the absence of other factors is controversial. One theory suggests that early childhood viral infections may be causally associated with the later development of asthma, whereas a contrary view suggests that respiratory infections during childhood protect against development of asthma by shifting the immunological profile of T-helper cells toward a T_H1 response (responsible for cellular defense) and away from a T_H2 response (which mediates allergic inflammation).

Airway Inflammation and Bronchial Hyperresponsiveness

Even though there is a significant association between asthma and allergies, this association is not universal. Many individuals with asthma have no other evidence of atopy and do not experience exacerbations as a result of antigen exposure. In this group, asthma attacks are often precipitated by other stimuli, as will be described later. However, the feature that both groups of patients—those with and those without an allergic background, sometimes referred to as "extrinsic" and "intrinsic" asthmatic patients, respectively—have in common is hyperresponsiveness of their airways to a variety of stimuli. When exposed to such stimuli, the airways often demonstrate bronchoconstriction, which can be measured as an increase in airway resistance or a decrease in forced expiratory flow rates.

Although many asthmatic patients have allergies, some do not, and the overall relationship between allergies and asthma is not clear.

The histologic feature that accompanies this hyperresponsiveness and is thought to be a critical component of its pathogenesis is *airway inflammation*. Airway inflammation, especially with eosinophils and lymphocytes, has been found on postmortem examination in persons with asthma who died of their disease, as well as on bronchial biopsy specimens obtained from patients with mild asthma. In addition, there is also often evidence of epithelial damage, with many areas of detached or absent epithelial cells, so that the basal cells or even the basement membrane becomes exposed. These histologic findings may be responsible for the hyperresponsiveness that can be documented in such persons with asthma, even when they are free of obvious bronchospasm.

Airway inflammation and epithelial injury may contribute to non-specific bronchial hyperresponsiveness.

No single factor or cell appears to be responsible for asthma, but rather there is a complex and interrelated series of events that likely culminate in airway hyperresponsiveness and episodes of airflow obstruction (Fig. 5-1). A variety of mediators released from inflammatory cells can alter the

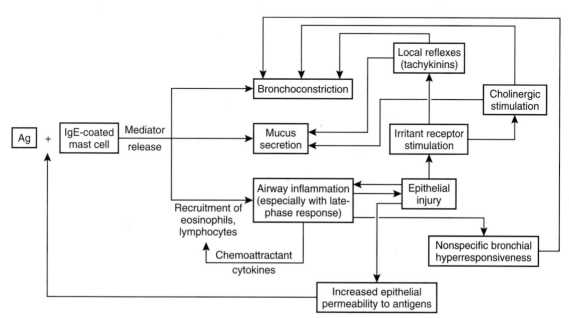

Figure 5-1 ■— Schematic diagram of events in pathogenesis of antigen-induced asthma. Hypothetical series of complex interactions is shown, focusing on bronchoconstriction, mucus secretion, and airway inflammation.

extracellular milieu of bronchial smooth muscle, increasing its responsiveness to bronchoconstrictive stimuli. Mediators that have been proposed to play such a role include prostaglandin and leukotriene products of arachidonic acid metabolism. Some cytokine mediators released from inflammatory cells have various effects on other inflammatory cells, thus perpetuating the inflammatory response. For example, lymphocytes of the T_H2 phenotype, which are thought to be a prominent component of the inflammatory response in asthma, release interleukin-5 (IL-5), which has a chemoattractant effect for eosinophils. IL-5 also stimulates the growth, activation, and degranulation of eosinophils. Another cytokine released from T_H2 lymphocytes—IL-4—exerts a different type of pro-inflammatory effect by activating B lymphocytes, enhancing synthesis of IgE, and promoting differentiation of T_H2 cells.

Mediators released from inflammatory cells may also produce tissue damage that contributes to the pathogenesis of asthma. For example, when eosinophils degranulate, they release several toxic proteins from their granules, such as major basic protein and eosinophil cationic protein. These and other eosinophil products may contribute to the epithelial damage that is a histologic feature of the asthmatic airway. Once the epithelium is injured or denuded, its barrier function is disrupted, allowing access of inhaled material to deeper layers of the mucosa. Additionally, the epithelial cells themselves may become actively involved in amplifying the inflammatory process (through production of cytokine and chemokine mediators) and in perpetuating airway edema (through vasodilation mediated by release of nitric oxide, leukotrienes, and prostaglandins). Finally, sensory nerve endings in the airway epithelial layer may become exposed, triggering a reflex arc and release of tachykinin mediators, such as substance P and neurokinin A, as shown in pathway 4 of Fig. 4-3. These peptide mediators, released at bronchial smooth muscle, submucosal glands, and blood vessels, are capable of causing bronchoconstriction and airway edema.

Mediators from inflammatory cells may recruit and activate other inflammatory cells and may promote epithelial injury.

Common Provocative Stimuli

For the asthmatic person, a substantial amount is known about the sequence of events from the time of exposure to a stimulus to the clinical response of bronchoconstriction. Considered here are four stimuli that can result in bronchoconstriction: (1) allergen (antigen) exposure, (2) inhaled irritants, (3) respiratory tract infection, and (4) exercise.

Common stimuli that precipitate bronchoconstriction in the asthmatic patient are the following:
1. *Exposure to an allergen*
2. *Inhaled irritants*
3. *Respiratory tract infection*
4. *Exercise*

Allergen Exposure

Allergens to which an asthmatic person may be sensitized are widespread throughout nature. Although patients and clinicians often first consider seasonal outdoor allergens, such as pollen, many indoor allergens may play a more critical role. These include antigens from house dust mites (*Dermatophagoides* and others), domestic animals, and cockroaches. When an asthmatic person has IgE antibody against a particular antigen, the antibody binds to high-affinity IgE receptors on the surface of tissue mast cells and circulating basophils (see Fig. 5-1). If that particular antigen is inhaled, it binds to and cross-links IgE antibody (against the antigen) bound to the surface of mast cells in the bronchial lumen. The mast cell is then activated, leading to release of preformed as well as newly synthesized mediators. The mediators released from the mast cell induce bronchoconstriction and increase the permeability of the airway epithelium, allowing the antigen access to the much larger population of specific IgE-containing mast cells that are deeper within the epithelium. The binding of antigen to antibody on this larger population of mast cells again initiates a sequence of events leading to release of chemical mediators capable of inducing bronchoconstriction and inflammation. Several mediators have been recognized (Table 5-1), but the discussion here is limited to the few that have been primarily implicated in the pathogenesis of allergic asthma. The major mediators include histamine and leukotrienes.

Histamine. This relatively small (MW 111) compound is found preformed within the mast cell and is released on exposure to the appropriate antigen. Histamine has several effects that may be important in asthma, including contraction of bronchial smooth muscle, augmentation of vascular permeability with formation of airway edema, and stimulation of irritant receptors (which can trigger a reflex neurogenic pathway via the vagus nerve, causing secondary bronchoconstriction). Despite these varied effects, the fact that the clinical manifestations of asthma do not respond to antihistamines suggests that histamine is not the most important chemical mediator involved.

Leukotrienes. The leukotrienes include a series of compounds (LTC_4, LTD_4, and LTE_4) that were formerly called slow-reacting substance of anaphylaxis (SRS-A). Unlike histamine, the leukotrienes are not preformed in the mast cell but are synthesized after antigen exposure and then released. To some extent, their actions are similar to those of histamine; they also have a direct bronchoconstrictor action on smooth muscle and can increase vascular permeability. The leukotrienes are synthesized from arachidonic acid (also the precursor for prostaglandins) but along a somewhat different pathway, involving a lipoxygenase enzyme as opposed to the cyclooxygenase enzyme used for prostaglandin synthesis (Fig. 5-2). LTC_4 and LTD_4, in particular, are extraordinarily potent bronchoconstrictors, and they may indeed have a crucial role in the pathogenesis of bronchial asthma. An interesting sidelight is provided by knowledge that some persons with asthma experience exacerbations of their disease after taking aspirin or other nonsteroidal anti-inflammatory drugs. These drugs are known to be inhibitors of the cyclooxygenase enzyme and may result in preferential shifting of the pathway shown in Figure 5-2 toward production of the bronchoconstrictor leukotrienes.

The role of the other mediators listed in Table 5-1 in the pathogenesis of asthma is less clear. It has been proposed that platelet-activating factor may play an important role in the recruitment of eosinophils to the lung. In addition, platelet-activating factor activates eosinophils, stimulating them to release proteins toxic to airway epithelial cells.

The Late-Phase Asthmatic Response. The airway response to antigen challenge, as measured by changes in forced expiratory volume in 1 second (FEV_1), appears to be more complicated and involves more than just the rapid,

Table 5-1
Potential Chemical Mediators in Asthma
Histamine Leukotrienes (LTC_4, LTD_4, LTE_4) Platelet-activating factor Prostaglandins (PGD_2) Eosinophil chemotactic factor of anaphylaxis Neutrophil chemotactic factor of anaphylaxis Bradykinin Serotonin Kallikrein

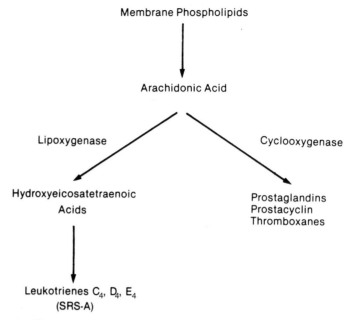

Figure 5-2 ■— Outline of pathway for formation of leukotrienes (SRS-A) and prostaglandins. Aspirin and other nonsteroidal anti-inflammatory drugs are inhibitors of the enzyme cyclooxygenase.

mediator-induced bronchoconstriction seen within the first half hour following exposure. In many patients, the return of FEV_1 to normal is followed by a secondary, delayed fall in FEV_1 occurring hours after antigen exposure and lasting up to days (Fig. 5-3). This delayed fall in FEV_1 is accompanied histologically by inflammatory changes in the airway wall. At the same time, bronchial hyperresponsiveness to nonspecific stimuli, such as histamine or methacholine, can be demonstrated.

It now appears that this "late-phase response," as it has been called, depends on the presence of antigen-specific IgE. Presumably, release of mediators after allergen binding to IgE-coated mast cells results in the influx of inflammatory cells, especially eosinophils, into the airway wall. Experimental data suggest that this airway inflammation is responsible for the nonspecific bronchial hyperresponsiveness seen at the time of the late-phase response.

Although the link between the episodic bronchoconstriction characteristic of asthma attacks and nonspecific bronchial hyperresponsiveness has not been clearly elucidated, it is reasonable to speculate that the clinically observed nonspecific bronchial hyperresponsiveness is a consequence of the inflammation associated with the late-phase asthmatic response.

Inhaled Irritants

Inhaled irritants, such as cigarette smoke, inorganic dusts, and environmental pollutants, are also common precipitants of bronchoconstriction in asthmatic persons. These airborne irritants appear to stimulate *irritant receptors* located primarily in the walls of the larynx, trachea, and large bronchi. Stimulation of the receptors initiates a reflex arc that travels to the central nervous system and back to the bronchi via the vagus nerve. This efferent vagal stimulation of the bronchi completes the reflex arc and induces bronchoconstriction. As mentioned in the discussion about chemical mediators, histamine is capable of stimulating irritant receptors, and at least part of its bronchocon-

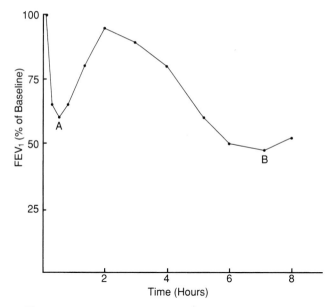

Figure 5-3 ■ Response of FEV₁ after antigen challenge in patient who demonstrates a biphasic response. Early bronchoconstrictive response is at A; slower onset, late-phase asthmatic response is at B.

strictive effect may be mediated indirectly via stimulation of the irritant receptors.

Respiratory Tract Infection

Respiratory tract infection is a factor for patients with nonallergic as well as allergic asthma. Viral infections are the most common ones in this category, but at times bacterial infections of the tracheobronchial tree can also be implicated. The mechanism by which respiratory infections precipitate bronchoconstriction in asthmatic persons is not entirely clear but is likely related to epithelial damage and airway inflammation. Potential consequences of the epithelial injury include release of mediators from inflammatory cells, stimulation of irritant receptors, and nonspecific bronchial hyperresponsiveness.

Exercise

Exercise can frequently provoke bronchoconstriction in patients with hyperreactive airways. The crucial factor in the pathogenesis appears to be heat movement from the airway wall, resulting in cooling of the airway. During exercise, individuals have a high minute ventilation, and the large amounts of relatively cool and dry inspired air must be warmed and humidified by the tracheobronchial mucosa. When the air is warmed and humidified, water evaporates from the epithelial surface, resulting in cooling of the airway epithelium. The phenomenon of exercise-induced bronchoconstriction can be reproduced by having an asthmatic person voluntarily breathe cold, dry air at a high minute ventilation. At the same minute ventilation, inhalation of warm, saturated air does not produce a similar effect. The mechanism that links airway cooling and drying with bronchoconstriction is less clear. Alteration of the ionic environment after drying of the mucosa, mediator release, hyperemia of the mucosa following airway rewarming, and stimulation of irritant receptors have all been proposed as mechanisms, but none is universally accepted.

Airway cooling is important in exercise-induced bronchoconstriction.

As might be expected from the above description of exercise-induced bronchoconstriction, inhalation of cold air during the winter months can be responsible for asthma exacerbations or worsening of symptoms in selected patients. The mechanism of airway narrowing in these patients following inhalation of cold air is also believed to be due to airway cooling and drying, and therefore is analogous to the mechanism of exercise-induced bronchoconstriction.

PATHOLOGY

Information about pathologic findings in asthma has often been obtained at autopsy studies and thus represents the consequences of particularly severe disease. In these cases, there is marked overdistention of the lungs, and the airways are occluded by thick, tenacious mucous plugs. Information has also become available regarding the histologic appearance of the airways in patients with stable, mild disease. Examination of the airways by microscopy demonstrates the following findings of variable severity that are apparent in both mild and in more severe disease:

1. Edema and cellular infiltrates within the bronchial wall, especially with eosinophils and lymphocytes
2. Epithelial damage, with a "fragile" appearance of the epithelium and with detachment of the surface epithelial cells from the basal cells
3. Hypertrophy and hyperplasia of the smooth muscle layer
4. Thickening of the epithelial basement membrane
5. Enlargement of the mucus-secreting apparatus, with hypertrophy of mucous glands and an increased number of goblet cells

The presence of these histologic abnormalities presumably contributes to the nonspecific bronchial hyperresponsiveness in such patients, even when they are free of an acute attack. In addition, the term airway remodeling is used to describe aspects of the histology such as items 3 through 5 above, which reflect more long-standing structural changes that contribute to persisting airflow obstruction.

PATHOPHYSIOLOGY

The pathophysiologic features of asthma largely follow from the pathologic abnormalities just described. Contraction of smooth muscle in the bronchial walls, mucosal edema, and secretions within the airway lumen all contribute to a decrease in airway diameter, which increases airway resistance. The pathologic changes are present at many levels of the tracheobronchial tree, from large airways down to the peripheral airways less than 2 mm in diameter.

As a result of narrowed airways with increased resistance, patients have difficulty with airflow during both inspiration and expiration. However, because intrathoracic airways are subjected to relatively negative external pressure (transmitted from negative pleural pressure) during inspiration, lumen size is larger during the inspiratory phase of the respiratory cycle. During expiration, relatively positive pleural pressure is transmitted to intrathoracic airways, thus decreasing their diameter. Therefore, greater difficulty with airflow on expiration than on inspiration is characteristic of asthma, as it is of any of the diseases that cause obstruction or narrowing of airways within the thorax. The greatest difficulty with expiration occurs when the patient is asked to perform a forced expiration; i.e., to breathe out as hard and

In asthma and other diseases associated with obstruction of intrathoracic airways, airflow is most compromised during expiration.

as fast as possible. With a forced expiration, pleural pressure becomes much more positive, thereby promoting airway closure and air trapping.

The effects of increased airway resistance are readily seen by measuring pulmonary function in asthmatic persons. During an attack, pulmonary function studies show decreases in forced expiratory flow rates as well as evidence of air trapping. On the forced expiratory spirogram, patients generally exhibit a decrease in both forced vital capacity (FVC) and forced expiratory volume in 1 second (FEV_1), with the decrease in FEV_1 usually more pronounced than the decrease in FVC. Hence, the ratio FEV_1/FVC, reflecting the proportion of the FVC that can be exhaled during the first second, is decreased. In addition, the maximal midexpiratory flow rate is also diminished.

Measurement of lung volumes shows evidence of air trapping, with increases in functional residual capacity (FRC), residual volume (RV), and sometimes total lung capacity (TLC). Of all these lung volumes, the most impressive increase is in RV, the volume left in the lungs at the end of a maximal exhalation, which may be greater than 200 percent of the predicted value. The increase in RV is believed to be due at least partly to premature airway closure as a result of smooth muscle constriction, mucous plugs, and inflammatory changes of the mucosa.

It is not entirely clear whether TLC truly increases or how this might occur. Two main factors determine TLC: (1) inspiratory muscles that act to expand the chest and (2) elastic recoil of the lung that acts to decrease lung volume. For reasons that are not certain, some evidence suggests that elastic recoil is decreased during acute asthma attacks, and it has also been suggested that inspiratory muscle strength (or the efficiency of contraction) may be increased.

FRC, the resting point of the lungs after a normal expiration, may also be increased for at least two reasons. First, because more time is required for expiration when airways are obstructed, patients may not have sufficient time before the next breath to fully exhale the volume from the previous breath. This phenomenon is sometimes called *dynamic hyperinflation* and is a problem particularly when the asthmatic person is breathing at a rapid respiratory rate. Another reason for the increase in FRC is related to persistent activity of the inspiratory muscles during expiration, maintaining lung volume at a higher than expected level throughout expiration.

The focus so far has been on the pulmonary function and physiologic abnormalities with a typical asthmatic attack. Between attacks, pulmonary function, as measured by FEV_1 and FVC, often returns to normal. However, even when a person is not having an acute attack, subtle abnormalities in pulmonary function may be present, such as a decrease in maximal midexpiratory flow rate and an increase in RV. These abnormalities may reflect some residual disease in the small airways of the lung, frequently the last region to become normal after an attack.

A subgroup of asthmatic persons, generally those with long-standing disease, have pulmonary function that does not return to normal; instead, they have easily demonstrable physiologic abnormalities (e.g., abnormal FEV_1 and FVC) persisting between attacks. Even though asthma is generally characterized by reversible episodes of airflow obstruction, these persons also appear to have a component of irreversible disease. Nevertheless, they still generally experience episodes of reversible airflow obstruction and worsening of expiratory flow rates superimposed upon whatever irreversible disease is present.

The increased resistance to airflow in asthma also exerts its toll on gas-exchange, which is generally disturbed during acute attacks. The most

Pulmonary function tests with asthma generally demonstrate a decreased FEV_1, FVC, and FEV_1/FVC ratio; air trapping and hyperinflation are demonstrated by increases in RV, FRC, and sometimes TLC.

common pattern of arterial blood gases consists of a low P_{O_2} accompanied by a low P_{CO_2} (respiratory alkalosis). The mechanism for the hypoxemia is ventilation-perfusion mismatch. The increased airways resistance in asthma is not evenly distributed, such that some airways are affected more than others. Therefore, inspired air is not distributed evenly but tends to go to less diseased areas. However, blood flow remains relatively preserved in the regions that are ventilating poorly. The regions of low ventilation-perfusion ($\dot{V}/\dot{Q}$) ratio contribute blood with a low P_{O_2} that cannot be compensated for by increases in the $\dot{V}/\dot{Q}$ ratio from other regions of the lung (see Chapter 1).

Despite the abnormality in P_{O_2}, persons are able to hyperventilate, and P_{CO_2} is usually low. When P_{CO_2} increases to normal or to a frankly elevated level, it often means worsening airflow obstruction or a tiring individual who is no longer able to maintain normal or high minute ventilation in the face of significant airflow obstruction. The stimulus or mechanism for the hyperventilation is not clear. During an acute asthma attack, it is possible that activation of irritant receptors stimulates ventilation or that other reflexes originating in the airways, lung, or chest wall may serve to stimulate ventilation.

> The most common pattern of arterial blood gases in asthma is a low P_{O_2} (due primarily to $\dot{V}/\dot{Q}$ mismatch) and a low P_{CO_2}.

CLINICAL FEATURES

The onset of asthma occurs most frequently during childhood and young adulthood, although asthma can also develop for the first time in older patients. In many patients, particularly those in whom asthma started before 16 years of age, the disease eventually regresses, and they are no longer subject to repeated episodes of reversible airway obstruction.

The symptoms most commonly noted by patients during an exacerbation of asthma are cough, dyspnea, wheezing, and chest tightness. Patients do not necessarily have a classic presentation with several or all of these complaints, but may merely have an unexplained cough or breathlessness on exertion. In some cases, patients can clearly identify a precipitating factor for an attack, such as exposure to an allergen, respiratory tract infection, exercise, exposure to cold air, emotional stress, or exposure to irritating dusts, fumes, or odors. In other cases, there is no identifiable precipitant. Exposures in the workplace, related to proteins or other chemicals to which the patient may be sensitized, are important precipitants in a subgroup of patients who are said to have *occupational asthma*. Some asthmatic persons are particularly sensitive to ingestion of aspirin, which perhaps favors production of leukotrienes from arachidonic acid. Some of these patients with aspirin sensitivity also have nasal polyps, leading to a well-recognized triad of asthma, aspirin sensitivity, and nasal polyposis. Other nonsteroidal anti-inflammatory drugs (which also inhibit the cyclooxygenase enzyme) can also produce bronchoconstriction in patients who are aspirin-sensitive.

On examination, patients experiencing an asthma attack usually have tachypnea and, on auscultation of the chest, prolonged expiration and evidence of wheezing. The wheezing is generally more prominent during expiration than inspiration, and may be triggered by having the patient exhale forcefully. Although the tendency is to equate wheezing and asthma, the presence of wheezing does not necessarily indicate a diagnosis of asthma. Wheezing reflects only airflow through narrowed airways; it can also be seen in such diverse disorders as congestive heart failure and chronic obstructive pulmonary disease or in the case of a foreign body in the airway. On the other hand, not all asthmatic persons wheeze. It is a common observation that

> Major symptoms during an acute asthma attack are the following:
> 1. Cough
> 2. Dyspnea
> 3. Wheezing
> 4. Chest tightness

> Despite its prominence, the presence of wheezing is not synonymous with asthma and merely reflects airflow through narrowed airways.

severe asthma may be associated with no wheeze at all if airflow is too impaired to generate an audible wheeze.

During a particularly severe attack that is refractory to treatment with bronchodilators, persons with asthma are said to be in *status asthmaticus*. These patients present difficult therapeutic challenges, may require assisted ventilation, and may even die as a result of the acute attack.

The overall severity of an individual's asthma can be characterized based on the frequency of exacerbations, nocturnal symptoms, and the magnitude of abnormality and variability in pulmonary function. The features used to define four categories of severity—mild intermittent asthma, mild persistent asthma, moderate persistent asthma, and severe persistent asthma—are shown in Table 5-2.

DIAGNOSTIC APPROACH

A clinical history of reversible episodes of bronchoconstriction is often crucial to the diagnosis of asthma. Helpful additional features in the history include other evidence for atopy (such as hay fever or eczema) or a family history of allergies or asthma. Physical examination during an attack often provides confirmatory evidence for airway obstruction.

The chest radiograph, although sometimes useful for ruling out other causes of wheezing or complications of asthma, is generally not particularly helpful in the diagnosis. It usually shows normal findings, but may demonstrate hyperinflation with relatively large lung volumes.

If the patient is producing sputum, microscopic examination frequently shows many eosinophils on the sputum smear. An increased percentage of eosinophils in peripheral blood is also common, even when the asthma has no clear relationship to allergies.

There is debate about the clinical usefulness of skin testing and inhalation testing with allergens in an attempt to identify antigens to which the patient is sensitized. Unfortunately, these tests do not necessarily correlate with each other and do not establish that antigens causing positive test results have been responsible for exacerbations of asthma.

Other types of provocation tests used to make a diagnosis of asthma rely on the principle that asthmatic persons have hyperreactive airways. Therefore, when tested with inhalation of methacholine (a cholinergic agent) or histamine, persons with asthma respond with bronchoconstriction to comparatively small doses of either agent. Inhalation of cold air at high minute ventilations with PCO_2 kept constant (termed *isocapneic hyperpnea*) can also be used as a challenge test to induce transient bronchoconstriction in patients in whom the diagnosis of asthma is uncertain.

Measurement of pulmonary function, especially FEV_1 and FVC, is particularly useful in the patient with suspected or known asthma. Documentation of reversible airflow obstruction, either during attacks or with the aforementioned challenge tests, is frequently sufficient to make the diagnosis. In practice, the diagnosis of asthma is most commonly made by the history of episodic dyspnea, wheezing, or cough, with documentation of reversible airflow obstruction by pulmonary function testing.

Patients can conveniently test their own pulmonary function through measurement of the peak expiratory flow rate. Such testing is particularly useful for monitoring the course of the disease and alerting the patient to adjust the medication regimen and/or seek attention from a physician. In

A diagnosis of asthma includes a history of episodic dyspnea, wheezing, or cough, along with reversible airflow obstruction documented by pulmonary function testing.

Table	5-2

Classification of Asthma by Severity: Clinical Aspects and Treatment

Asthma Severity	Clinical Features Before Treatment	Nighttime Symptoms	Lung Function	Treatment
Mild intermittent	• Symptoms ≤ twice per week • Asymptomatic and normal PEFR between exacerbations • Exacerbations brief	≤ twice per month	• FEV_1 or PEFR* ≥80% predicted • PEFR variability <20%	• Inhaled short-acting β_2-agonists as needed
Mild persistent	• Symptoms > twice per week but < once per day • Exacerbations may affect activity	> twice per month	• FEV_1 or PEFR ≥80% predicted • PEFR variability 20-30%	• Anti-inflammatory therapy (inhaled corticosteroid or cromoglycate) • Alternative: sustained-release theophylline or leukotriene modifier • Inhaled short-acting β_2-agonists as needed
Moderate persistent	• Daily symptoms • Daily use of inhaled short-acting β_2-agonist • Exacerbations affect activity • Exacerbations ≥ twice per week; may last days	> once per week	• FEV_1 or PEFR >60% and <80% predicted • PEFR variability >30%	• Anti-inflammatory therapy (increased dose of inhaled corticosteroid) • With or without addition of long-acting bronchodilator (long-acting β_2-agonist or sustained-release theophylline) • With or without addition of leukotriene modifier
Severe persistent	• Continual symptoms • Limited physical activity • Frequent exacerbations	Frequent	• FEV_1 or PEFR ≤60% predicted • PEFR variability >30%	• High-dose inhaled corticosteroids (± oral steroids) • Long-acting bronchodilator (long-acting β_2-agonist or sustained-release theophylline)

Adapted from Expert panel report II: guidelines for the diagnosis and management of asthma. National Asthma Education and Prevention Program, 1997.
*PEFR = peak expiratory flow rate

addition, the efficacy of treatment or changes in the therapeutic regimen can readily be assessed by serial measurement of the peak expiratory flow rate.

TREATMENT

The major categories of drugs used to treat asthma are those that dilate smooth muscle of the bronchial wall and those that have an anti-inflammatory action. Agents targeted at blocking production or activity of specific mediators are

Table	5-3			

Drug Therapy in Asthma

	Examples	Possible Routes of Administration	Mechanism of Action
Bronchodilators			
Sympathomimetics	Epinephrine Metaproterenol Terbutaline Albuterol Salmeterol Formoterol	Inhaled, oral, parenteral (depending on particular drug)	↑ cAMP via stimulation of adenylate cyclase
Xanthines	Theophylline Aminophylline	Oral Oral, parenteral	?↑cAMP via inhibition of phosphodiesterase; ? anti-inflammatory
Anticholinergics	Ipratropium	Inhaled	Blockade of cholinergic (bronchoconstrictor) effect on airways
Anti-inflammatory drugs			
Corticosteroids	Prednisone Methylprednisolone	Systemic (oral or parenteral, depending on particular drug)	Decreased inflammatory response in airways; ? additional mechanisms
	Beclomethasone Triamcinolone Flunisolide Fluticasone Budesonide	Inhaled	
Cromolyn		Inhaled	Inhibition of mediator release from mast cells; ? additional mechanisms
Nedocromil		Inhaled	? Similar to cromolyn
Drugs directed at specific targets			
5-Lipoxygenase inhibitors	Zileuton	Oral	Decreased production of leukotrienes
Leukotriene antagonists	Zafirlukast	Oral	Leukotriene D_4 receptor antagonism
Anti-IgE antibody (approval pending)	Omalizumab	Parenteral	Binds circulating IgE

also used, and a monoclonal antibody against IgE is the next agent on the horizon. The main categories of drugs used to treat asthma are shown in Table 5-3. Several of the drugs are also used for other types of pulmonary disease, particularly chronic obstructive pulmonary disease, and are mentioned in other chapters.

The most common bronchodilator agents in use for treatment of asthma are the sympathomimetic agents, which act on β_2-receptors to activate adenylate cyclase and increase intracellular cyclic adenosine monophosphate (cAMP). Increased levels of cAMP in bronchial smooth muscle, due specifically to stimulation of β_2-receptors, activate protein kinase A, which phosphorylates several regulatory proteins that mediate the bronchodilation. Beta stimulation also increases intracellular cAMP in mast cells, inhibiting release of chemical mediators that, secondarily, cause bronchoconstriction. Specific examples of available sympathomimetic drugs are listed in Table 5-3. Generally,

Sympathomimetic agents increase intracellular cAMP by activating adenylate cyclase; preferred agents preferentially stimulate β_2-receptors and decrease potential adverse cardiac effects caused by stimulation of β_1-receptors.

the preferred agents are those whose action is limited primarily to stimulation of β_2-receptors, in order to avoid some of the adverse cardiac effects induced by stimulation of β_1-receptors. Currently, the most commonly used β_2-specific agents are albuterol and salmeterol. Sympathomimetic agents can be given by several different routes, including oral or parenteral administration and inhalation. The inhaled agents are preferred because of fewer systemic side effects and direct delivery to the site of action in the airways.

Inhaled β_2-agonists are often used on an as-needed basis to reverse an acute episode of bronchoconstriction, and when such episodes are infrequent, they may be the only agents needed to control the patient's asthma. The newest β_2-agonists, salmeterol and formoterol, are long-acting (approximately 12 hours) and are not appropriate for as-needed use to treat acute symptoms. Also, β_2-agonist drugs may be used prophylactically before activities or exposure to stimuli that are known to precipitate bronchoconstriction. As the severity of asthma increases so that more frequent or regular use of an inhaled β_2-agonist is required, then addition of an anti-inflammatory agent (see the following third paragraph) is important.

The second class of bronchodilator agents, the methylxanthines, are generally believed to act by inhibiting the enzyme phosphodiesterase (PDE), which normally is responsible for the metabolic degradation of cAMP. When degradation is inhibited, the levels of cAMP in smooth muscle and mast cells increase, resulting again in bronchodilation and decreased mediator release from mast cells. However, the serum levels of methylxanthines needed to inhibit phosphodiesterase are higher than those actually achieved in patients, making it uncertain whether PDE inhibition is the major or exclusive mechanism of theophylline's action as a bronchodilator. In addition, theophylline may also have a component of anti-inflammatory activity, mediated by inhibition of the PDE IV isozyme in inflammatory cells. The most commonly used methylxanthines are theophylline and aminophylline. Theophylline is available only for oral administration, whereas aminophylline (a water-soluble salt of theophylline) can be given either orally or intravenously. Because methylxanthines can only be given systemically (as opposed to locally in the airway), systemic side effects—gastrointestinal, cardiac, and neurologic—are more problematic than with the inhaled sympathomimetic agents.

The third class of bronchodilator agents, used less frequently, consists of drugs that have an anticholinergic action. Ipratropium, available as an aerosol for inhalation, is the primary example of this class of agents, although it is formally approved in the United States only for use in chronic obstructive lung disease (see Chapter 6), not in asthma. By decreasing the bronchoconstrictor cholinergic tone to airways, the anticholinergic agents dilate bronchial smooth muscle. However, clinical studies have demonstrated that they are not as effective as the sympathomimetic agents in patients with asthma.

The second major category of drugs used to treat asthma includes the anti-inflammatory agents: corticosteroids, disodium cromoglycate (cromolyn), and nedocromil. Corticosteroids have been used for years for the treatment of asthma, acting to suppress the inflammatory response (by diminishing the number of eosinophils and lymphocytes infiltrating the airway) and to decrease the production of a number of inflammatory mediators. However, despite the general rationale for their use, many aspects of their anti-inflammatory action remain unknown. The glucocorticoids are thought to bind to a cytoplasmic receptor that is present in nearly all cell types. After the receptor binds to its glucocorticoid ligand, it moves to the cell nucleus, where it interacts with transcription factors, such as activator protein-1 (AP-1) and

Methylxanthines (aminophylline, theophylline) increase cAMP by inhibiting the enzyme phosphodiesterase, which degrades cAMP; this mechanism is arguably responsible for bronchodilation.

nuclear factor–kappa B, which regulate the transcription of other target genes. Important target genes whose transcription is suppressed by the action of glucocorticoids include a variety of inflammatory cytokines (e.g., IL-1, IL-3, IL-4, IL-5, IL-6, and tumor necrosis factor-α), the inducible form of nitric oxide synthase, and an inducible form of cyclooxygenase.

Because airway inflammation is believed to play an important role in the pathogenesis of asthma, particularly in the patient with more frequent attacks or more persistent airflow obstruction, corticosteroids have assumed a central role in the management of many cases of asthma. By decreasing airway inflammation, steroids are thought to ameliorate the underlying disease process in asthma, not just the bronchoconstriction resulting from airway inflammation.

Steroids have an important place both in management of acute asthma attacks and in maintenance therapy of disease requiring more than just infrequent use of a β_2-agonist bronchodilator. Frequently, steroids such as prednisone or methylprednisolone are started at high doses during an acute attack and then are tapered relatively rapidly. Because of the potential for significant adverse effects with long-term use of systemic (oral) steroids, chronic administration of oral steroids is avoided if the asthma can be managed with other modes of therapy. Foremost among these alternative forms of therapy are inhaled forms of corticosteroids, which deliver the drug locally to the airway and have minimal systemic absorption and side effects. Inhaled steroids are now the preferred form of "controller" or preventive therapy for patients with asthma not adequately managed with infrequent use of a β-agonist inhaler.

Systemic and inhaled corticosteroids have an important role in acute therapy and preventive management, respectively.

The other anti-inflammatory drugs that have been used for asthma are disodium cromoglycate (cromolyn) and nedocromil. Their mode of action has traditionally been thought to be inhibition of mediator release from mast cells. However, this mechanism has been disputed, and alternative mechanisms have been proposed, including inhibitory effects on other types of inflammatory cells or on the action of tachykinins. Both cromolyn and nedocromil are given in inhaled form. Neither is a bronchodilator, and neither is therefore useful for treatment of acute attacks. Rather, they are generally given as ongoing medication, with the goal of preventing future exacerbations.

Anti-inflammatory therapy is important when treatment of asthma requires more than infrequent use of an inhaled β_2-agonist.

More recently, agents have been developed that block the synthesis or action of a single type of mediator, specifically the leukotrienes. Interestingly, these agents only appear to be effective for some patients with asthma, and it is believed that underlying patient-related genetic factors affect the likelihood of a positive response. Specific agents that modify leukotrienes or leukotriene pathways include zafirlukast and montelukast, which antagonize the action of leukotriene D_4, and zileuton, which inhibits the enzyme 5-lipoxygenase. In addition, based on their mode of action, drugs that either block the synthesis of leukotrienes or antagonize their action have an important role in patients who are sensitive to aspirin or other nonsteroidal anti-inflammatory drugs.

The newest agent for asthma that is awaiting release is a monoclonal antibody to IgE. Based on the principle that IgE represents an important component of the pathobiology of allergic asthma, there is enthusiasm that antagonizing the effect of IgE will be an important therapeutic modality for selected cases of asthma. Because the drug is quite expensive, it is likely that its usage will be limited to particularly severe cases of asthma requiring chronic therapy with systemic corticosteroids.

At present, the overall strategy for management of asthma commonly proceeds in the following way. These general guidelines are also summarized in Table 5-2 according to the categories for clinical severity of disease. A patient with relatively infrequent attacks, with symptom-free periods, and with normal pulmonary function between attacks is managed with inhaled sympathomimetics. These are used both for management of bronchospasm once it occurs and also before exposure to stimuli often known to precipitate attacks—for example, exercise and allergen exposure.

When a patient's asthma cannot be managed successfully with infrequent use of a β_2-agonist inhaler, then an anti-inflammatory agent is generally added as maintenance (ongoing) therapy to suppress the underlying airway inflammation. Inhaled corticosteroids are used most frequently, although cromolyn and nedocromil are other alternatives, especially when allergens appear to have a prominent role in triggering exacerbations. Agents affecting leukotriene synthesis or action are increasingly being used, but their effectiveness in a given patient is at present unpredictable.

If therapy must be escalated beyond the above measures because of inadequate control, then regular use of inhaled β_2-agonists, addition of the methylxanthine theophylline, or both, are the major options. When patients have a significant acute attack or an attack that occurs despite adequate therapy as described, a short course of systemic steroids is generally effective. Particularly severe asthma exacerbations, i.e., *status asthmaticus,* often require high doses of intravenous corticosteroids along with aggressive bronchodilator therapy, and patients with respiratory failure may require intubation and mechanical ventilation.

Finally, for those patients in whom allergen exposure is an exacerbating factor for their asthma, allergen avoidance is a fundamental component of the management regimen. Environmental control measures to minimize allergen exposure include removal of carpets and encasing of mattresses and pillows in allergen-impermeable covers (to minimize dust mite exposure) and removal of pets from the home (to minimize exposure to animal antigens). Immunotherapy with repeated injections of antigen extract is sometimes used to desensitize the patient to the offending allergen, but its efficacy in patients with asthma is quite controversial and not generally accepted.

Because of the availability of effective forms of therapy, patients with asthma are generally capable of leading normal lifestyles with relatively little or no alteration in their daily activities. However, not all patients with asthma are so fortunate. Refractory disease, persistent airflow obstruction, and rapid development of life-threatening attacks are some of the extreme examples of asthma that pose a continuing challenge to physicians caring for these patients.

References

Reviews

Canadian Asthma Consensus Group: Canadian Asthma Consensus Report, 1999. CMAJ 161:S1-S61, 1999.
McFadden ER Jr and Gilbert IA: Asthma. N Engl J Med 327:1928-1937, 1992.
National Asthma Education and Prevention Program: Guidelines for the diagnosis and management of asthma. Expert Panel Report 2. NIH Publication No. 97-4051, 1997.
Woodruff PG and Fahy JV: Asthma: prevalence, pathogenesis, and prospects for novel therapies. JAMA 286:395-398, 2001.

Etiology and Pathogenesis

American Thoracic Society Workshop: Immunobiology of asthma and rhinitis. Pathogenic factors and therapeutic options. Am J Respir Crit Care Med 160:1778-1787, 1999.
Barnes PJ: Neurogenic inflammation in the airways. Respir Physiol 125:145-154, 2001.
Bousquet J et al: Asthma. From bronchoconstriction to airways inflammation and remodeling. Am J Respir Crit Care Med 161:1720-1745, 2000.

Busse WW and Lemanske RF Jr: Asthma. N Engl J Med 344:350-362, 2001.
Chung KF and Barnes PJ: Cytokines in asthma. Thorax 54:825-857, 1999.
Cookson WOC: Asthma genetics. Chest 121:7S-13S, 2002.
Gern JE and Busse WW: The role of viral infections in the natural history of asthma. J Allergy Clin Immunol 106:201-212, 2000.
Jacoby DB: Virus-induced asthma attacks. JAMA 287:755-761, 2002.
Los H, Koppelman GH, and Postma DS: The importance of genetic influences in asthma. Eur Respir J 14:1210-1227, 1999.
Nelson HS: The importance of allergens in the development of asthma and the persistence of symptoms. J Allergy Clin Immunol 105:S628-S632, 2000.
Oettgen HC and Geha RS: IgE in asthma and atopy: cellular and molecular connections. J Clin Invest 104:829-835, 1999.
Platts-Mills TA, Rakes G, and Heymann PW: The relevance of allergen exposure to the development of asthma in childhood. J Allergy Clin Immunol 105:S503-S508, 2000.
Wenzel SE (ed): The pathobiology of asthma: implications for treatment. Clin Chest Med 21:213-395, 2000.

Clinical Features and Diagnostic Approach

Cherniack RM: Physiologic diagnosis and function in asthma. Clin Chest Med 16:567-581, 1995.
Corrao WM, Braman SS, and Irwin RS: Chronic cough as the sole presenting manifestation of bronchial asthma. N Engl J Med 300:633-637, 1979.
Martin RJ: Nocturnal asthma: circadian rhythms and therapeutic interventions. Am Rev Respir Dis 147:S25-S28, 1993.
McFadden ER Jr: Exertional dyspnea and cough as preludes to acute attacks of asthma. N Engl J Med 292:555-559, 1975.
McFadden ER Jr and Gilbert IA: Exercise-induced asthma. N Engl J Med 330:1362-1367, 1994.
McFadden ER Jr, Kiser R, and DeGroot WJ: Acute bronchial asthma: relations between clinical and physiologic manifestations. N Engl J Med 288:221-225, 1973.
McFadden ER Jr and Lyons HA: Arterial–blood gas tension in asthma. N Engl J Med 278:1027-1032, 1968.
Naureckas ET and Solway J: Mild asthma. N Engl J Med 345:1257-1262, 2001.
Pratter MR and Irwin RS: The clinical value of pharmacologic bronchoprovocation challenge. Chest 85:260-265, 1984.
Rabatin JT and Cowl CT: A guide to the diagnosis and treatment of occupational asthma. Mayo Clin Proc 76:633-640, 2001.
Scanlon PD and Beck KC: Methacholine inhalation challenge. Mayo Clin Proc 69:1118-1119, 1994.

Treatment

Barnes PJ: Current therapies for asthma: promise and limitations. Chest 111: 17S-26S, 1997.
Barnes PJ: Inhaled glucocorticoids for asthma. N Engl J Med 332:868-875, 1995.
Barnes PJ: Pharmacology of airway smooth muscle. Am J Respir Crit Care Med 158:S123-S132, 1998.
Barrett TE and Strom BL: Inhaled β-adrenergic receptor agonists in asthma: more harm than good? Am J Respir Crit Care Med 151:574-577, 1995.
Busse WW: Long- and short-acting β_2-adrenergic agonists. Arch Intern Med 156:1514-1520, 1996.
Chang TW: The pharmacological basis of anti-IgE therapy. Nat Biotechnol 18:157-162, 2000.
Corbridge TC and Hall JB: The assessment and management of adults with *status asthmaticus*. Am J Respir Crit Care Med 151:1296-1316, 1995.
Drazen JM et al: Comparison of regularly scheduled with as-needed use of albuterol in mild asthma. N Engl J Med 335:841-847, 1996.
Fahy JV and Boushey HA: Controversies involving inhaled β_2-agonists and inhaled corticosteroids in the treatment of asthma. Clin Chest Med 16:715-733, 1995.
Horiuchi T and Castro M: The pathobiologic implications for treatment. Old and new strategies in the treatment of chronic asthma. Clin Chest Med 21:381-395, 2000.
Kamada AK et al: Issues in the use of inhaled glucocorticoids. Am J Respir Crit Care Med 153:1739-1748, 1996.
Leff AR: Regulation of leukotrienes in the management of asthma: biology and clinical therapy. Annu Rev Med 52:1-14, 2001.
Manthous, CA: Management of severe exacerbations of asthma. Am J Med 99:298-308, 1995.
Nelson HS: Beta-adrenergic bronchodilators. N Engl J Med 333:499-506, 1995.
Prussin C and Metcalfe DD: Update on the management of asthma. Adv Intern Med 46:31-50, 2001.
Salvi SS et al: The anti-inflammatory effects of leukotriene-modifying drugs and their use in asthma. Chest 119:1533-1546, 2001.
Silverman R: Treatment of acute asthma. A new look at the old and at the new. Clin Chest Med 21:361-379, 2000.
Weinberger M and Hendeles L: Theophylline in asthma. N Engl J Med 334:1380-1388, 1996.

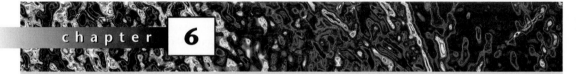

Chronic Obstructive Pulmonary Disease

The term *chronic obstructive pulmonary disease* (COPD) refers to chronic disorders that disturb airflow, whether the most prominent process is within the airways or within the lung parenchyma. The two disorders generally included in this category are chronic bronchitis and emphysema. Although the pathophysiology of airflow obstruction is different in these two disorders, patients frequently have features of both; thus it is appropriate to discuss them together. Although asthma could logically also be in this category, it is discussed in Chapter 5 because the term COPD, as commonly used, does not usually include bronchial asthma.

Other terms are synonymous with COPD—for example, chronic airflow limitation, chronic airflow obstruction (CAO), and chronic obstructive lung disease. Because COPD is the one in most common use, it is used here as well. Emphysema is discussed in this chapter, which is in the section of this text dealing with airways disease, even though the most obvious and visible pathologic manifestations of emphysema affect the lung parenchyma.

Chronic bronchitis is a diagnosis based on chronic cough and sputum production.

Chronic bronchitis is a clinical diagnosis used for patients with chronic cough and sputum production. It has certain pathologic features, but the diagnosis refers to the specific clinical presentation. For epidemiologic purposes, a more formal definition has been used, requiring that a chronic productive cough be present on most days during at least 3 months per year for 2 or more consecutive years. However, for clinical purposes, the physician does not necessarily adhere to this formal time requirement. Patients with chronic bronchitis frequently have periods of worsening or exacerbation, often precipitated by respiratory tract infection. Unlike patients with asthma, however, patients with pure chronic bronchitis usually have residual clinical disease even between exacerbations, and their disease is not primarily one of airways hyperreactivity. In those patients who have chronic bronchitis along with a prominent component of airways hyperreactivity, the diagnosis of *asthmatic bronchitis* is often given, because features of both disorders are present.

In contrast to the clinical diagnosis of chronic bronchitis, emphysema is formally a pathologic diagnosis, although certain clinical and laboratory features are also highly suggestive of the disease. Pathologically, emphysema is characterized by destruction of lung parenchyma and enlargement of air spaces distal to the terminal bronchiole. The region of the lung from the respiratory bronchioles down to the alveoli is involved, and determination of the particular type of emphysema depends on the pattern of destruction within the acinus. An antemortem diagnosis of emphysema obviously does not have the kind of confirmation offered by postmortem examination of the lung, but indirect support for the diagnosis is still useful and reasonably reliable.

Because chronic bronchitis and emphysema coexist to a variable extent in different patients, the broader term COPD is frequently more accurate. That these two disorders are tied so closely together is not surprising; a single etiologic factor—cigarette smoking—is primarily responsible for both processes. Inflammation induced by cigarette smoke, from the large airways down to the alveolar walls of the pulmonary parenchyma, is believed to be the common thread that ties together many of the varied manifestations of COPD. Throughout this chapter, specific reference is made to chronic bronchitis or to emphysema, because some of the clinical and pathophysiologic features are distinct enough to warrant separate consideration. However, patients do not necessarily fit neatly into these separate diagnostic categories.

The public health problems posed by COPD are enormous. It has been estimated that 16 million Americans have COPD, which is responsible for approximately 110,000 deaths per year in the United States. The morbidity, in terms of chronic symptoms, days lost from work, and permanent disability, is even more staggering. Unlike many diseases that the physician encounters, COPD is preventable in the majority of cases, because the main etiologic factor has been well established and is totally avoidable. Fortunately, since 1964, when the first Surgeon General's report on smoking and health was published, the prevalence of smoking in the United States has decreased from 40 percent to approximately 25 percent. Nevertheless, there are still more than 50 million current smokers and a large reservoir of former smokers who have placed themselves at high risk for COPD and other smoking-related diseases. Worldwide, an increasing prevalence of smoking in developing countries is contributing to the World Health Organization's prediction that COPD will be the third most common cause of death in the year 2020.

ETIOLOGY AND PATHOGENESIS

Several factors have been implicated in the cause of COPD, including smoking, environmental pollution, infection, and genetics. Of these four factors, smoking is clearly the most important and the one that will receive most attention here. Yet the fact that severe COPD develops in only about 15 percent of smokers suggests that other factors modify the risk. One other well-defined risk factor is discussed in detail in this section: the inherited deficiency of the protein α_1-antitrypsin. Other potential risk factors will be discussed briefly.

Smoking

Smoking affects the lung at multiple levels: the bronchi, the bronchioles, and the pulmonary parenchyma. In the larger airways—the bronchi—smoking has a prominent effect on the structure and function of the mucus-secreting

Emphysema is a diagnosis based on destruction of lung parenchyma and enlargement of air spaces distal to the terminal bronchiole.

Smoking is the key etiologic factor for chronic bronchitis; environmental pollutants and respiratory tract infection cause exacerbations but generally have an insignificant etiologic role.

apparatus, the bronchial mucous glands. An increase in the number and size of the glands is responsible for excessive mucus within the airway lumen. The airway wall becomes thickened, because of the hypertrophied and hyperplastic mucous glands as well as an influx of inflammatory cells (especially macrophages, neutrophils, and cytotoxic [CD8+] T lymphocytes) into the airway wall. Thickening of the wall diminishes the size of the airway lumen, and mucus within the lumen compromises its patency. Release of a variety of mediators from the inflammatory cells, including leukotriene B_4 (LTB_4), interleukin-8 (IL-8), and tumor necrosis factor-α (TNF-α), contributes to tissue damage and amplifies the inflammatory process in both the airways and the lung parenchyma. Similarly, oxidative stress, occurring as a result of reactive oxygen species present in cigarette smoke or released from inflammatory cells, contributes to the overall pathologic process.

At the same time that more mucus is produced in the larger airways, clearance of the mucus is altered by effects of cigarette smoke on the cilia lining the bronchial lumen. Structural changes in cilia have been well documented after long-term exposure to cigarette smoke, and functional studies have demonstrated impaired mucociliary clearance as a consequence of cigarette smoking.

The combined effects of smoking on mucus production, mucociliary clearance, and airway inflammation easily explain the epidemiologic data that demonstrate a significant correlation between cigarette smoking and the symptoms of chronic bronchitis: cough and sputum production. Pipe and cigar smoking are also predisposing factors in the development of chronic bronchitis, but the risk is significantly less than that from cigarette smoking, probably because pipe and cigar smoke is generally not inhaled.

Small airways—bronchioles less than approximately 2 mm in diameter—are also prominently affected by smoking. Smoking induces bronchiolar narrowing, inflammation, and fibrosis, with resulting airflow obstruction. As a later discussion will show, these changes in the small airways or bronchioles are believed to be responsible for much of the airflow obstruction demonstrable in patients with mild COPD.

> Cigarette smoking is responsible for most cases of emphysema; deficiency of serum α_1-antitrypsin is a predisposing factor for emphysema in a small proportion of cases.

In the pulmonary parenchyma, smoking results in the eventual development of emphysema. An understanding of the concepts about how smoking leads to the destruction of alveolar walls, which is characteristic of emphysema, requires familiarity with the *protease-antiprotease hypothesis*. According to this theory, emphysema results from destruction of the connective tissue matrix of alveolar walls by proteolytic enzymes—proteases—released by inflammatory cells in the alveoli. Studies in animals have demonstrated that injection of several proteolytic (i.e., capable of breaking down protein) enzymes into the airways of animals results in pathologic and physiologic changes similar to those of clinical emphysema.

The particular proteolytic enzymes thought to contribute to emphysema are those capable of breaking down elastin, a complex structural protein found in the walls of alveoli. Elastase, one of several enzymes within the category of serine proteases, appears to be the most important of these proteolytic enzymes. Neutrophils are the major source of elastase within the lungs, and therefore the enzyme is commonly called neutrophil elastase. If elastase were allowed to exert its proteolytic effect on elastin whenever it was released from a neutrophil, destruction of this important structural protein of the alveolar wall would ensue. Fortunately, there is an inhibitor of neutrophil elastase—usually called α_1-antitrypsin but also sometimes called α_1-antiprotease or α_1-protease inhibitor—normally present in the lung. It is believed that there is a balance between neutrophil elastase and its inhibitor so that wanton destruction of the alveolar wall does not occur. When this balance is disturbed, either by an increase in neutrophil elastase activity or by a decrease in antielastase activity, damage to elastin and to the alveolar wall can result, with the eventual production of emphysema.

In smokers, the balance between elastase and antielastase is thought to be disturbed in more than one way by cigarette smoke. First, an increased number of neutrophils can be found in the lungs of smokers, thus providing a source for increased amounts of neutrophil elastase. Second, there is evidence that oxidants derived from cigarette smoke and from inflammatory cells can oxidize a critical amino acid residue of α_1-antitrypsin at or near the site where the protease inhibitor binds to elastase. Oxidation of this amino acid interferes with the inhibitory activity of α_1-antitrypsin, again tipping the balance in favor of increased elastase activity. Hence, cigarette smoking may be a double-edged sword, increasing the amount of neutrophil elastase in the lung and decreasing the normal inhibitory mechanism that serves to limit uncontrolled elastin breakdown by the enzyme. This pathogenetic sequence hypothesized for the development of emphysema is summarized in Fig. 6-1.

In addition to degrading elastin in the alveolar wall, neutrophil elastase, when released in the airways, stimulates secretion of mucus. The primary defense against the action of neutrophil elastase in the airway is provided by a different antiprotease, secretory leukoprotease inhibitor, which is produced by airway epithelial and mucus-secreting cells.

However, elastase is not the only proteolytic enzyme that has been implicated in the development of smoking-related damage and emphysema. Recent interest has focused on an additional group of enzymes called the matrix metalloproteinases, which are produced by macrophages and neutrophils and are capable of breaking down a variety of structural components of the alveolar wall. Like the relationship between elastase and its inhibitor α_1-antitrypsin, the matrix metalloproteinases have a number of natural inhibitors, appropriately called tissue inhibitors of matrix metalloproteinases. Because of the influx of neutrophils and macrophages induced by cigarette smoke, it is believed that an increased burden of matrix metalloproteinases may result from smoking, potentially overwhelming the capability of the metalloproteinase inhibitors and contributing to the breakdown of alveolar walls.

Theories claim that proteolytic enzymes (especially elastase) are balanced by α_1-antitrypsin; disturbance of this balance in favor of proteolytic enzymes, either due to smoking or to a deficiency of α_1-antitrypsin, may result in emphysema.

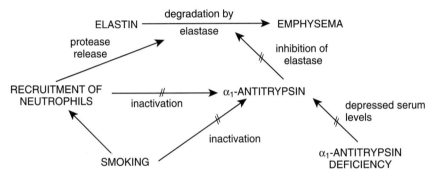

Figure 6-1 ■— Schematic diagram of hypothesized relationship between elastase and α_1-antitrypsin (also called α_1-protease inhibitor), indicating how smoking and α_1-antitrypsin deficiency alter the balance, leading to degradation of elastin.

Environmental Pollution

The other factors implicated in the pathogenesis of COPD—environmental pollution, infection, and genetics—are quantitatively much less important than smoking. Air pollution is important primarily because of its potential for causing exacerbations of preexisting disease, not for initiating COPD. However, occupational exposure to pollutants—for example, in the case of miners—does appear to be an important factor contributing to COPD, particularly chronic bronchitis. Additionally, in developing countries, environmental exposure to pollutants, as occurs with cooking in confined spaces, may play a role in the development of COPD.

Infection

Similarly, infections do not initiate the disease, but they do cause transient worsening of symptoms and pulmonary function in patients with preexisting COPD. Of the different types of respiratory tract infection, viral infection appears to be responsible for a large number of clinical exacerbations of symptoms. Bacterial infections probably play a less important role but can cause superinfection of patients already harboring an acute viral infection.

An interesting additional role for infection is suggested by data indicating that childhood respiratory tract infections may increase the risk for subsequent development of COPD. This may be one of the factors helping to explain why the development of COPD is not uniform in all smokers. A possible way in which childhood respiratory infection might contribute to the later risk for development of COPD is by affecting lung growth and function during childhood. The smoker who starts with a lower level of function because of childhood respiratory infections may be more likely in later life to suffer functionally important consequences from heavy smoking.

Genetic Factors

Genetic factors presumably contribute to the risk for development of COPD, but the nature of any such predisposition remains to a large extent poorly defined. The one hereditary factor that has been best established as predisposing to emphysema is deficiency of the serum protein α_1-antitrypsin. α_1-antitrypsin is a glycoprotein, with a molecular weight of 54,000, that is made in the liver and normally circulates in blood. Minor changes in the gene coding for α_1-antitrypsin produce alterations in the structure of the protein that can be detected by biochemical methods, and more than 75 alleles of α_1-antitrypsin have been identified. Each of these alleles has a name, preceded by the letters *Pi* for "protease inhibitor." Everybody has two genes coding for α_1-antitrypsin, one of maternal and one of paternal origin. The normal (and most common) allele is termed *Pi M,* and the normal complement of two *M* genes is called *Pi MM.* A person with the *Pi MM* genotype has approximately 200 mg/dL of the *M* type of protease inhibitor circulating in the blood. With one of the variant *Pi* types, termed *Pi Z,* the amino acid sequence of the protein is slightly altered, impairing transport of the protein from its site of production in the liver. Hence, the abnormal protein remains in globules in the liver, where it may result in liver disease, and only small amounts enter the blood. Individuals who are homozygous for the *Z* gene *(Pi ZZ)* have circulating levels of α_1-antitrypsin that are approximately 15 percent of normal, or 30 mg/dL. Heterozygotes, with one *M* and one *Z* gene *(Pi MZ),* have intermediate levels of circulating α_1-antitrypsin, in the range of 50 to 60 percent of normal levels.

The most important form of α_1-antitrypsin deficiency is *Pi ZZ.*

Having the *Pi ZZ* genotype is a strong risk factor for the premature development of emphysema, particularly if the individual is also a smoker. Emphysema frequently develops as early as the third or fourth decade of life in persons with the *Pi ZZ* genotype (who are commonly said to have α_1-antitrypsin deficiency because of the low serum levels). As mentioned already, the structural integrity of alveolar walls appears to depend on the balance between elastin degradation by elastase and protection from this destruction afforded by α_1-antitrypsin. In patients with α_1-antitrypsin deficiency, lack of the elastase inhibitor is believed to permit elastase action to proceed in an unchecked fashion, and the early development of emphysema is the consequence.

Another factor of interest, one that is presumably at least partially genetically determined, is the degree of the patient's preexisting bronchial hyperresponsiveness. There are data to support the hypothesis that there is an accelerated decline in lung function in patients who have greater levels of bronchial responsiveness. However, the potential for smoking to induce changes in bronchial responsiveness makes it difficult to determine cause and effect relationships, making this an area of controversy.

PATHOLOGY

Much of the pathology in chronic bronchitis relates to mucus and to the mucus-secreting apparatus in the airways. As mentioned in Chapter 4, mucus-secreting glands and goblet cells are responsible for the production of bronchial secretions, but the mucous glands are the more important source. In chronic bronchitis, there is enlargement (hypertrophy and hyperplasia) of the mucus-secreting glands, which has been objectively assessed by comparing the relative thickness of the mucous glands with the total thickness of the airway wall. This ratio, known as the *Reid index*, is increased in patients with chronic bronchitis. In general, the number of goblet cells in the airways is increased as well, and these particular cells are also abundant in airways more peripheral than usual. As a result of these alterations in the mucus-secreting apparatus, the quantity of airway mucus is increased, and it is likely that the composition may be altered as well. In practice, the secretions found in these patients are often thick and apparently more viscous than usual. The bronchial walls also demonstrate evidence of an inflammatory process, with cellular infiltration and variable degrees of fibrosis.

> Chronic bronchitis is characterized by enlargement of the mucus-secreting glands and an increased number of goblet cells.

In the smaller airways (i.e., bronchioles), inflammation, fibrosis, intraluminal mucus, and an increase in goblet cells all contribute to a decrease in luminal diameter. Because the resistance of airways varies inversely with the fourth power of the radius, even small changes in bronchiolar size may result in major impairment to airflow at the level of the small airways. It is thought that these pathologic changes in the small airways are the primary cause of airflow obstruction in patients with mild COPD.

In patients with severe chronic airflow obstruction, the most important process responsible for the airflow obstruction is emphysema. As mentioned earlier, the pathology of emphysema is characterized by destruction of alveolar walls and enlargement of terminal air spaces (Fig. 6-2). Several types of emphysema have distinct pathologic features, primarily dependent on the distribution of the lesions. The most important types are panacinar (panlobular) emphysema and centriacinar (centrilobular) emphysema (Fig. 6-3). Panacinar emphysema is characterized by a more or less uniform involvement of the

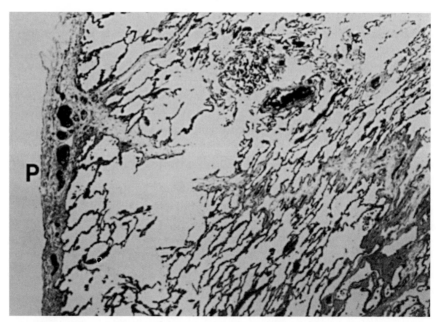

Figure 6-2 ■— Low-power photomicrograph shows localized region of emphysema in left half of figure, adjacent to pleural surface (P). Because emphysema here is localized, destruction of alveolar walls and enlargement of terminal air spaces can be contrasted with appearance of normal lung in right half of figure. (Courtesy Dr. Earl Kasdon.)

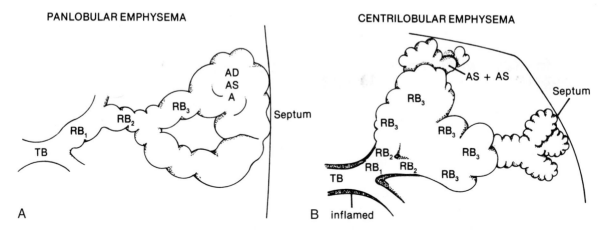

PANLOBULAR EMPHYSEMA   CENTRILOBULAR EMPHYSEMA

Figure 6-3 ■— Diagram of panlobular (*A*) and centrilobular (*B*) emphysema. In panlobular (panacinar) emphysema, the enlargement of air spaces is relatively uniform throughout acinus. In centrilobular (centriacinar) emphysema, enlargement of air spaces is primarily at level of respiratory bronchioles. TB = terminal bronchiole; RB$_1$ through RB$_3$ = three generations of respiratory bronchioles; AD = alveolar duct; AS = alveolar sac; A = alveolus. (From Thurlbeck WM: Chronic obstructive lung disease. *In* Sommers SC [ed]: Pathology Annual, vol. 3. New York, Appleton-Century-Crofts, 1968.)

Pathologic changes from smoking often start in small airways, predating the advanced findings associated with chronic bronchitis and emphysema.

acinus—the region beyond the terminal bronchiole, including respiratory bronchioles, alveolar ducts, and alveolar sacs. Examination of a section of lung with panacinar emphysema shows that the damage in an involved area is relatively diffuse (Fig. 6-4). Typically, the lower zones of the lung are more involved than the upper zones. Panacinar emphysema is the usual type of emphysema described in patients who have α_1-antitrypsin deficiency, although it is not limited to this clinical setting.

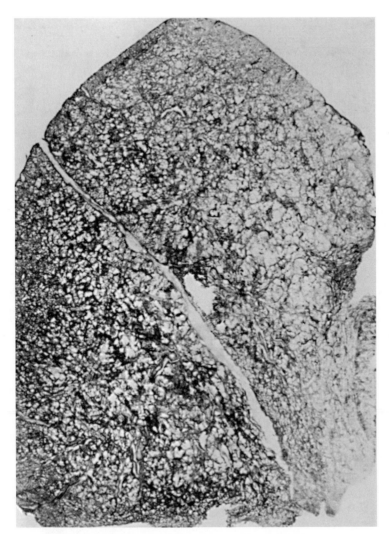

Figure 6-4 ▬— Mounted section of whole lung shows diffuse involvement seen with panacinar emphysema. (From Thurlbeck WM: Chronic Airflow Obstruction in Lung Disease. Philadelphia, WB Saunders Co., 1976.)

In centrilobular emphysema, the predominant involvement and dilatation are found in the proximal part of the acinus, namely the respiratory bronchiole. The appearance of a lung section with centrilobular emphysema is different from that with panacinar emphysema. In centrilobular emphysema, the involvement in an affected area seems to be more irregular, with apparently spared alveolar tissue between the dilated respiratory bronchioles at the center of the acinus (Fig. 6-5). This type of emphysema is the typical form in smokers. It is reasonable to speculate that the prominent involvement focused around the respiratory bronchiole is a consequence of an extension of the bronchiolar inflammation in mild COPD.

PATHOPHYSIOLOGY

Underlying a discussion of the pathophysiology of COPD is the fact that cigarette smoking affects the large airways, the small airways, and the pulmonary parenchyma. The pathophysiologic consequences resulting from disease at

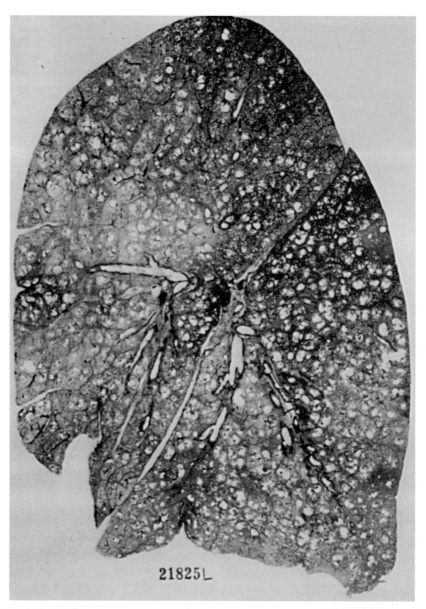

Figure 6-5   ■—   Mounted section of whole lung shows centrilobular emphysema. Adjacent to emphysematous spaces (which represent dilated respiratory bronchioles) are spared areas of lung parenchyma (representing alveolar ducts and alveolar spaces). (From Thurlbeck WM: Internal surface area and other measurements in emphysema. Thorax 22:483-496; 1967. BMJ Publishing Group.)

each of these levels contribute to the overall clinical picture of COPD. In addition, the degree of airway reactivity, which is probably determined by genetic and environmental factors, appears to modify the clinical expression of disease in a given patient. This section simplifies, summarizes, and places into a conceptual framework some of the information regarding structure-function correlations for each of these aspects of COPD.

Functional Abnormalities in Airways Disease

In the larger airways—the bronchi—an increase in the mucus-secreting apparatus and in the amount of mucus produced results in the symptoms of excessive cough and sputum production that are characteristic of chronic bronchitis. Although a decrease in the size of the large airways as a result of secretions, an increase in the mucus-secreting apparatus, and inflammation might be expected to correlate well with the degree of airflow obstruction, this does not necessarily appear to be the case. Some patients with typical symptoms of chronic bronchitis do not exhibit abnormally high resistance or changes in other measurements of airflow. When airflow obstruction exists, there generally are additional pathologic factors—either in the small airways (inflammation and fibrosis) or in the pulmonary parenchyma (emphysema)— that are critical for its presence. In relatively mild airflow obstruction associated with chronic bronchitis, disease in the small airways often makes an important contribution to airflow obstruction. When airflow obstruction is more marked, coexisting emphysema is often the primary reason responsible for the obstruction.

> Coexistent small airway disease or emphysema, or both, contributes significantly to decreased expiratory flow rates in chronic bronchitis.

In those patients who have a component of airways hyperreactivity contributing to their disease, the clinical expression is often more that of asthmatic bronchitis. Airway smooth muscle constriction adds more reversible airflow obstruction than is typically seen in the patient without airways hyperreactivity.

The common problem produced by the aforementioned processes that affect airways is a decrease in the overall cross-sectional area of the airways. Airways resistance, commonly abbreviated R_{aw}, is potentially increased by anything that compromises the lumen of the airways: intraluminal secretions; bronchospasm; or thickening of the airway wall by edema, inflammatory cells, fibrosis, or enlargement of the mucus-secreting apparatus. When disease is primarily in the peripheral airways and is mild, the functional consequences may be relatively subtle. As these peripheral airways contribute only about 10 to 20 percent of the overall airways resistance, total resistance is preserved unless the small airways disease is considerable or there is additional disease affecting the larger airways.

As another potential consequence of airways disease, expiratory flow rates, including forced expiratory volume in 1 second (FEV_1), FEV_1/forced vital capacity (FVC) ratio, and maximal midexpiratory flow rate (MMFR), are generally decreased. After the use of inhaled bronchodilators, there may or may not be a significant improvement in flow rates. Those patients with asthmatic bronchitis and greater airways reactivity generally have the most striking improvement in flow rates after receiving an inhaled bronchodilator.

Before a discussion of how lung volumes change in patients with the airways disease associated with COPD, it is useful to review the factors that determine the major lung volumes, namely total lung capacity (TLC), functional residual capacity (FRC), and residual volume (RV). TLC is the point at which the force of the inspiratory muscles acting to expand the lungs is equaled by the elastic recoil of the respiratory system (primarily lung recoil) resisting expansion. At FRC, the resting point of the respiratory system, there is a balance between the elastic recoil of the lungs and the elastic recoil of the chest wall, which are acting in opposite directions—the lungs inward and the chest wall outward. The determinants of RV depend to some extent on age. In a normal young person, RV is the point at which the relatively stiff chest wall can be compressed no further by the expiratory muscles. With increasing age, a sufficient number of airways close at low lung volumes to limit further expiration, and airway closure is an important determinant of RV. In disease states in which airways are likely to close at low lung volumes, airway closure is associated with an elevated RV, even if the patient is young.

In patients with pure airways disease,TLC theoretically remains relatively close to normal, because neither the elastic recoil of the lung nor inspiratory muscle strength is altered. Similarly, FRC should remain normal because the recoil of the lung and the recoil of the chest wall are unchanged. However, if expiration is prolonged and the respiratory rate is quite high, then the patient may not have sufficient time during expiration to reach the normal resting end-expiratory point. In this case, FRC is increased. RV is generally also increased with these processes that involve airways, because the narrowing and occlusion of small airways by secretions and inflammation result in air trapping during expiration.

Functional Abnormalities in Emphysema

Although emphysema—destruction of alveolar walls—leads to decreased expiratory flow rates, the pathophysiology is somewhat different from the situation in pure airways disease. The primary problem in emphysema is the loss of elastic recoil, i.e., loss of the lung's natural tendency to resist expansion. One of the consequences of decreased elastic recoil is a decreased driving pressure that expels air from the alveoli during expiration. A simple analogy is a balloon filled with air, in which the elastic recoil is the "stiffness" of the balloon. With a given volume of air inside an unsealed balloon, a stiffer balloon will expel air more rapidly than will a less stiff balloon. An emphysematous lung is like a less stiff balloon: a smaller than normal force drives air out of the lungs during expiration.

Loss of driving pressure is not the only consequence of emphysema. There is also an indirect effect on the collapsibility of airways. Normally, traction is exerted on the walls of airways by a supporting structure of tissue from the lung parenchyma. When the alveolar tissue is disrupted, as in emphysema, the supporting structure for the airways is diminished, and less radial traction is exerted to prevent airway collapse (Fig. 6-6). During a forced expiration, the strongly positive pleural pressure promotes collapse; airways lacking an adequate supporting structure are more likely to collapse (and have diminished flow rates and air trapping) than are normally supported ones.

The decrease in elastic recoil in emphysema also alters the compliance curve of the lung and the measured lung volumes. The compliance curve, as discussed in Chapter 1, relates transpulmonary pressure and the associated volume of gas within the lung. Because an emphysematous lung has less elastic recoil (is less stiff), it resists expansion less than does its normal

In emphysema, decreased expiratory flow rates are largely due to loss of elastic recoil of the lung, resulting in the following:

1. A lower driving pressure for expiratory airflow
2. Loss of radial traction on the airways provided by supporting alveolar walls, thus promoting airway collapse during expiration

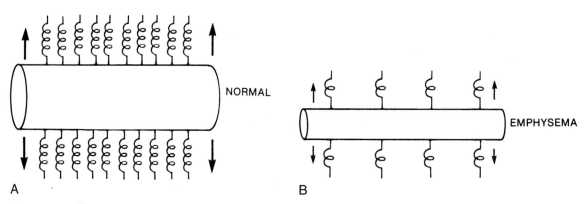

Figure 6-6 ■— Schematic diagram of radial traction exerted by alveolar walls (represented as springs), acting to keep airways open. The normal situation is shown in *A*, and loss of radial traction, as seen in emphysema, is shown in *B*.

counterpart. Therefore, the compliance curve is shifted upward and to the left, and the lung has more volume at any particular transpulmonary pressure (Fig. 6-7). TLC is increased, because loss of elastic recoil results in a smaller force opposing the action of the inspiratory musculature. FRC is also increased, because the balance between the outward recoil of the chest wall and the inward recoil of the lung is shifted in favor of the chest wall. As in bronchitis, RV is also substantially increased in emphysema, because poorly supported airways are more susceptible to closure during a maximal expiration.

Mechanisms of Abnormal Gas-Exchange

In obstructive lung disease, many of the observed pathologic changes affecting airflow are not uniformly distributed. For example, in chronic bronchitis some airways are extensively affected by secretions and plugging, and others remain relatively uninvolved. Therefore, ventilation is not uniformly distributed throughout the lung; regions of the lung supplied by more diseased airways receive diminished ventilation in comparison with regions supplied by less diseased airways. Although there may be a compensatory decrease in blood flow to underventilated alveoli, the compensation is not totally effective, and inequalities and mismatching of ventilation and perfusion result. As discussed earlier, this type of ventilation-perfusion disturbance, with some areas of lung having low ventilation-perfusion ratios and contributing desaturated blood, leads to arterial hypoxemia.

In obstructive lung disease, nonuniformity of the disease process results in $\dot{V}/\dot{Q}$ mismatch and hypoxemia.

Carbon dioxide elimination is also impaired in some patients with obstructive lung disease. The mechanism of alveolar hypoventilation and CO_2

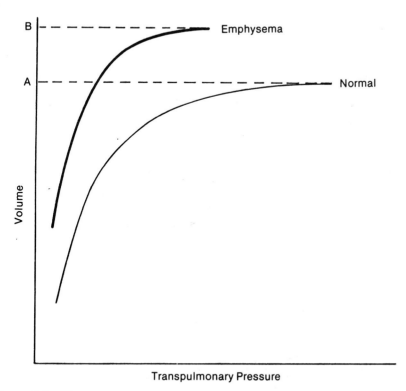

Figure 6-7 ▬ Compliance curve of lung in emphysema compared with that of normal lung. In addition to shift of curve upward and to left, it can be seen that TLC in emphysema (point B on volume axis) is greater than normal TLC (point A). In pure chronic bronchitis without emphysema, compliance curve is normal.

Mechanisms that contribute to alveolar hypoventilation and CO_2 retention in obstructive lung disease are the following:

1. Increased work of breathing
2. Abnormalities of ventilatory drive
3. $\dot{V}/\dot{Q}$ mismatch
4. Decreased effectiveness of the diaphragm

retention, however, is less clear than the mechanism of hypoxemia. Several factors probably contribute, including increased work of breathing (resulting from impaired airflow), abnormalities of central ventilatory drive, and ventilation-perfusion mismatch creating some areas with high ventilation-perfusion ratios that effectively act as dead space.

An additional problem, fatigue of inspiratory muscles, has received attention as a factor contributing to acute CO_2 retention when affected patients are in respiratory failure (see Chapter 19). The importance of diaphragmatic fatigue in the stable patient with chronic hypercapnia is less certain. However, it is clear that contraction of the diaphragm, the major muscle of inspiration, is less efficient and less effective in patients with obstructive lung disease. When FRC is increased, the diaphragm is lower and flatter, and its fibers are shortened even before the initiation of inspiration. A shortened, flattened diaphragm is at a mechanical disadvantage compared with a longer, curved diaphragm, and it is less effective as an inspiratory muscle.

Pulmonary Hypertension

A potential complication of COPD is the development of pulmonary hypertension—high pressures within the pulmonary arterial system. Long-standing pulmonary hypertension puts an added workload onto the right ventricle, which hypertrophies and may eventually fail. The term used to describe disease of the right ventricle secondary to lung disease (either COPD or other forms of lung disease) is *cor pulmonale*, a topic that is discussed in Chapter 14. The primary feature of COPD that leads to pulmonary hypertension and eventually to cor pulmonale is hypoxia. A decrease in Po_2 is a strong stimulus to constriction of pulmonary arterioles (see Chapter 12). With correction of the hypoxia, the pulmonary vasoconstriction may be reversible.

The major cause of pulmonary hypertension in COPD is hypoxia; additional factors include hypercapnia, polycythemia, and destruction of the pulmonary vascular bed.

Several additional but less important factors may contribute to elevated pulmonary artery pressure: hypercapnia, polycythemia, and reduction in area of the pulmonary vascular bed. Hypercapnia, like hypoxia, is also capable of causing pulmonary vasoconstriction; to a large extent, this effect may be mediated by the change in pH resulting from an increase in Pco_2. An elevation in hematocrit—polycythemia—is often found in the chronically hypoxemic patient, producing an increased blood viscosity and contributing to an elevated pulmonary artery pressure. Finally, in emphysema, the destruction of alveoli is accompanied by a loss of pulmonary capillaries. Therefore, in extensive disease, the limited pulmonary vascular bed may result in a high resistance to blood flow and consequently an increase in pulmonary artery pressure.

Two Types of Presentation

Two presentations of obstructive lung disease are the *pink puffer* (type A) and the *blue bloater* (type B), but a clear distinction between their underlying processes is an oversimplification.

In practice, clinicians have often distinguished two pathophysiologic types of COPD, termed *type A* and *type B*, or, more colloquially, *pink puffer* and *blue bloater*, respectively. Originally, type A (pink puffer) physiology was associated with underlying emphysema, and type B (blue bloater) physiology was equated with chronic bronchitis. Although the association with a particular pathologic process appears to be an oversimplification, the pathophysiologic types of presentation can provide a helpful conceptual framework and are sometimes useful clinically. In most cases a patient does not fall clearly into one category or the other but has some features suggestive of both.

The patient with type A disease is referred to as a pink puffer because (1) arterial Po_2 tends to be reasonably well preserved, so that the patient is "pink," i.e., not cyanotic and (2) dyspnea and high minute ventilation are prominent features, with the patient appearing to be working hard to get air, i.e., "puffing." Not only is the P_{O_2} not markedly decreased, but the P_{CO_2} also is not abnormally high. On the basis of the general (although oversimplified) concept that emphysema is the primary process in these patients, relative preservation of the P_{O_2} may be related to a simultaneous and matched loss of ventilation and perfusion when alveolar walls are destroyed. Because gas-exchange abnormalities are not a striking feature of patients with type A disease, no prominent stimulus of hypoxia leads to pulmonary hypertension. In addition, an elevation of the hematocrit value, often a result of hypoxemia, is not seen.

The patient with type B disease, on the other hand, is characterized by major problems with gas-exchange, namely hypoxemia and hypercapnia. This patient is termed a blue bloater because (1) cyanosis can result from significant hypoxemia and (2) the patient frequently is obese and can have peripheral edema resulting from right ventricular failure. Again, on the basis of the oversimplified concept that patients with type B disease have primarily chronic bronchitis, it is reasonable to attribute hypoxemia to ventilation-perfusion mismatch. Presumably, regions of lung supplied by diseased airways are underventilated, while perfusion is relatively preserved. Ventilation-perfusion mismatch results in arterial hypoxemia because of desaturated blood coming from areas with a low ventilation-perfusion ratio. As discussed earlier, several mechanisms may contribute to the development of CO_2 retention, although the primary differences explaining why type A patients do not retain CO_2 and type B patients often do are not entirely clear. As a consequence of the gas-exchange abnormalities (particularly hypoxemia) in type B patients, pulmonary hypertension, cor pulmonale, and elevations in the hematocrit value (secondary polycythemia) commonly accompany the clinical picture.

Despite the common association of type B pathophysiology with the symptoms of chronic bronchitis, these patients frequently also have pathologic evidence of emphysema, particularly of the centrilobular variety. How much of the clinical picture is secondary to bronchitis and how much is secondary to coexisting centrilobular emphysema are difficult to determine.

CLINICAL FEATURES

Symptoms most commonly experienced by patients with COPD include dyspnea and cough, frequently with sputum production. Dyspnea is the most prominent symptom in those patients with type A pathophysiology; type B patients generally complain of chronic cough and sputum production. Many patients have features of both, whereas some patients with COPD are symptom-free, with a diagnosis based on pulmonary function tests.

Frequently, patients have a certain level of chronic symptoms, but their disease course is then punctuated by periods of exacerbation. The precipitating factor producing an exacerbation is often a respiratory tract infection, particularly of viral origin. In addition, bacteria also may be chronically present in the tracheobronchial tree, which should normally be sterile, and an acute bacterial infection can sometimes be implicated in acute exacerbations. Other factors that cause acute deterioration in these patients include exposure to air pollutants, bronchospasm (particularly if patients have a superimposed asthmatic component to their disease), and congestive heart failure, to name

The precipitating factor for an exacerbation of COPD is often a viral infection.

just a few. When exacerbations are severe, patients may go into frank respiratory failure, a complication that is discussed in Chapter 27.

In addition to chronic symptoms of dyspnea or cough, or both, which may worsen during periods of acute exacerbation, patients also may experience secondary cardiovascular complications of their lung disease—cor pulmonale. As mentioned, the patient with type B physiology is more susceptible to this complication than is the type A patient.

On physical examination, patients with type A physiology often appear thin (if not cachectic), and they frequently may be leaning forward and resting on extended arms. This position allows fixation of one end of the shoulder and neck muscles, allowing them to function more effectively as accessory muscles of respiration. These patients are not cyanotic and do not demonstrate peripheral edema characteristic of right ventricular failure. In contrast, patients with type B disease are often obese and sometimes cyanotic but generally appear to be in less respiratory distress than the type A counterpart.

Examination of the chest often discloses an increase in the anteroposterior diameter, indicating hyperinflation of the lungs. Patients may be using accessory muscles of respiration, such as the sternocleidomastoid and trapezius muscles, and the intercostal muscles may retract with each inspiration. When diaphragmatic excursion is assessed by percussion of the lung bases during inspiration and expiration, diminished movement is noted. Breath sounds are generally decreased in intensity, and expiration is prolonged. Wheezing may also be heard but unfortunately does not necessarily reflect reversible bronchospasm. Although some patients do not wheeze on their normal tidal breathing, they exhibit this finding when asked to give a forced exhalation. In those patients with chronic bronchitis and profuse airway secretions, rhonchi are frequently heard. When cor pulmonale is present, with or without frank right ventricular failure, patients have the cardiac findings that are described in Chapter 14.

Smoking is not only the primary factor that initiates COPD; it is also a major risk factor that determines the prognosis of a patient's illness. Those patients who continue to smoke appear to have the greatest further deterioration of pulmonary function over time, whereas respiratory tract infections, although they may cause acute deterioration, do not appear to affect the rate at which pulmonary function is lost.

A wide spectrum of severity is characteristic of COPD, and therefore the morbidity that patients experience from their disease varies tremendously. Patients with mild disease are able to continue their usual work and lifestyle with minimal, if any, changes. Those with severe disease are quite limited in their capacity for any exertion, are subject to frequent hospitalizations, and may have a life expectancy of less than 5 years.

Continuation of smoking is a major risk factor affecting the prognosis in COPD.

DIAGNOSTIC APPROACH

In most cases, the diagnosis of COPD is made with a combination of history and physical examination. As mentioned earlier, chronic bronchitis is actually a clinical diagnosis, and it is here that the history is particularly crucial. Although emphysema is formally a pathologic diagnosis, a lung biopsy is not performed to make this diagnosis. Pathologic confirmation is generally obtained only at postmortem examination, if one is performed.

A valuable study on a macroscopic level for assessing the lungs of patients with COPD is the chest radiograph. Patients with chronic bronchitis alone frequently have a normal chest radiograph. Minor changes of increased markings through the lungs may be present, but it is difficult to know whether these can be attributed to coexisting emphysema (the "increased markings" pattern of emphysema is discussed later). When cor pulmonale develops in these patients, secondary cardiac changes may also be seen, indicative of right ventricular hypertrophy or dilatation.

In patients with emphysema, two radiographic patterns are well described. In the first, which is the type most frequently recognized, patients have hyperinflation, with large lung volumes, flat diaphragms, and an increase in the anteroposterior diameter (seen on the lateral view). In addition, a paucity of vascular markings in the lung results from destruction of alveolar septa and enlargement of alveolar spaces. This pattern is known as the *arterial deficiency* pattern of emphysema because of the changes in vascular markings and is often associated with underlying panacinar emphysema (Fig. 6-8). In patients with α_1-antitrypsin deficiency and early onset of emphysema, the arterial deficiency pattern is quite striking in the lower lobes, where there may be almost a complete loss of vascular markings.

The other radiographic pattern in patients with emphysema is termed the *increased markings* pattern. In this pattern, the radiograph demonstrates prominent lung markings and may also give evidence of pulmonary hypertension and cor pulmonale. Patients with this type of presentation often have clinical chronic bronchitis and type B physiology, and their radiographic findings are probably related to coexistent centrilobular emphysema.

High-resolution computed tomography is recognized as a more sensitive imaging method for detecting emphysema. However, because it is expensive

Characteristic radiographic findings in the more frequently recognized arterial deficiency pattern of COPD are the following:

1. Large lung volumes
2. Flat diaphragms
3. Increased anteroposterior diameter
4. Loss of vascular markings

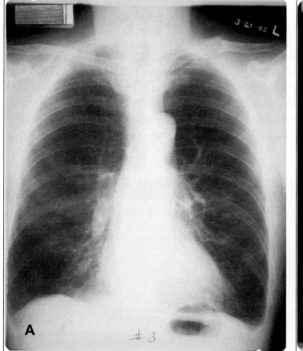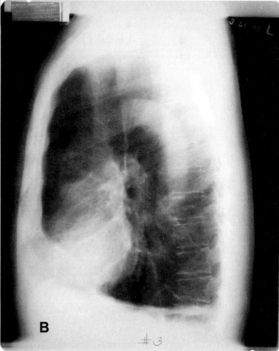

Figure 6-8 ━━ Chest radiograph of patient with severe COPD, showing arterial deficiency pattern of emphysema. Lungs are hyperinflated, diaphragms are low and flat (in this case they are actually inverted on lateral film), and there is paucity of vascular markings. *A*, Posteroanterior and *B*, lateral views.

Pulmonary function tests in
COPD show the following:

1. Airflow obstruction
   (decreased FVC, FEV$_1$,
   FEV$_1$/FVC, MMFR)
2. Air trapping (increased
   RV, FRC, and often TLC)
3. Diffusing capacity
   generally decreased in
   emphysema, normal in
   chronic bronchitis

and rarely changes the management plan in this setting, it should not be considered part of the usual diagnostic evaluation for these patients.

The most useful physiologic adjuncts in evaluating patients with COPD are pulmonary function tests and arterial blood gas analysis. Pulmonary function tests demonstrate airflow obstruction, with a decrease in FVC, FEV$_1$, the FEV$_1$/FVC ratio, and MMFR. The tests generally give evidence of air trapping, with an elevation in RV. In patients whose lung compliance is increased, that is, those with emphysema, TLC is generally elevated. FRC is elevated either as a result of increased compliance (decreased elastic recoil) in emphysema or as a consequence of insufficient expiratory time in the face of significant airflow obstruction. Whether emphysema is present can be indirectly assessed by measuring the diffusing capacity for carbon monoxide. In patients with emphysema, in whom the surface area for gas-exchange is lost, the diffusing capacity is typically decreased. In pure airways disease—for example, chronic bronchitis without emphysema—the diffusing capacity is generally normal.

The results of arterial blood gas analysis depend to a large extent on the pathophysiologic type of disease, and in fact the blood gas determination is an important criterion for classifying the patient in one of the two pathophysiologic categories. Patients with type A pathophysiology have a normal or mildly decreased arterial Po$_2$, with a normal or slightly decreased arterial Pco$_2$. Those with type B physiology have more strikingly abnormal blood gas values and, often, marked hypoxemia as well as CO$_2$ retention. With chronic elevation in the Pco$_2$, the kidneys retain bicarbonate in an attempt to compensate and return the pH toward normal. With acute exacerbations of COPD, the hypoxemia frequently becomes even worse and the CO$_2$ retention more pronounced, so that the pH may drop from the stable compensated value.

Type B patients are more
hypoxemic than are type A
patients and often have
hypercapnia.

Many of the clinical features characterizing patients with type A and those with type B pathophysiology are summarized in Table 6-1.

TREATMENT

Several modalities of treatment are available for the patient with COPD, the usefulness of each varying from patient to patient. Although bronchoconstriction in patients with COPD is considerably less than that in patients with bronchial asthma, bronchodilators remain an important part of the treatment of many patients with COPD. The agents used are identical to the ones dis-

Table 6-1		
Clinical Distinctions Between Type A and Type B Pathophysiology		
Feature	**Type A**	**Type B**
Commonly used name	Pink puffer	Blue bloater
Disease association	Predominant emphysema	Predominant bronchitis
Major symptom	Dyspnea	Cough and sputum
Appearance	Thin, wasted, not cyanotic	Obese, cyanotic
Po$_2$	↓	↓↓
Pco$_2$	Normal or ↓	Normal or ↑
Elastic recoil of lung	↓	Normal
Diffusing capacity	↓	Normal
Hematocrit	Normal	Often ↑
Cor pulmonale	Infrequent	Common

cussed in Chapter 5, including sympathomimetic agents, methylxanthines, and anticholinergic drugs. Anticholinergic drugs, especially inhaled ipratropium, have been used with much greater frequency during the past several years, with many physicians believing they are now the first-line agents for use in patients with COPD. Data on these patients suggest that ipratropium is at least as effective as the inhaled β-agonists, and side effects are minimal.

When acute respiratory tract infections develop in patients with COPD, or even when these patients have an exacerbation of their disease without a clear precipitant, they are often treated with antibiotics. The primary usefulness of antibiotics is against bacterial infections; however, a bacterial cause is difficult to document with certainty, and many exacerbations are thought to be either noninfectious or triggered by viral respiratory infections. In practice, patients are frequently treated with antibiotics when there is a change in the quantity and/or nature of their chronic sputum production, even though a bacterial infection may or may not be present. Of the potential bacterial pathogens, the ones most frequently implicated are *Streptococcus pneumoniae*, *Haemophilus influenzae*, and *Moraxella catarrhalis*. As a result, the choice of antibiotic often allows coverage for these organisms.

The use of corticosteroids for the treatment of these patients is controversial and dependent on the clinical setting. A short course of systemic corticosteroids is frequently given at the time of an acute exacerbation, and most studies suggest a benefit in this setting of improving pulmonary function and reducing treatment failure. On the other hand, only a minority of patients with chronic, stable, but severe disease show improved pulmonary function after being placed on a regimen of oral corticosteroids. The utility of inhaled corticosteroids in COPD is even less clear. These agents have no role in the treatment of acute exacerbations, and, in contrast to their benefit in chronic asthma, have limited usefulness in chronic, stable COPD.

Modalities available for treatment of COPD are the following:

1. *Bronchodilators*
2. *Antibiotics*
3. *Corticosteroids*
4. *Supplemental oxygen*
5. *Exercise rehabilitation*
6. *Chest physiotherapy*
7. *Surgery (selected cases)*

An important adjunct to therapy is the administration of supplemental O_2 to those patients with significant hypoxemia (i.e., arterial Po_2 of 55 torr or less). Fortunately, the Po_2 of hypoxemic patients with COPD usually responds quite well to even relatively small amounts of supplemental O_2 (in the range of 24 to 28 percent O_2). A low flow rate of O_2 (1 to 2 L/min), given by nasal prongs, is an effective and well-tolerated method for achieving these concentrations of inspired O_2. Oxygen is particularly important in those patients with pulmonary hypertension and in those with secondary polycythemia, because each of these complications is largely caused by and responsive to treatment for hypoxemia. Evidence also suggests that survival of hypoxemic patients with COPD can be improved by the administration of supplemental O_2. This is actually the first demonstration of a form of therapy capable of altering the natural history and improving the long-term survival of these patients.

The goal of O_2 therapy is to shift the Po_2 into the range in which hemoglobin is almost fully saturated, i.e., a Po_2 greater than 60 to 65 torr. Ideally, O_2 saturation should be well maintained on a continuous basis, throughout the day and night. In some patients with COPD who are not significantly hypoxemic during the day, a substantial drop in their Po_2 and O_2 saturation can occur at night; in these patients, nocturnal O_2 may theoretically be of benefit, although this has not been proved.

For those patients in whom airway secretions cause significant symptoms, chest physiotherapy and postural drainage are sometimes used to help mobilize and clear the secretions. These techniques utilize percussion of the chest wall to loosen secretions and induce cough, followed by positional changes to allow gravity to aid in drainage of the secretions. However, the utility of chest physiotherapy and postural drainage is not generally accepted, as outcome studies have not clearly supported their benefit.

In the small subgroup of patients with COPD who have α_1-antitrypsin deficiency, therapy is available in the form of α_1-antitrypsin prepared from pooled human plasma. The rationale for this therapy is to replace the deficient protease inhibitor and to try to inhibit or prevent unchecked proteolytic destruction of alveolar tissue. Although it has been demonstrated that intravenous infusions of α_1-antitrypsin do increase concentrations of this antiprotease in alveolar epithelial lining fluid, it is not definitively known if such replacement therapy alters the accelerated decline in pulmonary function.

In patients with impaired exercise tolerance secondary to COPD, a rehabilitation program focusing on education and a regimen of exercise training is often quite beneficial. Most patients entering such a program report an improved sense of well-being at the same time they experience an improvement in their exercise tolerance. Education of the patient in the importance of smoking cessation is also obviously a critical part of any comprehensive therapeutic program, and pharmacologic assistance to ameliorate the effects of nicotine withdrawal, using nicotine replacement therapy and/or the drug bupropion, is often valuable. Vaccination against influenza and pneumococcus is indicated in all patients as a preventive strategy and a component of the overall therapeutic regimen.

Two surgical approaches have been used for patients with severe COPD who remain markedly symptomatic despite optimal therapy. One of these, *lung volume reduction surgery*, initially sounds counterintuitive, because it involves removing portions of both lungs from patients whose pulmonary reserve is marginal at best. However, there are two interesting pathophysiologic rationales underlying this approach. First, removal of some lung tissue diminishes overall intrathoracic volume, allowing the flattened and foreshortened diaphragm to return toward its normal position and resume its usual curved configuration. A flattened, foreshortened diaphragm is an inefficient respiratory muscle, and the changes in its position and shape following surgery facilitate its effectiveness during inspiration. Second, when the most diseased regions of lung are selectively removed, i.e., the regions with the least elastic recoil, the overall elastic recoil of the lung improves. Lung elastic recoil is an important determinant of expiratory flow and airway collapse, and improving the elastic recoil has secondary benefits on airway patency and expiratory flow. Although lung volume reduction surgery is an intriguing approach, it is still relatively new, and its overall benefit and the long-term outcome are being investigated.

The other surgical approach to end-stage COPD is *lung transplantation*. However, because of the resources needed, the shortage of donor organs, and the age of the patients, this is not a practical approach for large numbers of patients. Those whose emphysema is due to α_1-antitrypsin deficiency, in whom the disease occurs at an early age, may be a particularly appropriate subgroup to consider for lung transplantation.

Finally, when acute respiratory failure supervenes as a part of COPD, mechanical ventilation may be necessary for supporting gas-exchange and maintaining acceptable arterial blood gas values. Such ventilatory assistance with intermittent positive pressure may be delivered via either a mask (noninvasive positive pressure ventilation) or an endotracheal tube. More detailed information about the treatment of acute respiratory failure superimposed on chronic disease of the obstructive variety is covered in Chapter 27. A discussion of mechanical ventilation is found in Chapter 29.

References

Reviews

American Thoracic Society: Standards for the diagnosis and care of patients with chronic obstructive pulmonary disease. Am J Respir Crit Care Med 152:S77–S120, 1995.

Barnes PJ: Chronic obstructive pulmonary disease. N Engl J Med 343:269-280, 2000.

Pauwels RA et al: Global strategy for the diagnosis, management, and prevention of chronic obstructive pulmonary disease. NHLBI/WHO global initiative for chronic obstructive lung disease (GOLD) workshop summary. Am J Respir Crit Care Med 163:1256-1276, 2001.

The COPD Guidelines Group of the Standards of Care Committee of the BTS: BTS guidelines for the management of chronic obstructive pulmonary disease. Thorax 52:S1–S28, 1997.

Thurlbeck WM: Chronic Airflow Obstruction in Lung Disease. Philadelphia, WB Saunders Co., 1976.

Etiology and Pathogenesis

Antó JM, Vermeire P, Vestbo J, and Sunyer J: Epidemiology of chronic obstructive pulmonary disease. Eur Respir J 17:982-994, 2001.

Burchfiel CM et al: Effects of smoking and smoking cessation on longitudinal decline in pulmonary function. Am J Respir Crit Care Med 151:1778-1785, 1995.

Carrell RW and Lomas DA: Alpha$_1$-antitrypsin deficiency—a model for conformational diseases. N Engl J Med 346:45-53, 2002.

Cosio MG and Cosio Piqueras MG: Pathology of emphysema in chronic obstructive pulmonary disease. Monaldi Arch Chest Dis 55:124-129, 2000.

Hogg JC and Senior RM: Pathology and biochemistry of emphysema. Thorax 57:830-834, 2002.

Mahadeva R and Lomas DA: Alpha$_1$-antitrypsin deficiency, cirrhosis and emphysema. Thorax 53:501-505, 1998.

O'Connor GT, Sparrow D, and Weiss ST: The role of allergy and nonspecific airway hyperresponsiveness in the pathogenesis of chronic obstructive pulmonary disease. Am Rev Respir Dis 140:225-252, 1989.

Saetta M et al: Cellular and structural bases of chronic obstructive pulmonary disease. Am J Respir Crit Care Med 163:1304-1309, 2001.

Shaheen SO, Barker DJP, and Holgate ST: Do lower respiratory tract infections in early childhood cause chronic obstructive pulmonary disease? Am J Respir Crit Care Med 151:1649-1652, 1995.

Shapiro SD: Evolving concepts in the pathogenesis of chronic obstructive pulmonary disease. Clin Chest Med 21:621-632, 2000.

Viegi G et al: Epidemiology of chronic obstructive pulmonary disease (COPD). Respiration 68: 4-19, 2001.

Clinical Features

Black LF: Early diagnosis of chronic obstructive pulmonary disease. Mayo Clin Proc 57:765-772, 1982.

Burrows B, Bloom JW, Traver GA, and Cline MG: The course and prognosis of different forms of chronic airways obstruction in a sample from the general population. N Engl J Med 317:1309-1314, 1987.

Cleverley JR and Müller NL: Advances in radiologic assessment of chronic obstructive pulmonary disease. Clin Chest Med 21:653-663, 2000.

Diener CF and Burrows B: Further observations on the course and prognosis of chronic obstructive lung disease. Am Rev Respir Dis 111:719-724, 1975.

Fletcher C and Peto R: The natural history of chronic airflow obstruction. Br Med J 1:1645-1648, 1977.

George RB: Course and prognosis of chronic obstructive pulmonary disease. Am J Med Sci 318:103-106, 1999.

Müller NL and Coxson H: Imaging the lungs in patients with chronic obstructive pulmonary disease. Thorax 57:982-985, 2002.

Sherk PA and Grossman RF: The chronic obstructive pulmonary disease exacerbation. Clin Chest Med 21:705-721, 2000.

White AJ, Gompertz S, and Stockley RA: The aetiology of exacerbations of chronic obstructive pulmonary disease. Thorax 58:73-80, 2003.

Treatment

Alsaeedi A, Sin DD, and McAlister FA: The effects of inhaled corticosteroids in chronic obstructive pulmonary disease: a systematic review of randomized placebo-controlled trials. Am J Med 113:59-65, 2002.

Barnes PJ: New therapies for chronic obstructive pulmonary disease. Thorax 53:137-147, 1998.

Brochard L et al: Noninvasive ventilation for acute exacerbations of chronic obstructive pulmonary disease. N Engl J Med 333:817-822, 1995.

Celli BR: Pulmonary rehabilitation in patients with COPD. Am J Respir Crit Care Med 152:861-864, 1995.

Ferguson GT: Update on pharmacologic therapy for chronic obstructive pulmonary disease. Clin Chest Med 21:723-738, 2000.

Ferguson GT and Cherniack RM: Management of chronic obstructive pulmonary disease. N Engl J Med 328:1017-1022, 1993.

Flaherty KR and Martinez FJ: Lung volume reduction surgery for emphysema. Clin Chest Med 21:819-848, 2000.

Gross NJ: Ipratropium bromide. N Engl J Med 319:486-494, 1988.

McCrory DC, Brown C, Gelfand SE, and Bach PB: Management of acute exacerbations of COPD. A summary and appraisal of published evidence. Chest 119:1190-1209, 2001.

McEvoy CE and Niewoehner DE: Corticosteroids in chronic obstructive pulmonary disease. Clinical benefits and risks. Clin Chest Med 21:739-752, 2000.

Murciano D, Auclair M-H, Pariente R, and Aubier M: A randomized, controlled trial of theophylline in patients with severe chronic obstructive pulmonary disease. N Engl J Med 320:1521-1525, 1989.

Saint S, Bent S, Vittinghoff E, and Grady D: Antibiotics in chronic obstructive pulmonary disease exacerbations. JAMA 273:957-960, 1995.

Singh JM, Palda VA, Stanbrook MB, and Chapman KR: Corticosteroid therapy for patients with acute exacerbations of chronic obstructive pulmonary disease. Arch Intern Med 162:2527-2536, 2002.

Snow V et al: The evidence base for management of acute exacerbations of COPD. Clinical practice guideline, part 1. Chest 119:1185-1189, 2001.

Stoller JK: Acute exacerbations of chronic obstructive pulmonary disease. N Engl J Med 346:988-994, 2002.

Tarpy SP and Celli BR: Long-term oxygen therapy. N Engl J Med 333:710-714, 1995.

Wilson R: Bacteria, antibiotics and COPD. Eur Respir J 17:995-1007, 2001.

chapter 7

Miscellaneous Airway Diseases

BRONCHIECTASIS
Etiology and Pathogenesis
Pathology
Pathophysiology
Clinical Features
Diagnostic Approach
Treatment
CYSTIC FIBROSIS
Etiology and Pathogenesis
Pathology

Pathophysiology
Clinical Features
Diagnostic Approach
Treatment
UPPER AIRWAY DISEASE
Etiology
Pathophysiology
Clinical Features
Diagnostic Approach
Treatment

In this chapter, a few additional selected disorders that affect airways are considered, chosen because of their clinical or physiologic importance. The first of these, bronchiectasis, is a disease that used to be much more common. The availability of effective antibiotics for the control of respiratory tract infections has made this problem less prevalent and has also diminished its clinical consequences. The second disorder, cystic fibrosis, is a genetic disease that generally manifests in childhood and is notable for the often devastating clinical consequences that ensue. Finally, a brief consideration of abnormalities of the upper airway (which for our purposes here includes the airway at or above the level of the trachea) is presented to acquaint the reader with the physiologic principles that allow detection of these disorders.

BRONCHIECTASIS

Bronchiectasis is an irreversible dilation of airways caused by inflammatory destruction of airway walls. Because the most common etiologic factor is infection, which triggers the destructive inflammatory process, the extent of the bronchiectasis in a particular patient depends upon the location and extent of the underlying infection. In some cases, bronchiectasis is localized to a specific region of the lung; in other cases, the process may involve more than one area or may even be widespread, involving a large portion of both lungs.

Etiology and Pathogenesis

Infection and obstruction are the two underlying problems that contribute to the development of dilated or bronchiectatic airways. The responsible infection(s) in a given patient may have been viral or bacterial; some years ago, measles and pertussis (whooping cough) pneumonia were common problems

Prior infection or obstruction, or both, are the most common problems leading to bronchiectasis.

resulting in bronchiectasis. Currently, a variety of other viral and bacterial infections are often responsible, with tuberculosis being one important example. At times, fungal infections may be responsible, as with *allergic bronchopulmonary aspergillosis*. This condition, found almost exclusively in patients with underlying asthma, is characterized by colonization of airways with *Aspergillus* organisms and by thick mucous plugs and bronchiectasis in relatively proximal airways.

When obstruction of an airway is associated with bronchiectasis behind the obstruction, a superimposed infection may also contribute to destruction of the airway wall. Tumors, thick mucus, or foreign bodies are commonly the cause of bronchial obstruction resulting in bronchiectasis.

An additional factor that plays a role in some patients is a defect in the ability of the airway to clear itself of, or protect itself against, bacterial pathogens (see Chapter 22). Such a defect predisposes a person to recurrent infections and eventually to airway dilation and bronchiectasis. The abnormality may involve inadequate humoral immunity and insufficient antibody production (hypogammaglobulinemia) or defective leukocyte function. Another problem that has received significant attention is dyskinetic cilia syndrome, in which ciliary dysfunction affects the ability of the ciliary blanket that lines the airway to clear bacteria and to protect the airway against infection. The ciliary dysfunction is not limited to the lower airways; it also affects the nasal mucosa and, in males, may affect sperm motility and hence fertility. Pathologically, the dynein arms that are a characteristic feature of the ultrastructure of cilia are frequently absent in this disorder. One specific syndrome associated with bronchiectasis and ciliary dysfunction is *Kartagener's syndrome,* which includes a triad of sinusitis, bronchiectasis, and situs inversus (discovered by the presence of dextrocardia).

Abnormalities of ciliary structure and function can result in recurrent infections and bronchiectasis.

Pathology

The primary pathologic feature of bronchiectasis is evident on gross inspection of the airways, which are markedly dilated in the involved region (Fig. 7-1). Three specific patterns of dilation have been described: cylindrical, varicose, and saccular bronchiectasis. The dilated airways are generally filled with a considerable amount of secretions, which may be grossly purulent. Microscopic changes of the bronchial wall epithelium, consisting of ulceration and squamous metaplasia, are also seen.

As a result of the exuberant inflammatory changes in the bronchial wall, the blood supply, provided by the bronchial arteries, is increased. The arteries enlarge and increase in number, and new anastomoses may form between the bronchial and pulmonary artery circulations. Inflammatory erosion or mechanical trauma at the site of these vascular changes is often responsible for the hemoptysis seen so frequently in patients with bronchiectasis.

Coexisting disease in the remainder of the tracheobronchial tree is not at all uncommon. Either other areas of bronchiectasis may be present or there may be generalized changes of chronic bronchitis, as described in Chapter 6.

Vessels from the bronchial arterial circulation supplying a bronchiectatic region are often a source of bleeding and hemoptysis.

Pathophysiology

Once the airways have become irreversibly dilated, their defense mechanisms against infection are disturbed. The normal propulsive action of cilia is lost in the involved area, even if it was intact before the development of bronchiectasis. Bacteria colonize the enlarged airways, and secretions pool in the dilated sacs of patients with saccular bronchiectasis. In many cases the relationship

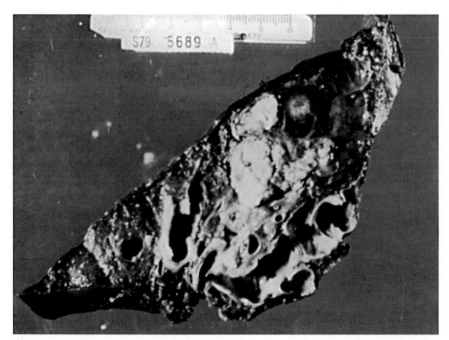

Figure 7-1 ■— Surgically removed specimen of lung shows extensive bronchiectasis. Some of the grossly dilated airways are filled with large amounts of mucoid and purulent material.

established between the colonizing bacteria and the host is relatively stable over time, but the course may be punctuated by acute exacerbations of the airway infection.

Functionally, patients with a localized area of bronchiectasis are not impaired in the same way as other patients with generalized obstructive lung disease. Measurement of their pulmonary function may reveal surprisingly few, if any, abnormalities. When seen, functional abnormalities are either the result of extensive bronchiectasis involving a large area of one or both lungs or the result of coexistent generalized airway disease, primarily chronic bronchitis.

Clinical Features

The most prominent symptom in patients with bronchiectasis is generally cough and copious sputum production. The sputum may be frankly purulent, and it is often the profuse amount of yellow or green sputum production that raises the physician's suspicion of bronchiectasis. However, not all patients with bronchiectasis have significant sputum production. It has been estimated that approximately 10 to 20 percent of patients are free of copious sputum production, and these patients are said to have "dry" bronchiectasis.

The other frequent symptom in patients with bronchiectasis is hemoptysis, which may be impressive in amount. The hypertrophied bronchial artery circulation to the involved area is probably responsible for this symptom in the majority of cases.

Physical examination of the patient with bronchiectasis may reveal few abnormalities, even over the area of involvement. On the other hand, the examiner may hear strikingly abnormal findings in a localized area, such as rales or rhonchi. Clubbing is frequently present. Although the mechanism is not clear, clubbing is thought to be associated with the chronic suppurative process.

Common clinical features of bronchiectasis are the following:

1. Cough
2. Copious and purulent sputum
3. Hemoptysis
4. Localized rales or rhonchi
5. Clubbing

Whether arterial blood gas values are abnormal in these patients often depends on the extent of involvement and the presence or absence of underlying chronic bronchitis. With well-localized disease, both P_{O_2} and P_{CO_2} may be normal. At the other extreme, patients may have the blood gas changes seen in the type B pattern of chronic obstructive lung disease, namely hypoxemia and hypercapnia, and the complication of cor pulmonale may also develop.

Diagnostic Approach

The diagnosis of bronchiectasis is usually suggested by a history of copious sputum production or hemoptysis, or both. Evaluation on a macroscopic level generally includes a chest radiograph, the findings of which are often nonspecifically abnormal in the involved area. The radiograph may show an area of increased markings, crowded vessels, or "ring" shadows corresponding to dilated or saccular airways. However, none of the findings on the routine radiograph is considered diagnostic of bronchiectasis. In the past the definitive diagnosis depended on bronchography, a radiographic procedure in which an opaque contrast material was used to outline part of the tracheobronchial tree (Fig. 7-2). More recently, computed tomography (CT) has become the initial procedure often used to define the presence, location, and extent of bronchiectasis (Fig. 7-3). High-resolution CT (with sections 1 to 2 mm thick) provides excellent detail and is particularly useful for detecting subtle bronchiectasis. As a result, bronchography is now rarely performed.

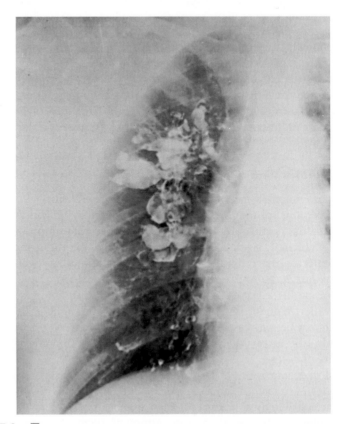

Figure 7-2 ■— Bronchogram of patient with extensive saccular bronchiectasis, primarily in right upper lobe.

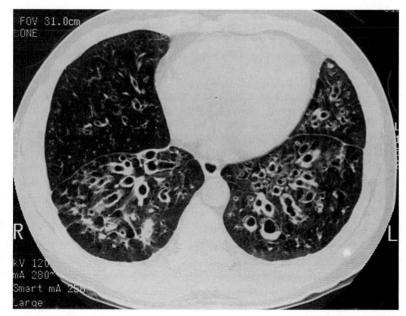

Figure 7-3 ■— High-resolution CT scan of bronchiectasis showing dilated airways in both lower lobes and in the lingula. When seen in cross section, the dilated airways have a ring-like appearance.

Evaluation on a microscopic level does not offer much help for the patient with presumed bronchiectasis, except for examination of the sputum for microorganisms, particularly during an acute exacerbation of the disease. Patients with bronchiectasis frequently become colonized and infected with *Pseudomonas aeruginosa,* and the finding of this otherwise relatively unusual pathogen may be a clue to the presence of underlying bronchiectasis. The findings on functional evaluation were discussed in the Pathophysiology and Clinical Features sections.

Treatment

The three major aspects of treatment of the patient with bronchiectasis are antibiotics, bronchopulmonary drainage (clearance of airway secretions), and bronchodilators. Antibiotics are used in various ways in these patients. Sometimes, patients are treated only when there is a clear change in the quantity or appearance of the sputum. In other cases, patients are given a regimen of intermittent or even continuous antibiotics in an attempt to keep a chronic infection under control. Agents such as amoxicillin and trimethoprim-sulfamethoxazole, which are effective against the organisms *Streptococcus pneumoniae* and *Haemophilus influenzae,* are often used in patients with bronchiectasis. When these patients are infected with *Pseudomonas* organisms, treatment is generally more difficult. Oral ciprofloxacin has become useful for therapy of *Pseudomonas* infection as an alternative to parenteral antibiotics, but secondary development of resistance to this oral antibiotic is common. Chest physical therapy and positioning to allow better drainage of secretions (postural drainage) are frequently used for the patient with copious sputum; alternatively, inflatable vests or mechanical vibrators on the chest are increasingly being used to facilitate clearance of secretions. Bronchodilators may be useful in patients who have coexisting airway obstruction that is at least partially reversible.

Treatment of bronchiectasis includes bronchopulmonary drainage, antibiotics, and bronchodilators; surgical therapy with resection of the diseased area is infrequent.

In the past, surgery was used for many patients with localized bronchiectasis. Because medical therapy is frequently effective in limiting symptoms and impairment, resection of the diseased area is now performed much less frequently. In general, surgery is reserved for selected patients who have significant, poorly controlled symptoms attributable to a single localized area and who do not have other areas of bronchiectasis or significant evidence of generalized chronic obstructive pulmonary disease.

CYSTIC FIBROSIS

Cystic fibrosis, the most common lethal genetic disease affecting the white population, is inherited as an autosomal recessive trait and is present in approximately 1 in 2,500 live births. Onset of the disease is often in childhood, although cases are being recognized in adults, and children with the disease are living longer into adulthood. The clinical presentation is dominated by severe lung disease and by pancreatic insufficiency, resulting from thick and tenacious secretions produced by exocrine glands.

Etiology and Pathogenesis

Major defects in cystic fibrosis are the following:

1. Production of thick, tenacious secretions from exocrine glands
2. Elevated concentrations of sodium, chloride, and potassium in sweat

Two major abnormalities have been recognized that are responsible for the clinical expression of cystic fibrosis. The first abnormality relates to the quality of the secretions produced by various exocrine glands. These secretions are thick and tenacious and block the tubes into which the secretions are normally deposited (especially airways and pancreatic ducts). Second, abnormal electrolyte composition has been observed in the sweat produced by affected patients, specifically elevated concentrations of sodium, chloride, and potassium. These abnormalities in the composition of sweat have proved to be crucial in the diagnosis of the disorder.

The techniques of molecular biology have identified the basic genetic defect in the majority of patients with cystic fibrosis. On the long arm of chromosome 7 resides the gene coding for a 1,480–amino acid protein called the *cystic fibrosis transmembrane conductance regulator* (CFTR). This protein appears to play a critical role in normal chloride transport across the apical surface of epithelial cells. Because of a 3-nucleotide deletion in most patients with cystic fibrosis, a single phenylalanine residue is missing at position 508 (called the ΔF508 deletion), resulting in abnormal chloride transport across cell membranes. Working by mechanisms that have not yet been fully elucidated, this impermeability of epithelial cells to chloride transport is thought to be responsible for both the high electrolyte concentrations in sweat and the abnormally thick secretions produced by exocrine glands. Although the ΔF508 mutation is responsible for approximately 70 percent of cases of cystic fibrosis, more than 800 different cystic fibrosis mutations have been identified.

Pathology

The pathologic findings in cystic fibrosis appear to result from obstruction of ducts or tubes by tenacious secretions. In the pancreas, this obstruction of the ducts eventually produces fibrosis, atrophy of the acini, and cystic changes. In the airways, thick mucous plugs appear in the bronchi, obstructing both airflow and the normal drainage of the tracheobronchial tree. Early in the course of the disease, the airway changes are found predominantly in the bronchioles, which are plugged and obliterated by the secretions. Later, the findings are more extensive, superimposed areas of pneumonitis appear, and frank bronchiectasis and areas of abscess formation may be found. Cardiac complications of cor pulmonale frequently occur, and pathologic examination of the heart shows evidence of right ventricular hypertrophy.

Pathophysiology

In the pancreas, the pathologic process leads to pancreatic insufficiency, with maldigestion and malabsorption of foodstuffs, particularly fat. In the lung, the major problem is with recurrent episodes of tracheobronchial infection and bronchiectasis resulting from bronchial obstruction and from defective mucociliary transport. In addition, evidence suggests that the CFTR mutation may contribute to airway infection by altering the binding and clearance of microorganisms by airway epithelial cells, and by impairing activity of antimicrobial peptides in the airway (especially human β-defensin-1). The major organisms that eventually colonize the airways are *Staphylococcus aureus* and *Pseudomonas aeruginosa*. Difficulty with these organisms seems to be entirely a result of the local (airway) host defense mechanisms; the humoral immune system—the ability to form antibodies—appears to be intact.

As a result of airways obstruction, functional changes develop that are characteristic of obstructive airways disease and air trapping. These patients also exhibit the pathophysiologic changes seen in type B patients with chronic obstructive pulmonary disease, that is, ventilation-perfusion mismatch, hypoxemia (sometimes with CO_2 retention), pulmonary hypertension, and cor pulmonale.

> Major clinical problems from cystic fibrosis are the following:
> 1. Pancreatic insufficiency
> 2. Recurrent episodes of tracheobronchial infection
> 3. Bronchiectasis

Clinical Features

The first clinical problem in approximately 10 to 20 percent of patients with cystic fibrosis develops in the neonatal period, with intestinal obstruction from thick meconium. This obstruction is called *meconium ileus*. The remainder of patients usually have a childhood presentation with pancreatic insufficiency or recurrent bronchial infections, or both. Occasionally, patients are first diagnosed as adults. Almost all males with the disease are sterile. Females are capable of having children, although their fertility rate is decreased.

The physical examination of patients with cystic fibrosis reveals the findings to be expected with severe airflow obstruction and with plugging of airways by secretions. Wheezing and coarse rales or rhonchi occur frequently, and clubbing is common.

Several complications may develop as a result of this disease. Pneumothorax and hemoptysis, which may be massive, can be major problems in management. Eventually, frank respiratory insufficiency and cor pulmonale develop. Although patients certainly may live into adult life when good care has been provided, their life span is significantly reduced.

> Serious complications of cystic fibrosis are the following:
> 1. Pneumothorax
> 2. Massive hemoptysis
> 3. Respiratory insufficiency
> 4. Cor pulmonale

Diagnostic Approach

Definitive diagnosis of cystic fibrosis is made by analysis of sweat electrolytes. The concentrations of sodium, chloride, and potassium are elevated in sweat from these patients, and a sweat chloride concentration greater than 60 mEq/L is generally considered diagnostic. Only individuals homozygous for the cystic fibrosis gene demonstrate this abnormality, inasmuch as heterozygous carriers have normal sweat electrolytes. Identification of heterozygotes (i.e., carriers

> Diagnosis of cystic fibrosis is made by demonstration of an elevated concentration of sweat chloride.

of the cystic fibrosis gene) and in utero detection of homozygotes have now become possible with DNA probe techniques.

The chest radiograph (Fig. 7-4) often demonstrates an increase in markings, along with the findings of bronchiectasis that were described in the previous section. There may also be evidence of focal pneumonitis at times during the course of the disease.

Early in the disease, functional assessment of these patients shows evidence of obstruction of small airways. As the disease progresses, there is evidence of more generalized airway obstruction (decreased forced expiratory volume in 1 second [FEV_1], forced vital capacity [FVC], and FEV_1/FVC ratio), and air trapping (increased residual volume [RV]/total lung capacity [TLC] ratio) is evident. The elastic recoil of the lung is generally preserved, and TLC is most commonly within the normal range. Because (1) emphysematous changes generally are not seen in patients with cystic fibrosis and (2) the alveolar-capillary interface remains relatively preserved, most frequently the diffusing capacity is also normal. Arterial blood gas values often demonstrate hypoxemia, and hypercapnia also may be seen as the disease progresses.

Treatment

Therapy for cystic fibrosis is based on an attempt to diminish the clinical consequences and to manage complications when they occur. The principles of therapy are similar to those used for bronchiectasis: bronchopulmonary drainage (using chest physical therapy and postural drainage, a flutter valve, or a vibrating vest), antibiotics, and bronchodilators. Agents used to decrease

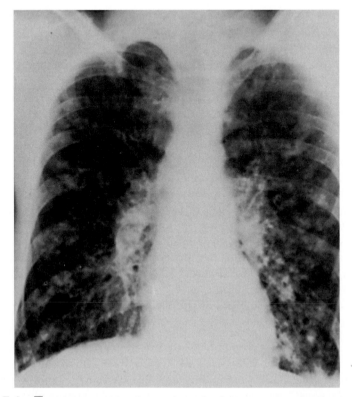

Figure 7-4 ■— Posteroanterior chest radiograph of patient with cystic fibrosis, showing diffuse increase in markings throughout both lungs. These findings represent extensive fibrotic changes and bronchiectasis. (Courtesy of Dr. Mary Ellen Wohl.)

the viscosity of the sputum appear to offer benefit in some patients. In particular, because DNA released from inflammatory cells contributes significantly to the viscosity of mucus, inhalation of recombinant deoxyribonuclease (DNase) has been used to degrade DNA, decrease mucus viscosity, and improve clearance of secretions. Although current forms of therapy have significantly improved prognosis in cystic fibrosis, the natural history is still one of progressive pulmonary dysfunction and eventual death as a result of the disease or its complications. Despite initial concern about using lung transplantation in these patients because of their chronic pulmonary infection, experience with bilateral lung transplantation suggests post-transplantation survival is similar to that of other patients undergoing lung transplantation.

Now that the genetic basis for the disease in the majority of patients has been identified, there has been hope that gene therapy may provide a means for reversing the primary defect as well as the characteristic abnormality in airway secretion. Unfortunately, initial enthusiasm for gene therapy as a "cure" for cystic fibrosis has been tempered by difficulty finding an effective and non-toxic method (vector) for delivering the gene to the airway and achieving sufficient and durable expression of the normal gene.

UPPER AIRWAY DISEASE

So far, the obstructive diseases that have been considered primarily affect the airways below the level of the main carina, i.e., the bronchi and the bronchioles. In contrast to disease of these lower airways, a variety of other disorders affect the pharynx, larynx, and trachea and produce what is termed *upper airway obstruction.* The discussion of these disorders will be limited and will include a brief consideration of representative etiologic factors as well as a discussion of some of the tests used to make the diagnosis. In particular, the use of the flow-volume loop to define the location of upper airway obstruction is considered.

Etiology

The upper airway may be affected by either acute problems or those that have followed a more subacute or chronic course. On an acute basis, the larynx is probably the major area subject to obstruction. Potential causes include infection (epiglottitis, which is often due to *Haemophilus influenzae*), thermal injury and the resulting laryngeal edema from smoke inhalation, aspiration of a foreign body, and laryngeal edema from an allergic (anaphylactic) reaction.

On a chronic basis, the upper airway may be partially obstructed by hypertrophy of the tonsils, by tumors (particularly of the trachea), by strictures of the trachea (often resulting from previous instrumentation of the trachea), or by vocal cord paralysis. Some patients are also subject to recurrent episodes of upper airway obstruction during sleep; this entity is one variety of what is termed *sleep apnea syndrome,* which is considered further in Chapter 18.

Pathophysiology

The resistance of a tube to airflow varies inversely as the fourth power of the radius, and hence even small changes in airway size may produce dramatic changes in resistance and in the work of breathing. If the airways under consideration were always stiff, or if a disorder did not allow any flexibility in the size of the airway, then inspiration and expiration would be impaired by the same amount, and the flow rate generated during inspiration would be essentially identical to the flow rate during expiration. This type of obstruction is termed a *fixed* obstruction.

If, on the other hand, airway diameter changes during the respiratory cycle, then the greatest impairment to airflow occurs during the time that airway diameter is smallest. This type of obstruction is termed a *variable* obstruction. If the obstruction is within the thorax, then changes in pleural pressure during the respiratory cycle affect the size of the airway and therefore the magnitude of the obstruction. During a forced expiration, the positive pleural pressure causes airway narrowing, making the obstructing lesion more critical. In contrast, during inspiration, the airways increase their diameter, and the effects of a partial obstruction are less pronounced (see Fig. 3-20).

If the obstruction is above the level of the thorax (i.e., outside the thorax), then changes in pleural pressure are not directly transmitted to the airway in question. Rather, the negative airway pressure during inspiration tends to create a vacuum-like effect on extrathoracic upper airways, narrowing them and therefore augmenting the effect of any partial obstruction. During expiration the pressure generated by the flow of air from the intrathoracic airways tends to widen the extrathoracic airways and to decrease the net effect of a partially obstructing lesion (see Fig. 3-20).

The location and respiratory variability of an upper airway obstruction affect the appearance of the flow-volume curve and the findings on physical examination.

Clinical Features

In terms of symptoms, patients with upper airway obstruction may have dyspnea or cough; on physical examination they may have evidence of flow through narrowed airways. If the lesion is variable and intrathoracic, the primary difficulty with airflow occurs during expiration, and patients demonstrate expiratory wheezing. If it is variable and extrathoracic, obstruction is more marked during inspiration, and patients frequently manifest inspiratory stridor, a high-pitched continuous inspiratory sound often best heard over the trachea. With acute upper airway obstruction, such as that seen with inhalation of a foreign body, anxiety and respiratory distress are often apparent, signaling a medical emergency. In patients with epiglottitis, respiratory distress is often accompanied by sore throat, change in voice, dysphagia, and drooling.

Diagnostic Approach

In the evaluation of suspected disorders of the upper airway, radiography and direct visualization provide the most useful information about the macroscopic appearance of the airway. Lateral neck radiographs or CT scans of the upper airway may reveal the localization, extent, and character of a partially obstructing lesion. A CT scan may offer particularly useful information by providing a cross-sectional view of the airways from the larynx down to the carina. Direct visualization of the upper airway may be obtained by laryngoscopy or bronchoscopy, during which the physician may observe whether edema, vocal cord paralysis, or an obstructing lesion such as a tumor is present. However, direct visualization of the airways by these techniques is not entirely without risk: the instrument used occupies part of the already compromised airway and may induce airway spasm that further obstructs the airway.

The functional assessment of the patient with presumed upper airway obstruction can be useful in quantifying and localizing the obstruction, because the functional consequences of a fixed versus a variable obstruction and an extrathoracic versus an intrathoracic obstruction are quite different. To understand these differences, the flow-volume loop and the principles discussed in the Pathophysiology section must be understood. This type of physiologic evaluation is appropriate for chronic upper airway obstruction, not for acute, life-threatening obstruction.

With a fixed lesion causing a relatively critical obstruction, the maximum flow rates generated during inspiration and expiration are approximately equal, and a "plateau" marks both the inspiratory and expiratory parts of the flow-volume curve. When the lesion is variable, the effect of the obstruction depends on whether it is intrathoracic or extrathoracic. With an intrathoracic obstruction, the critical narrowing occurs during expiration, and the expiratory part of the flow-volume curve displays a plateau. With an extrathoracic obstruction, the expiratory part of the loop is preserved, and the inspiratory portion displays the plateau. A schematic diagram of the flow-volume loops observed in these types of upper airway obstruction is shown in Figure 3-21.

Treatment

Because many different types of disorders result in upper airway obstruction, treatment varies greatly, depending on the underlying problem, particularly in terms of its acuteness and its severity. In acute, severe upper airway obstruction, emergency procedures such as endotracheal intubation or tracheostomy may be necessary to maintain a patent airway. Discussion of each disorder and further consideration of emergency management may be found in other textbooks and in some of the articles in the following list of references.

References

Bronchiectasis

Barker AF: Bronchiectasis. Semin Thorac Cardiovasc Surg 7:112-118, 1995.
Barker AF: Bronchiectasis. N Engl J Med 346:1383-1393, 2002.
Barker AF and Bardana EJ Jr: Bronchiectasis: update of an orphan disease. Am Rev Respir Dis 137:969-978, 1988.
Cartier Y et al: Bronchiectasis: accuracy of high-resolution CT in the differentiation of specific diseases. AJR Am J Roentgenol 173:47-52, 1999.
Cohen M and Sahn SA: Bronchiectasis in systemic disease. Chest 116:1063-1074, 1999.
Keistinen T, Saynajakangas O, Tuuponen T, and Kivela SL: Bronchiectasis: an orphan disease with a poorly-understood prognosis. Eur Respir J 10:2784-2787, 1997.
Kumar NA, Nguyen B, and Maki D: Bronchiectasis: current clinical and imaging concepts. Semin Roentgenol 36:41-50, 2001.
Lillington GA: Dyskinetic cilia and Kartagener's syndrome. Bronchiectasis with a twist. Clin Rev Allergy Immunol 21:65-69, 2001.
Pasteur MC et al: An investigation into causative factors in patients with bronchiectasis. Am J Respir Crit Care Med 162:1277-1284, 2000.

Cystic Fibrosis

Davis PB, Drumm M, and Konstan MW: Cystic fibrosis. Am J Respir Crit Care Med 154:1229-1256, 1996.
Fiel SB (ed): Cystic fibrosis. Clin Chest Med 19:423-567, 1998.
Huang NN et al: Clinical features, survival rate, and prognostic factors in young adults with cystic fibrosis. Am J Med 82:871-879, 1987.
Kotloff RM and Zuckerman JB: Lung transplantation for cystic fibrosis. Chest 109:787-798, 1996.
Lion TG et al: Survival effect of lung transplantation among patients with cystic fibrosis. JAMA 286:2683-2689, 2001.
Pier GB et al: Role of mutant CFTR in hypersusceptibility of cystic fibrosis patients to lung infections. Science 271:64-67, 1996.
Pitt BR: CFTR trafficking and signaling in respiratory epithelium. Am J Physiol Lung Cell Mol Physiol 281:L13-L15, 2001.
Ramsey BW: Management of pulmonary disease in patients with cystic fibrosis. N Engl J Med 335:179-188, 1996.
Robinson P: Cystic fibrosis. Thorax 56:237-241, 2001.

Rubin BK: Emerging therapies for cystic fibrosis lung disease. Chest 115:1120-1126, 1999.

di Sant'Agnese PA and Davis PB: Cystic fibrosis in adults: 75 cases and a review of 232 cases in the literature. Am J Med 66:121-132, 1979.

Stern RC: The diagnosis of cystic fibrosis. N Engl J Med 336:487-491, 1997.

Webb AK and David TJ: Clinical management of children and adults with cystic fibrosis. Br Med J 308:459-462, 1994.

Wine JJ: The genesis of cystic fibrosis lung disease. J Clin Invest 103:309-312, 1999.

Upper Airway Disease

Acres JC and Kryger MH: Upper airway obstruction. Chest 80:207-211, 1981.

Kryger M, Bode F, Antic R, and Anthonisen N: Diagnosis of obstruction of the upper and central airways. Am J Med 61:85-93, 1976.

Limper AH and Prakash UBS: Tracheobronchial foreign bodies in adults. Ann Intern Med 112:604-609, 1990.

MayoSmith MF, Hirsch PJ, Wodzinski SF, and Schiffman FJ: Acute epiglottitis in adults. N Engl J Med 314:1133-1139, 1986.

Miller WT: Obstructive diseases of the trachea. Semin Roentgenol 36:21-40, 2001.

Proctor DF: The upper airways—II: the larynx and trachea. Am Rev Respir Dis 115:315-342, 1977.

Rafanan AL and Mehta AC: Stenting of the tracheobronchial tree. Radiol Clin North Am 38:395-408, 2000.

Shapiro J, Eavey RD, and Baker AS: Adult supraglottitis: a prospective analysis. JAMA 259:563-567, 1988.

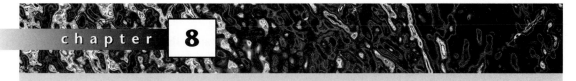

Anatomic and Physiologic Aspects of the Pulmonary Parenchyma

ANATOMY
PHYSIOLOGY

Chapters 8 through 11 focus on the region of the lung directly involved in gas-exchange, often called the *pulmonary parenchyma*. This region includes the alveolar walls and spaces (with the alveolar-capillary interface) at the level of the alveolar sacs, ducts, and respiratory bronchioles. Although the broad group of disorders involving these structures have traditionally been described under the rubric of *interstitial lung disease*, the term *diffuse parenchymal lung disease* is increasingly being used and more accurately reflects the breadth of the pathologic involvement.

Before specific diseases are discussed in Chapters 9 through 11, this chapter provides a description of the normal anatomy of the gas-exchanging region of the lung and some aspects of its normal physiology. In Chapters 9 through 11, the primary focus is on those disorders, generally subacute or chronic, whose main pathologic features appear to reside within the alveolar wall. The deliberate exclusion of pneumonia, acute pulmonary injury (acute respiratory distress syndrome), and diseases of the pulmonary vasculature is due to their different pathologic appearance, and they are considered separately in other parts of this text.

Chapter 9 provides an overview of the diffuse parenchymal lung diseases, emphasizing how disturbances in alveolar structure are closely linked with aberrations in function. Although a wide variety of disorders affect the alveolar wall, many of the pathophysiologic features are common to a large number of individual diseases. Knowledge of these general pathophysiologic features and their effects on the normal function of the lung is useful for understanding the consequences of the individual disease entities. For specific diseases with special characteristics, a consideration of these individual features is included.

ANATOMY

For the lung to function efficiently as a gas-exchanging organ, it makes sense that a large surface area should be available where O_2 can be taken up and CO_2 released. At the alveolar wall, where this gas-exchange occurs, an extensive network of capillaries coursing through and coming into close contact with alveolar gas facilitates this exchange. In the normal lung the capillaries are closely apposed to the alveolar lumen, and there is little tissue extraneous to the gas-exchanging process (Fig. 8-1).

The surface of the alveolar walls—the region bordering the alveolar lumen—is lined by a continuous layer of epithelial cells. Two different types of these lining epithelial cells, called *type I* and *type II cells*, can be identified. Type I cells are less numerous than type II cells, but they have impressively long cytoplasmic extensions that line more than 95 percent of the alveolar surface (Fig. 8-2). The type I cells have very few cytoplasmic organelles, and they appear to function primarily as a barrier preventing the free movement of material such as fluid from the alveolar wall into the alveolar lumen.

In contrast, the more numerous type II cells do not have long cytoplasmic extensions, but they do have many cytoplasmic organelles (mitochondria, rough endoplasmic reticulum, Golgi apparatus), which indicate an important synthetic role for these cells. The product of the type II cells is a material of high lipid content called *surfactant.* Specific inclusion bodies within the type II cells, termed *lamellar inclusions,* appear to be the packaged form of surfactant that is eventually released into the alveolar lumen. Surfactant acts like

Type I alveolar epithelial cells have long cytoplasmic processes that line almost the entire alveolar surface.

Type II cells produce surfactant and are important in the reparative process for type I cells.

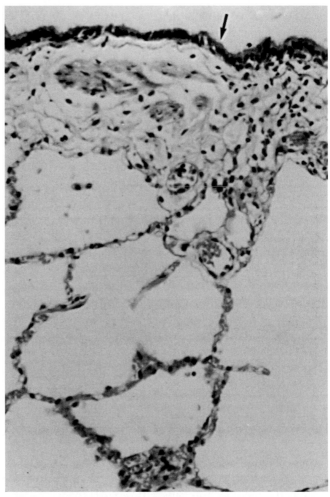

Figure 8-1 ■— Photomicrograph of alveolar walls showing normal thin, lacy appearance. At top of photo is bronchial lumen, lined by bronchial epithelial cells (*arrow*). Peribronchial tissue lies between bronchial epithelium and alveolar walls. (Courtesy of Dr. Earl Kasdon.)

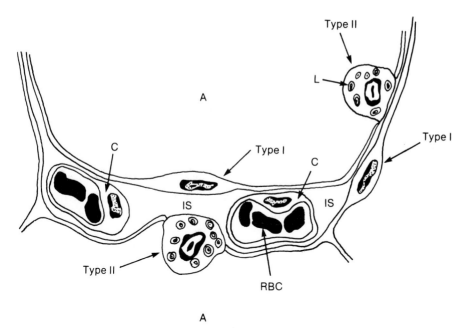

Figure 8-2 ━━■━ Schematic diagram of normal alveolar structure. Type I and type II epithelial cells are shown lining alveolar wall. Type I cells are relatively flat and are characterized by long cytoplasmic processes. Type II cells are cuboidal. Two capillaries are shown. C = capillary endothelial cells; RBC = erythrocytes in the capillary lumen; IS = interstitial space (relatively acellular region of the alveolar wall); L = type II cell cytoplasmic lamellar bodies, the source of surfactant; A = alveolar space.

a detergent to reduce the surface tension of the alveoli. It "stabilizes" the alveolus in the same way that a bubble is prevented from collapsing by a detergent material, and it therefore prevents microatelectasis (collapse on a microscopic level). The type II epithelial cells have a cuboidal shape and are often seen to bulge into the alveolar lumen. However, because they do not have long cytoplasmic extensions, they cover less than 5 percent of the alveolar surface.

Type II cells have an additional function relating to maintenance and repair of the injured alveolar epithelium. Type I epithelial cells are quite susceptible to a variety of injurious agents, whether the agents reach the alveolar wall via the airways or via the blood stream. When type I cells are damaged, the reparative process involves hyperplasia of the type II cells and eventual differentiation into cells with the characteristics of type I cells.

Pulmonary capillaries course through the alveolar walls as part of an extensive network of intercommunicating vessels. Unlike the alveolar epithelial cells, which are quite impermeable under normal circumstances, junctions between capillary endothelial cells permit passage of small-molecular-weight proteins. The importance of the permeability features of the alveolar epithelial and capillary endothelial cells will become apparent in the discussion of acute respiratory distress syndrome in Chapter 28, because this disorder is characterized by increased permeability and leakage of fluid and protein into alveolar spaces.

The alveolar epithelial and capillary endothelial cells rest on a basement membrane. At some regions of the alveolar wall, nothing stands between the epithelial and endothelial cells other than their basement membranes, which are fused to form a single basement membrane. At other regions, a space called the *interstitial space,* consisting of relatively acellular material (see Fig. 8-2), intervenes. The major components of the interstitial space are collagen, elastin, proteoglycans, a variety of macromolecules involved with cell-cell and cell-matrix interactions, some nerve endings, and some fibroblast-like cells. There are also small numbers of lymphocytes as well as cells that appear to be in a transition state between blood monocytes and alveolar macrophages (which are derived from circulating monocytes).

Within the alveolar lumen a thin layer of liquid covers the alveolar epithelial cells. This extracellular alveolar lining layer is composed of an aqueous phase immediately adjacent to the epithelial cells, covered by a surface layer of lipid-rich surfactant produced by the type II epithelial cells. Within the alveolar lining layer are also alveolar macrophages, a type of phagocytic cell important in protecting the distal lung against bacteria and in clearing inhaled dust particles.

PHYSIOLOGY

Although some of the physiologic principles relating to the pulmonary parenchyma are covered briefly in Chapter 1, this chapter further discusses two topics that are important in the pathophysiologic abnormalities of diffuse parenchymal lung disease. In this section, a review of gas-exchange at the alveolar-capillary level is followed by a discussion of how disturbances within the pulmonary parenchyma affect the mechanical properties of the lung.

Gas-exchange between the alveolus and the capillary depends on the passive diffusion of gas from a region of higher to one of lower partial pressure. The PO_2 in the alveolus is normally in the range of 100 torr, and the blood entering the pulmonary capillary has a PO_2 of approximately 40 torr. This difference gives rise to a driving pressure for O_2 to diffuse from the alveolus to the pulmonary capillary, where it binds with hemoglobin in the erythrocyte. The barrier to diffusion—which includes the thin cytoplasmic extension of the type I cell, the basement membrane of the type I and capillary endothelial cells, and the capillary endothelial cell itself—is extremely thin, measuring approximately 0.5 μm. In some areas of the alveolar wall, there is also a thin layer of interstitium, but presumably diffusion and gas-exchange occur preferentially at the thinnest region where the interstitium is sparse or absent.

Although the rate of gas transfer across the alveolar-capillary interface depends on the thickness of the barrier, O_2 uptake by the blood is usually completed early during the transit through the capillaries. The total time spent by a red blood cell traveling through the pulmonary capillaries is approximately 0.75 second, and equilibration with O_2 occurs within the first third of this time. Therefore, extra time is available for diffusion should there be disease affecting the alveolar-capillary interface and impairing the normal process of diffusion. Carbon dioxide diffuses even more readily than does O_2; therefore, there is also reserve time available for its diffusion.

Consequently, although the diffuse parenchymal lung diseases do affect gas-exchange, impaired diffusion across an abnormal alveolar-capillary interface is not a primary contributor to this disturbance in gas-exchange, at least when the patient is not exercising. This issue is considered further in Chapter 9 as part of the discussion of abnormalities in gas-exchange in patients with diseases affecting the alveolar wall.

Another important aspect of physiology relating to the lung parenchyma is that of compliance, or more simply, the stiffness of the lung. As stated in

Oxygen uptake and CO_2 elimination at the alveolar-capillary interface are completed early during transit of an erythrocyte through the pulmonary vascular bed.

Chapter 1, the lung is elastic and behaves like a balloon or a rubber band in terms of resisting expansion. Therefore, pressure must be exerted through the airway to inflate a lung; or, conversely, negative pressure can also be applied around the lung to cause it to expand. For any given volume of air in the lungs, a certain pressure is required to achieve this degree of inflation, and a curve can be drawn relating volume on the Y axis to pressure on the X axis (see Fig. 1-3A). Because the net pressure producing expansion is the difference between the pressure exerted on the alveoli (via the airway) and the absolute pressure outside the lung, the term *transpulmonary pressure* is used to describe this distending pressure. In vivo, when the lung is sitting within the chest, pressure outside the lung is the pleural pressure. If a lung is removed and dealt with in isolation, the pressure outside the lung would be atmospheric pressure.

The normal compliance relationship between volume and pressure in the lung is a curve that flattens out at high distending pressures when the lung reaches its upper limit of expansion. At this point the elastic tissues of the lung can be stretched no further, and additional pressure does not add extra volume to the lung.

Diseases affecting the alveolar walls commonly disturb this pressure-volume relationship, making the lung either stiffer (more resistant to expansion) or less stiff (easier to expand). For the stiffer, less compliant lung, the compliance curve is shifted to the right, i.e., a lower volume is achieved for any given transpulmonary pressure. Most of the diseases covered in this section, which are included in the category of diffuse parenchymal lung disease, affect the compliance of the lung in this way (Fig. 8-3). In contrast,

> The compliance curve of the lung in interstitial lung disease is shifted downward and to the right.

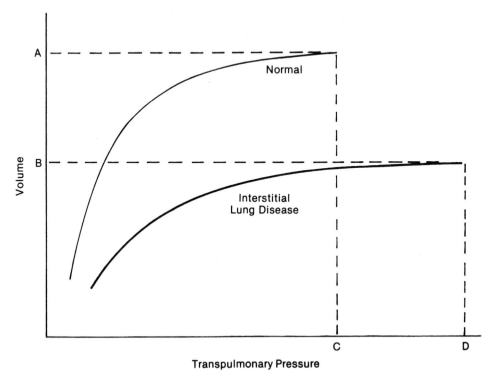

Figure 8-3 ■— Compliance curve of lung in interstitial lung disease compared with that of normal lung. In addition to shift of curve downward and to right, it can be seen that TLC in interstitial lung disease (point B on volume axis) is characteristically less than normal TLC (point A). Maximal pressure at TLC is called maximal static recoil pressure (Pst_{max}), represented for normal lung and lung with interstitial disease by points C and D, respectively. Compare with Figure 6-7.

as discussed in Chapter 6 and illustrated in Figure 6-7, patients with emphysema, whose lungs are less resistant to expansion (i.e., more compliant), have compliance curves that are shifted to the left. This principle of compliance is an important one in pulmonary physiology. Chapters 1 and 6 have alluded to the role compliance plays in determining lung volumes measured in pulmonary function testing, particularly total lung capacity and functional residual capacity. This principle is cited again in the next chapter in discussing the pathophysiology of diseases that affect the alveolar walls.

References

Anatomy

Gail DB and Lenfant CJM: Cells of the lung: biology and clinical implications. Am Rev Respir Dis 127:366-387, 1983.

Rooney SA: The surfactant system and lung phospholipid biochemistry. Am Rev Respir Dis 131:439-460, 1985.

Schneeberger EE: Alveolar type I cells. *In* Crystal RG, West JB, Weibel ER, and Barnes PJ (eds): The Lung: Scientific Foundations, 2nd ed. Philadelphia, Lippincott-Raven, 1997, pp 535-542.

Weibel ER: The Pathway for Oxygen. Cambridge, MA, Harvard University Press, 1984.

Weibel ER and Crystal RG: Structural organization of the pulmonary interstitium. *In* Crystal RG, West JB, Weibel ER, and Barnes PJ (eds): The Lung: Scientific Foundations, 2nd ed. Philadelphia, Lippincott-Raven, 1997, pp 685-695.

Whitsett JA and Weaver TE: Hydrophobic surfactant proteins in lung function and disease. N Engl J Med 347:2141-2148, 2002.

Physiology

Leff AR and Schumacker PT: Respiratory Physiology: Basics and Applications. Philadelphia, WB Saunders Co., 1993.

West JB: Respiratory Physiology—The Essentials, 6th ed. Baltimore, Lippincott Williams & Wilkins, 2000.

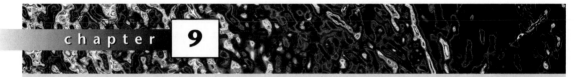

chapter 9

Overview of the Diffuse Parenchymal Lung Diseases

PATHOLOGY
    Pathology of the Idiopathic
       Interstitial Pneumonias
    End-Stage Diffuse Parenchymal
       Lung Disease
PATHOGENESIS
PATHOPHYSIOLOGY
    Decreased Compliance
    Decrease in Lung Volumes

    Impairment of Diffusion
    Abnormalities in Small Airways
       Function
    Disturbances in Gas-Exchange
    Pulmonary Hypertension
CLINICAL FEATURES
DIAGNOSTIC APPROACH
TREATMENT

A large group of disorders affects the alveolar wall in a fashion that may ultimately lead to diffuse scarring or fibrosis. As mentioned in Chapter 8, these disorders have traditionally been referred to as the *interstitial lung diseases,* although the term is somewhat of a misnomer. The interstitium formally refers only to the region of the alveolar wall exclusive of and separating the alveolar epithelial and the capillary endothelial cells. These diseases, on the other hand, affect all components of the alveolar wall: epithelial cells, endothelial cells, and the cellular and noncellular components of the interstitium. In addition, the disease process often extends into the alveolar spaces and is therefore not limited just to the alveolar wall. As a result, the expression *diffuse parenchymal lung disease* is now preferred by many authors and is the term we will generally use in this book. For practical purposes, however, the reader should recognize that the expressions *diffuse parenchymal lung disease* and *interstitial lung disease* are typically referring to the same group of disorders causing inflammation and fibrosis of alveolar structures.

There are more than 150 diffuse parenchymal lung diseases. Table 9-1 lists the most common of these disorders, grouped by broad categories based on whether the underlying etiology of the disease is currently known or unknown. A third category of "mimicking disorders" is included, in recognition of the fact that a number of additional well-defined clinical problems can produce diffuse parenchymal abnormalities on chest radiograph. Even though these mimicking disorders are often not included among the traditional list of diffuse parenchymal lung diseases, the clinician must remember to consider these mimicking disorders in the appropriate clinical settings.

As it is difficult even for the pulmonary specialist to know about all these diseases, it is obviously inappropriate for the novice in pulmonary medicine to worry about amassing knowledge regarding each individual entity. Rather, the reader is urged first to develop an understanding of the pathologic, pathogenetic, pathophysiologic, and clinical features that these disorders have in

Table	9-1	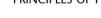

Classification of Selected Diffuse Parenchymal Lung Diseases

Known Etiology
Due to inhaled inorganic dusts (pneumoconiosis, e.g., asbestosis, silicosis)
Due to organic antigens (hypersensitivity pneumonitis)
Iatrogenic (drugs, radiation pneumonitis)

Unknown Etiology
Idiopathic interstitial pneumonias
Associated with connective tissue (systemic rheumatic) disease
Sarcoidosis
Less common
   Pulmonary Langerhans' cell histiocytosis
   Lymphangioleiomyomatosis
   Goodpasture's syndrome
   Wegener's granulomatosis*
   Chronic eosinophilic pneumonia
   Bronchiolitis obliterans with organizing pneumonia*
   Pulmonary alveolar proteinosis

Mimicking Disorders
Congestive heart failure
Disseminated carcinoma ("lymphangitic carcinomatosis")
Pulmonary infection (e.g., Pneumocystis, viral pneumonia)

*Typically associated with focal or multifocal rather than diffuse disease.

common. This chapter, which covers these areas, refers to individual diseases only when necessary. The focus of the next two chapters is on the major types of diffuse parenchymal lung disease. Chapter 10 includes those disorders associated with an identifiable etiologic agent. Perhaps 35 percent of patients with diffuse parenchymal lung disease are in this category. Chapter 11 deals with diseases for which a specific etiologic agent has not been identified. The majority of patients with diffuse parenchymal lung disease belong in this second category. These chapters cover only a small number of the described types of diffuse parenchymal disease; the goal throughout is to consider those disorders the reader is most likely to encounter. Included in our discussion of diseases of unknown etiology in Chapter 11 are several disorders that affect the lung parenchyma but do not characteristically have diffuse findings on chest radiograph. Examples of diseases in which the findings are more typically focal (or multifocal, with more than one area of involvement) include Wegener's granulomatosis and bronchiolitis obliterans with organizing pneumonia.

The diseases covered in these three chapters are primarily *chronic* (or sometimes *subacute*) diseases affecting the alveolar structures. An additional group of diseases is associated with acute injury to various components of the alveolus. These latter disorders are of clinical importance as causes of acute respiratory failure, and they are discussed in Chapter 28.

PATHOLOGY

Diffuse parenchymal (interstitial) lung diseases are characterized pathologically by alveolitis and fibrosis.

Typically, the diffuse parenchymal lung diseases, regardless of cause, have two major pathologic components: an inflammatory process in the alveolar wall and alveolar spaces (sometimes called an *alveolitis*) and a scarring or fibrotic process (Fig. 9-1). Both features generally occur simultaneously, although the relative proportions of inflammation and fibrosis vary with the particular

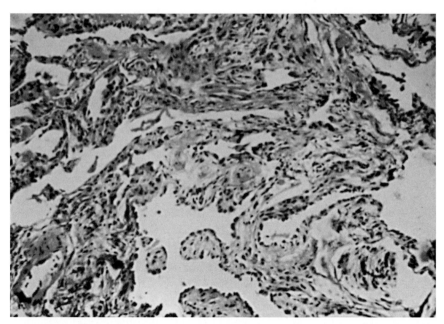

Figure 9-1 ■— Photomicrograph of interstitial lung disease shows markedly thickened alveolar walls. Cellular inflammatory process and fibrosis are present. Compare with appearance of normal alveolar walls in Figure 8-1.

cause and duration of the disease. The presumption has generally been that active inflammation is the primary process and that fibrosis follows as a secondary feature. However, the concept has recently been proposed that fibrosis itself, representing abnormal wound repair, is the primary process rather than alveolar inflammation in at least one of these diseases, idiopathic pulmonary fibrosis (see section on Pathogenesis).

When an active alveolitis is present, a variety of inflammatory cells infiltrate the alveolar wall—macrophages, lymphocytes, neutrophils, eosinophils, and plasma cells. Individual types of diffuse parenchymal lung disease may be associated with a prominence of a particular one of these cell types, e.g., eosinophils in chronic eosinophilic pneumonia. In addition to the presence of inflammatory cells, other characteristic pathologic features that help define a specific disorder may be associated with the alveolitis. These individual patterns are useful in, and in many cases critical to, the diagnosis of a specific pathologic entity.

One of the most important of the pathologic features associated with several of the diffuse parenchymal lung diseases is the *granuloma*. A granuloma is a localized collection of cells called *epithelioid histiocytes,* which are essentially tissue cells of the phagocytic or macrophage series (Fig. 9-2). These are generally accompanied by T lymphocytes within and often forming a rim around the granuloma. The granuloma typically also has multinucleated giant cells, which result from a fusion of several phagocytic cells into a single large cell with abundant cytoplasm and many nuclei (see Fig. 9-2). Examples of diffuse parenchymal lung disease in which granulomas are part of the pathologic process include sarcoidosis and hypersensitivity pneumonitis. Granulomas are often considered to reflect some underlying immune process, specifically an immune reaction to an exogenous agent. In the case of hypersensitivity pneumonitis, many such agents have been identified. However, in the case of sarcoidosis, no specific exogenous agent has been identified.

Interstitial diseases with granulomas include sarcoidosis and hypersensitivity pneumonitis.

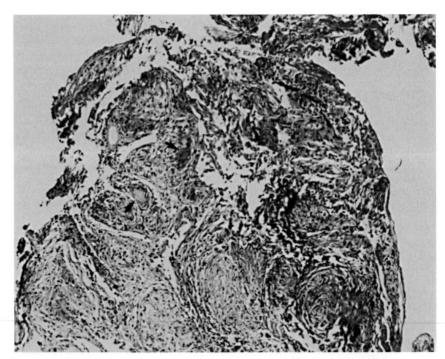

Figure 9-2 ▪▬— Low-power photomicrograph of transbronchial lung biopsy sample from patient with sarcoidosis. Numerous confluent granulomas throughout entire specimen obliterate normal pulmonary architecture. Two multinucleated giant cells are marked by arrows. (Courtesy of Dr. Earl Kasdon.)

Granulomas in the lung have many other causes (e.g., tuberculosis, certain fungal infections, and foreign bodies), but these are not covered here because the granulomas are generally not associated with diffuse parenchymal lung disease.

Pathology of the Idiopathic Interstitial Pneumonias

Pathologists and clinicians have spent considerable time and effort trying to refine the description and categorization of a subgroup of diffuse parenchymal lung diseases often called the *idiopathic interstitial pneumonias*. These disorders display variable amounts of nonspecific inflammation and fibrosis, and they lack granulomas or other specific pathologic features characteristic of other, previously well-defined diseases. There has been uncertainty and confusion about how to classify the idiopathic interstitial pneumonias, and whether the various pathologic appearances represent different diseases or different stages or parts of the spectrum of a single disease. Although this is still an evolving field, we will attempt to present a simplified framework based on current pathologic and clinical concepts about these disorders.

Some of the pathologic categories subsumed under the idiopathic interstitial pneumonias include:
1. Usual interstitial pneumonia (UIP)
2. Desquamative interstitial pneumonia (DIP)
3. Nonspecific interstitial pneumonia (NSIP)
4. Acute interstitial pneumonia (AIP)

We will discuss four pathologic entities subsumed under the broad term idiopathic interstitial pneumonias. These are: (1) usual interstitial pneumonia (UIP); (2) desquamative interstitial pneumonia (DIP); (3) nonspecific interstitial pneumonia (NSIP); and (4) acute interstitial pneumonia (AIP). In this section we will briefly describe the pathologic characteristics defining these four entities, and in Chapter 11 we will focus on a broader consideration of the more important clinical counterparts of some of these pathologic entities. According to one recently proposed classification scheme, several other pathologic entities are also included as idiopathic interstitial pneumonias, and the interested reader should consult the relevant references listed at the end of this chapter for further details and discussion.

Usual interstitial pneumonia (UIP) is characterized by patchy areas of interstitial inflammation and fibrosis interspersed between areas of relatively preserved lung tissue (Fig. 9-3). Fibrosis is a prominent component of the pathology, with focal collections of proliferating fibroblasts called "fibroblastic foci." The fibrosis is often associated with *honeycombing,* representing cystic air spaces that result from retraction of the surrounding fibrotic lung tissue. The inflammatory process in the alveolar walls is nonspecific and typically composed of a variety of cell types, including lymphocytes, macrophages, and plasma cells. There is also hyperplasia of type II pneumocytes (alveolar epithelial cells), presumably reflecting an attempt to replenish damaged type I cells. The most important of the clinical disorders associated with the histopathologic pattern of UIP is *idiopathic pulmonary fibrosis* (IPF), and the terms are often used synonymously. However, the pathologic appearance of UIP can also result from exposure to certain inhaled dusts (especially asbestos), from a number of drug-induced lung diseases, and as a form of parenchymal lung disease associated with a number of systemic rheumatic ("connective tissue") diseases.

Desquamative interstitial pneumonia (DIP) is a more homogeneous-appearing process than UIP, characterized by large numbers of intra-alveolar mononuclear cells. Although originally thought to represent desquamated alveolar epithelial cells (hence the name DIP), these cells are now known to be intra-alveolar macrophages. A less prominent component of the histology is inflammation within alveolar walls, and there is minimal associated fibrosis. Based on a strong association of this histologic pattern with a history of

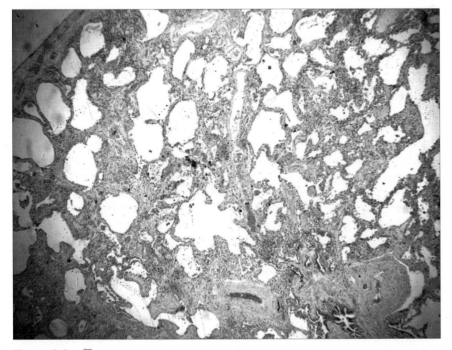

Figure 9-3 ■— Low-power photomicrograph of usual interstitial pneumonia, demonstrating the heterogeneity of the fibrotic and inflammatory process. (Courtesy of Dr. Olivier Kocher.)

smoking, as well as an apparent overlap with smoking-induced inflammation of respiratory bronchioles with pigmented macrophages, it is thought that smoking may be an important underlying etiology for this pathologic pattern.

The most prominent histopathologic component of *nonspecific interstitial pneumonia* (NSIP) is a mononuclear cell infiltrate within the alveolar walls. In contrast to UIP, the process appears relatively uniform; fibrosis, although variable, is generally less apparent. In the past, this pattern was often not separated from UIP, and its inclusion in many clinical studies of IPF served to confound our understanding of the natural history and treatment of IPF. The histologic pattern of NSIP can be idiopathic, but it can also occur in association with a number of the connective tissue diseases.

Acute interstitial pneumonia (AIP) is believed to represent the organizing or fibrotic stage of diffuse alveolar damage, which is the histologic pattern seen in acute respiratory distress syndrome (ARDS) (see Chapter 28). However, in most cases of ARDS, an inciting cause is apparent; in AIP, no initiating trigger for ARDS can be identified. The histology shows fibroblast proliferation and type II pneumocyte hyperplasia in the setting of what appears to be organizing diffuse alveolar damage.

End-Stage Diffuse Parenchymal Lung Disease

When diffuse parenchymal lung disease has been present for a fairly long time and is associated with significant fibrosis, often any distinctive features of a prior alveolitis are lost. For example, any of the granulomatous lung diseases may no longer demonstrate the characteristic granulomas after sufficient time has elapsed and a substantial degree of fibrosis has developed. Therefore, at a certain point all the interstitial lung diseases, if sufficiently severe and chronic, follow a final common pathway toward *end-stage* interstitial lung disease. Along with severe fibrosis, the lung at end-stage exhibits a great deal of distortion that can be seen both grossly and microscopically, with areas of contraction and other areas showing formation of cystic spaces. In many cases, the result is honeycomb lung, in which the dense scarring and intervening cystic regions may make areas of the lung resemble a honeycomb (Fig. 9-4).

PATHOGENESIS

There has been a great deal of research during the last two decades attempting to clarify the pathogenetic sequence of events in various types of diffuse parenchymal lung disease. Yet, in most cases, what initiates these diseases is still not known, and our understanding of the cellular and biochemical events producing inflammation and fibrosis remains at a descriptive level. This section outlines the general scheme of events thought to be operative in the production of parenchymal inflammation and fibrosis. In Chapters 10 and 11, in which specific diseases are discussed, additional information, which is believed to be relevant to the pathogenesis of each disease, is presented. The general scheme outlined here has features similar to that of other forms of lung injury described elsewhere in this book—for example, emphysema (in Chapter 6) and acute respiratory distress syndrome (in Chapter 28). A fundamental but as yet unanswered question is what determines whether an injurious agent eventually leads to emphysema, acute lung injury (with acute respiratory distress syndrome), or chronic parenchymal inflammation and fibrosis.

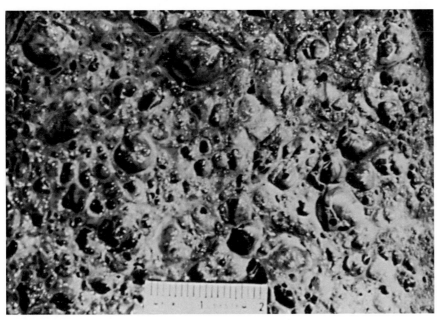

Figure 9-4 ■— Appearance of honeycomb lung from patient with severe interstitial lung disease. There are many cystic areas between bands of extensively scarred and retracted pulmonary parenchyma.

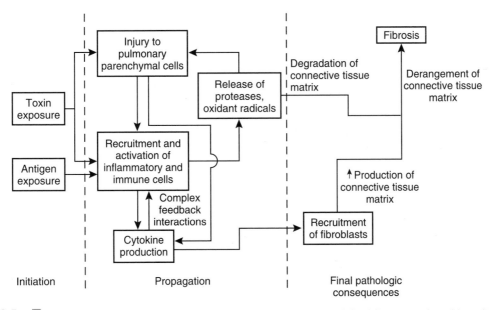

Figure 9-5 ■— Schematic diagram illustrates general aspects of pathogenesis of the diffuse parenchymal lung diseases.

Figure 9-5 summarizes the general sequence of events presumed to be common to many of the diffuse parenchymal lung diseases. These events can be divided into three stages: initiation, propagation, and final pathologic consequences. Each of these stages will be considered in turn.

The initiating stimulus for the diffuse parenchymal lung diseases is generally believed to be either a toxin or an antigen. The most obvious presumed toxins include some of the inhaled inorganic dusts—for example, asbestos—responsible for producing the pneumoconioses. Inhaled antigens have been

Pathogenetic features of interstitial lung disease are the following:

1. Initiation—by antigens, toxins
2. Propagation—with inflammatory cells, proteases, cytokines
3. Final pathologic consequence—fibrosis

best identified as the cause of chronic hypersensitivity pneumonitis. In sarcoidosis and perhaps in idiopathic pulmonary fibrosis, exposure to one or more antigens may initiate the disease, but no specific antigens have yet been identified.

Once there has been exposure to an initiating stimulus, a complex series of interrelated events is responsible for propagation of the disease. At the microscopic level the consequence of these propagating events is inflammation, a hallmark of many of the diffuse parenchymal lung diseases. Toxins may be directly injurious to pulmonary parenchymal (alveolar epithelial) cells, whereas either toxins or antigens may result in activation and recruitment of inflammatory and immune cells. Inflammatory cells can release a variety of mediators, such as proteolytic enzymes or toxic oxygen radicals, that can secondarily further injure pulmonary parenchymal cells. In addition, a wide variety of cytokine mediators, produced by inflammatory and immune cells, have been identified. These cytokines have complex secondary effects on other inflammatory and immune cells, often acting either to amplify or to diminish the inflammatory response.

Some of the cytokines, such as transforming growth factor-β and platelet-derived growth factor, have the capability of recruiting and stimulating the replication of fibroblasts, which are critical for the eventual production of new connective tissue. Action of proteases from inflammatory cells may also be responsible for degradation of connective tissue components. The combination of new synthesis and degradation of connective tissue defines the derangement of the connective tissue matrix that is seen histologically as fibrosis, the final pathologic consequence of interstitial lung disease. In idiopathic pulmonary fibrosis, the most recent (and now prevailing) concept is that alveolar epithelial injury results in epithelial cell expression of cytokine mediators which promote fibrogenesis, and that inflammation, although present in variable degrees, is not the critical trigger for the development of fibrosis.

PATHOPHYSIOLOGY

With minor exceptions and variations, the pathophysiologic features of the chronic diffuse parenchymal lung diseases are similar and therefore are discussed here as a single group. As a result of the inflammation and fibrosis affecting the alveolar walls, the following abnormalities are generally seen (Fig. 9-6): (1) decreased compliance (increased stiffness) of the lung, (2) a generalized decrease in lung volumes, (3) impairment of diffusion, (4) abnormalities in small airways function without generalized airflow obstruction, (5) disturbances in gas-exchange, usually consisting of hypoxemia without CO_2 retention, and (6) in some cases pulmonary hypertension. Each of these features is briefly considered in turn.

Decreased Compliance

The distensibility of the lungs is altered significantly by processes involving inflammation and fibrosis of the alveolar walls. The lungs become much stiffer, have a greatly increased elastic recoil, and therefore require greater distending (transpulmonary) pressures to achieve any given lung volume. The pressure-volume or compliance curve is shifted to the right, as shown in Figure 8-3, and at total lung capacity (TLC) a much higher elastic recoil

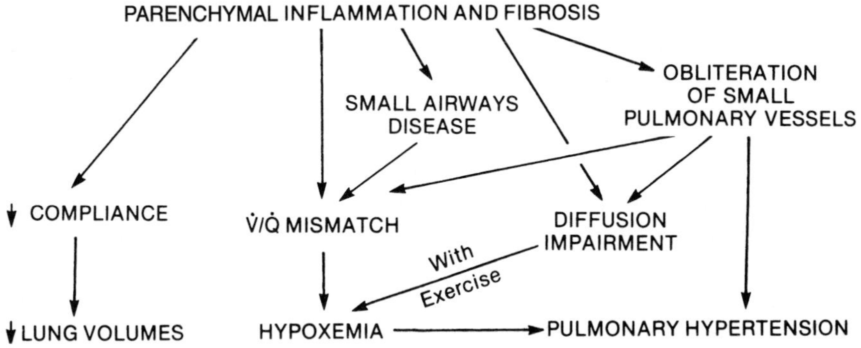

Figure 9-6 ■— Schematic diagram illustrates interrelationships between various pathologic and physiologic features of interstitial lung disease.

pressure is found than in normal lungs. This maximal pressure at TLC is termed the *maximum static recoil pressure of the lung* (Pst_{max}). Because wider swings in transpulmonary pressure are required to achieve a normal tidal volume during inspiration, the patient's work of breathing is increased. As a result, patients with diffuse parenchymal lung disease tend to breathe with smaller tidal volumes in order to expend less energy while increasing respiratory frequency to maintain adequate alveolar ventilation.

Compliance curves in diffuse parenchymal lung disease are shifted downward and to the right, reflecting increased stiffness of the lung.

Decrease in Lung Volumes

Early in the course of diffuse parenchymal lung disease, the lung volumes may be normal. However, in most cases some reduction in lung volumes will be seen shortly, including a reduction in TLC, vital capacity (VC), functional residual capacity (FRC), and, to a lesser extent, residual volume (RV). The decreases in TLC and FRC are a direct consequence of the change in compliance of the lung. At TLC, the force generated by the inspiratory muscles is balanced by the inward elastic recoil of the lung. Because the recoil pressure is increased, this balance is achieved at a lower lung volume or lower TLC. At FRC, the outward recoil of the chest wall is balanced by the inward elastic recoil of the lung. The balance will be achieved at a lower lung volume or lower FRC because of the greater elastic recoil of the lung.

Lung volumes are characteristically decreased in interstitial lung disease.

Impairment of Diffusion

Measurement of diffusion by the usual techniques involving carbon monoxide typically shows a decrease in the diffusing capacity. Although thickening of the alveolar-capillary interface (because of interstitial inflammation and fibrosis) might be expected to be responsible for this decrease, it is not the major factor. Rather, the processes of inflammation and fibrosis destroy a portion of the alveolar-capillary interface and reduce the surface area available for gas-exchange. This decrease in surface area appears to be mainly responsible for the observed diffusion abnormality.

Diffusing capacity is reduced, with destruction of a portion of the alveolar-capillary interface and reduced surface area for gas-exchange.

Abnormalities in Small Airways Function

Large airways generally function normally in these patients, and the forced expiratory volume in 1 second to forced vital capacity ratio is usually normal or even increased. However, frequently the pathologic process occurring in the alveolar walls also affects small airways within the lung. Light microscopy commonly demonstrates inflammation and fibrosis in the peribronchiolar regions,

Small airways function is often disturbed in interstitial lung disease; large airways function is generally preserved.

with narrowing of the lumen of the small airways or bronchioles. Tests of small airways function often show the physiologic effects of this narrowing. The clinical importance of small airways dysfunction in the absence of larger airways abnormalities is uncertain, but it is certainly possible that ventilation-perfusion ($\dot{V}/\dot{Q}$) mismatching and hypoxemia may be a consequence. In a few of the disorders causing diffuse parenchymal lung disease, evidence of more significant airflow obstruction may be seen. This relatively infrequent problem sometimes results from severe fibrosis and airway distortion.

Disturbances in Gas-Exchange

The gas-exchange consequences of diffuse parenchymal lung disease most frequently consist of hypoxemia without CO_2 retention or, in fact, with hypocapnia. Although a diffusion block was once proposed as the cause of the hypoxemia, most evidence supports $\dot{V}/\dot{Q}$ mismatch as the major contributor to hypoxemia. The pathologic process in the alveolar walls is an uneven one, and the normal matching of ventilation and perfusion is disrupted. In patients with small airways disease, dysfunction at this level probably also contributes to the $\dot{V}/\dot{Q}$ mismatch and to hypoxemia. Characteristically, patients with interstitial lung disease become even more hypoxemic with exercise. Although the entire mechanism of the fall in PO_2 on exercise is complex, diffusion limitation does appear to be a contributing factor. The combination of impaired diffusion and decreased transit time of the red blood cell during exercise may prevent complete equilibration of the PO_2 in pulmonary capillary blood with alveolar PO_2. Despite the often profound hypoxemia in patients with severe pulmonary fibrosis, PCO_2 is generally normal or low, inasmuch as patients are able to increase their minute ventilation sufficiently to compensate for a decrease in tidal volume and for any additional dead space.

Pulmonary Hypertension

Eventually, pulmonary hypertension and cor pulmonale often develop in patients with severe interstitial lung disease. Rarely, the cause of the pulmonary hypertension is a primary process affecting pulmonary vessels as well as alveolar walls. More frequently, the process in the alveolar walls is the cause of the pulmonary hypertension. There are two main contributing factors: (1) hypoxemia and (2) obliteration of small pulmonary vessels by the fibrotic process in the alveolar walls. During exercise the pulmonary hypertension becomes even more marked. This is due partly to worsening hypoxemia and partly to limited ability of the pulmonary capillary bed to distend and recruit new vessels to handle the exercise-induced increase in cardiac output.

CLINICAL FEATURES

Patients with diffuse parenchymal lung disease most commonly have dyspnea as their presenting symptom. The dyspnea is noticed initially on exertion but with severe disease may be experienced even at rest. Cough, usually nonproductive, may also be present. On physical examination, auscultation of the chest characteristically reveals dry crackles or rales, which are often most prominent at the bases of the lungs. Clubbing may be present, particularly with certain types of interstitial lung disease. If cor pulmonale develops, cardiac physical findings may be associated with pulmonary hypertension and right ventricular hypertrophy.

Arterial blood gases in interstitial lung disease generally show hypoxemia (resulting from $\dot{V}/\dot{Q}$ mismatch) and a normal or decreased PCO_2; with exercise the PO_2 falls even further.

Pulmonary hypertension is common in severe interstitial lung disease; it is a result of hypoxemia and obliteration of small pulmonary vessels.

Chest examination is often notable for crackles, particularly at the lung bases.

DIAGNOSTIC APPROACH

The chest radiograph is certainly the most important means for making the initial macroscopic assessment of diffuse parenchymal lung disease. The characteristic radiographic picture is an interstitial pattern, described as either *reticular* (increased linear markings) or *reticulonodular* (increased linear and small nodular markings) (see Fig. 3-6). This pattern is believed to reflect a process involving the alveolar walls, although histopathology often indicates that the process extends into alveolar spaces as well. Absence of radiographic abnormalities does not exclude the presence of interstitial disease: Entirely normal chest radiographic findings have been reported in up to 10 percent of such patients. The pattern on chest radiograph is not particularly useful for gauging the relative amounts of inflammation versus fibrosis, each of which may result in a similar pattern. The reticular or reticulonodular changes are frequently diffuse throughout both lung fields, although individual causes of interstitial lung disease may be more likely to result in either an upper or a lower lung field predominance of the abnormal markings. In addition to the interstitial pattern, certain diseases may reveal other associated findings on chest radiograph, such as hilar adenopathy or pleural disease. These additional features noted with some diseases are discussed in Chapters 10 and 11.

> A reticular or reticulonodular pattern on chest radiograph is characteristic of interstitial lung disease; however, up to 10 percent of patients may have normal radiographic findings.

With long-standing and severe disease, the lungs may become grossly distorted; in addition, there may be regions of cyst formation between scarred and retracted areas of lung (see Fig. 9-4). A corresponding pattern of honeycombing on chest radiograph may also be apparent. Cor pulmonale may be suspected on chest radiograph by the presence of right ventricular enlargement, best seen on the lateral view.

High-resolution computed tomography of the chest has been assuming an increasing role in the evaluation of diffuse parenchymal lung disease (see Fig. 3-9). Because of the quality of images of the pulmonary parenchyma, early changes of interstitial lung disease that are not evident on routine chest radiography can sometimes be seen. In addition, the specific pattern of abnormality on a high-resolution computed tomographic scan may be suggestive of a particular underlying diagnosis and may perhaps help to distinguish inflammation from fibrosis.

Despite the importance of the macroscopic evaluation, making a diagnostic distinction between the different types of diffuse parenchymal lung disease usually requires investigation at the microscopic or histologic level. A variety of biopsy procedures have been used to obtain tissue specimens from the lung, which are then subjected to several routine staining techniques. The most frequently used biopsy procedures for this purpose are the thoracoscopic lung biopsy and the transbronchial biopsy (via fiberoptic bronchoscopy). Thoracoscopic biopsy often is the more appropriate of the two procedures in order to obtain a sufficient piece of tissue for examination. As will be seen, however, when sarcoidosis (or certain other forms of interstitial disease) is suspected, transbronchial biopsy is a particularly suitable initial procedure.

Another way of sampling the cell population of the alveolitis is by a procedure called *bronchoalveolar lavage*. A fiberoptic bronchoscope is placed as distally as possible into an airway, and an irrigation or lavage of fluid through the bronchoscope allows cells from the alveolar spaces to be collected. These cells are thought to be representative of the cell populations that are responsible for the alveolitis. Although this technique has been useful as a relatively noninvasive means of obtaining cells for research studies on interstitial lung disease, its clinical utility for making a diagnosis or for sequential evaluation of disease activity is limited.

The findings on functional assessment of the patient with interstitial lung disease were basically reviewed in the Pathophysiology section of this chapter. Briefly, patients have a restrictive pattern on pulmonary function testing, with decreased lung volumes and preserved airflow. Diffusing capacity is usually reduced, indicative of loss of surface area for gas exchange. Hypoxemia is usually (although not necessarily) present, and the Po_2 falls even further with exercise. Hypercapnia is rarely a feature of the disease. When it occurs, hypercapnia usually reflects preterminal disease or an additional, unrelated process.

TREATMENT

Corticosteroids are used for decreasing the inflammatory component of a number of the diffuse parenchymal lung diseases.

Treatment considerations vary from disease to disease. In general, patients with interstitial disease either do not respond well to any form of treatment or respond to corticosteroids to a variable extent. The rationale for corticosteroid therapy is to reduce the alveolitis component of the disease, whereas the fibrosis is generally considered irreversible. In some cases, cytotoxic therapy (e.g., cyclophosphamide) has been used in addition to (or instead of) corticosteroids, but objective data for the utility of cytotoxic agents are scanty and vary with the particular disease. Other interesting therapeutic approaches involve targeting specific growth factors, cytokines, or oxidants that are involved in the inflammatory and fibrotic process within the lungs; however, these approaches are investigational at present. Specific aspects of treatment are covered in the discussion of individual diseases in Chapters 10 and 11.

References

American Thoracic Society and European Respiratory Society: Idiopathic pulmonary fibrosis: diagnosis and treatment. Am J Respir Crit Care Med 161:646-664, 2000.
American Thoracic Society and European Respiratory Society: American Thoracic Society/European Respiratory Society international multidisciplinary consensus classification of the idiopathic interstitial pneumonias. Am J Respir Crit Care Med 165:277-304, 2002.
British Thoracic Society: The diagnosis, assessment and treatment of diffuse parenchymal lung disease in adults. Thorax 54 (Suppl 1):S1-S30, 1999.
Colten HR and Krause JE: Pulmonary inflammation—a balancing act. N Engl J Med 336:1094-1096, 1997.
Demedts M, du Bois RM, Nemery B, and Verleden GM (eds): Interstitial lung diseases: a clinical update. Eur Respir J 18 (Suppl 32):1s-133s, 2001.
Gibson GJ: Interstitial lung diseases: pathophysiology and respiratory function. Eur Respir Mon 5 (Monograph 14):15-28, 2000.
Glaspole I, Conron M, and du Bois RM: Clinical features of diffuse parenchymal lung disease. Eur Respir Mon 5 (Monograph 14):1-14, 2000.
Katzenstein ALA and Myers JL: Idiopathic pulmonary fibrosis. Clinical relevance of pathologic classification. Am J Respir Crit Care Med 157:1301-1315, 1998.
Lynch DA: Imaging of diffuse infiltrative lung disease. Eur Respir Mon 5 (Monograph 14):29-54, 2000.
Ryu JH, Olson EJ, Midthun DE, and Swensen SJ: Diagnostic approach to the patient with diffuse lung disease. Mayo Clin Proc 77:1221-1227, 2002.
Schwarz MI and King TE Jr (eds): Interstitial Lung Disease, 3rd ed. Hamilton, Ontario, BC Decker, 1998.
Selman M, King TE Jr, and Pardo A: Idiopathic pulmonary fibrosis: prevailing and evolving hypotheses about its pathogenesis and implications for therapy. Ann Intern Med 134:136-151, 2001.
Wolff G and Crystal RG: Biology of pulmonary fibrosis. In Crystal RG, West JB, Weibel ER, and Barnes PJ (eds): The Lung: Scientific Foundations, 2nd ed. Philadelphia, Lippincott-Raven, 1997, pp 2509-2524.

chapter 10

Diffuse Parenchymal Lung Diseases Associated with Known Etiologic Agents

DISEASES CAUSED BY INHALED INORGANIC DUSTS Silicosis Coal Worker's Pneumoconiosis Asbestosis Berylliosis	**HYPERSENSITIVITY PNEUMONITIS** **DRUG-INDUCED PARENCHYMAL LUNG DISEASE** **RADIATION-INDUCED LUNG DISEASE**

The focus in this chapter is on a few of the major categories of diffuse parenchymal (interstitial) lung disease for which an etiologic agent has been identified. The general principles discussed in Chapter 9 apply to most of these conditions, and the features emphasized here are those peculiar to or characteristic of each cause. Considering the vast number of diffuse parenchymal lung diseases, this chapter only scratches the surface of information available. When one is confronted with a patient having a particular type of interstitial lung disease, it is best to learn or relearn the details of the disease at that time.

DISEASES CAUSED BY INHALED INORGANIC DUSTS

Many types of interstitial lung disease caused by inhalation of inorganic dusts have been identified, for which the term *pneumoconiosis* is used. Examples of the many responsible agents include silica, asbestos, coal, talc, mica, aluminum, and beryllium. In most cases, contact has occurred for a prolonged time as a result of occupational exposure. In some of these diseases, the parenchymal process is known to progress even in the absence of continued exposure.

For an inhaled inorganic dust to initiate an alveolitis, it must be deposited at an appropriate area of the lower respiratory tract. If particle size is too large or too small, deposition tends to be in the upper airway or in the larger airways of the tracheobronchial tree. Particles with a diameter of approximately 0.5 to 5 μm are the ones for which deposition in the respiratory bronchioles or the alveoli is most likely.

Unfortunately, no effective treatment is available for interstitial lung disease caused by most inhaled inorganic dusts. Therefore, the important issues facing physicians are recognition and prevention of these disorders. Total avoidance of exposure is obviously the optimal form of prevention, but

Particles with a diameter of 0.5 to 5 μm are the ones most likely to be deposited in respiratory bronchioles or alveoli.

when exposure is necessary, appropriate precautions with effective masks are essential.

Four types of pneumoconiosis are briefly considered here: silicosis, coal worker's pneumoconiosis, asbestosis, and berylliosis. For information about the numerous other agents, consult the more detailed references at the end of this chapter.

Silicosis

Silicosis is the interstitial lung disease resulting from exposure to silica (silicon dioxide). Of several crystalline forms of silica, quartz is the one most frequently encountered, usually as a component of rock or sand. Persons at risk include sandblasters, rock miners, quarry workers, and stonecutters. In most cases, development of disease requires at least 20 years of exposure, but with particularly heavy doses of inhaled silica, as are found in sandblasters, much shorter periods are sufficient.

Although the pathogenesis of silicosis is not known with certainty, theories have centered around the potential toxicity of silica for macrophages. Silica particles in the lower respiratory tract are engulfed and ingested by alveolar macrophages. In this process, the macrophages are thought to be activated and eventually destroyed by the silica particles. With their activation and destruction, the macrophages release chemical mediators that may initiate or perpetuate an alveolitis, eventually leading to development of fibrosis. When destroyed, the macrophages also release the toxic silica particles, which are now capable of repeating the process after being reingested by other macrophages. Pathologically, the inflammatory process is initially localized around the respiratory bronchioles but eventually becomes more diffuse throughout the parenchyma. Generally, there is also a characteristic acellular nodule, called a *silicotic nodule*, which is composed of connective tissue (Fig. 10-1). At first the nodules are small and discrete; on progression of the disease they become larger and may coalesce.

> The pulmonary effects of silica may be related to a toxic effect on alveolar macrophages.

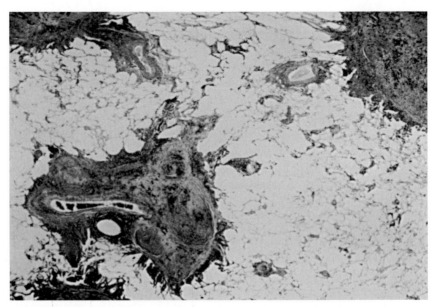

Figure 10-1 ■— Low-power view of silicotic lung shows characteristic appearance of silicotic nodules. (From Morgan WKC and Seaton A: Occupational Lung Diseases. Philadelphia, WB Saunders Co., 1975.)

Initially, the radiographic appearance of silicosis is notable for small, rounded opacities or nodules. At this point the patient is said to have *simple pneumoconiosis*. When the nodules become larger and coalescent, the pneumoconiosis is *complicated*, for which the term *progressive massive fibrosis* has also been used (Fig. 10-2). As a general rule, in patients with silicosis the upper lung zones are more heavily affected than are the lower zones.

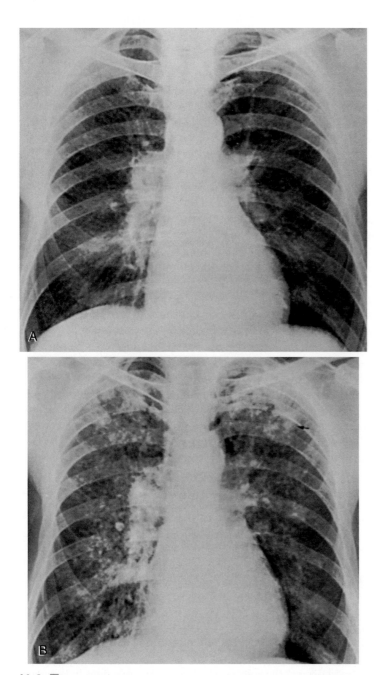

Figure 10-2 ━ Radiographic appearance of (*A*) simple and (*B*) complicated silicosis in same patient. In *A*, there are small nodules throughout both lungs, particularly in the upper zones, with a reticular component as well. In *B*, nodules have become larger and are coalescent in upper zones. One of the confluent shadows on left shows cavitation (*arrow*). Interval between radiographs *A* and *B* is 11 years. (From Fraser RG et al: Diagnosis of Diseases of the Chest, vol III, 3rd ed. Philadelphia, WB Saunders Co., 1990.)

There may also be enlargement of the hilar lymph nodes, which frequently calcify.

In addition to the potential problem of progressive pulmonary involvement and eventual respiratory failure, patients with silicosis are particularly susceptible to infections with mycobacteria, perhaps because of impaired macrophage function. The specific organisms may be either *Mycobacterium tuberculosis*, the etiologic agent for tuberculosis, or other species of mycobacteria, often called *atypical* or *nontuberculous mycobacteria* (see Chapter 24).

Silicosis is a predisposing factor for secondary infections by mycobacteria.

Coal Worker's Pneumoconiosis

Individuals who have worked as part of the coal mining process and have been exposed to large amounts of coal dust are at risk for the development of *coal worker's pneumoconiosis* (CWP). In comparison with silica, coal dust is a less fibrogenic material, and the tissue reaction is much less marked for equivalent amounts of dust deposited in the lungs.

Tissue reaction to inhaled coal dust is much less than that to silica.

The pathologic hallmark of CWP is the coal macule, which is a focal collection of coal dust surrounded by relatively little tissue reaction, in terms of either cellular infiltration or fibrosis (Fig. 10-3). The initial lesions tend to be distributed primarily around respiratory bronchioles. Small associated regions of emphysema, termed *focal emphysema*, may also be seen.

As with silicosis, the disease is often separated into *simple* and *complicated* forms. In simple CWP the chest radiograph consists of relatively small and discrete densities that are usually more nodular than linear. In this phase of the disease, patients have little in the way of symptoms, and pulmonary function is usually relatively preserved. In later stages of the disease, to which fortunately only a small minority of individuals progress, chest radiographic findings and clinical symptoms become more pronounced. With extensive disease and coalescent opacities on chest radiograph, the patients are said to have complicated disease, also called *progressive massive fibrosis.*

Symptoms and pulmonary function changes in CWP occur primarily in patients with progressive massive fibrosis.

Why complicated disease develops in some patients with CWP is not entirely clear. At one time, it was speculated that patients with progressive massive fibrosis had also been exposed to toxic amounts of silica and that the simultaneous silica exposure was responsible for most of the fibrotic process. However, although some patients do have a mixed form of pneumoconiosis from both coal dust and silica exposure, it appears that progressive massive fibrosis can result from coal dust in the absence of concomitant exposure to silica.

Asbestosis

Asbestos, formerly utilized widely because of its thermal and fire resistance, is actually a fibrous derivative of silica, termed a *fibrous silicate*. Among the health hazards it presents are the development of diffuse interstitial fibrosis and the potential for inducing several types of neoplasm, particularly bronchogenic carcinoma and mesothelioma. These latter problems are discussed in Chapters 20 and 21, respectively. The term *asbestosis* should be reserved for the interstitial lung disease that occurs as a result of asbestos exposure.

Individuals at risk for development of asbestosis include insulation, shipyard, and construction workers as well as persons who have been exposed by working with brake linings. Even though the health hazards of asbestos have been well recognized and its use consequently curtailed, workers may still be exposed in the course of remodeling or reinsulating pipes or buildings in which asbestos had been used. The duration of exposure necessary for

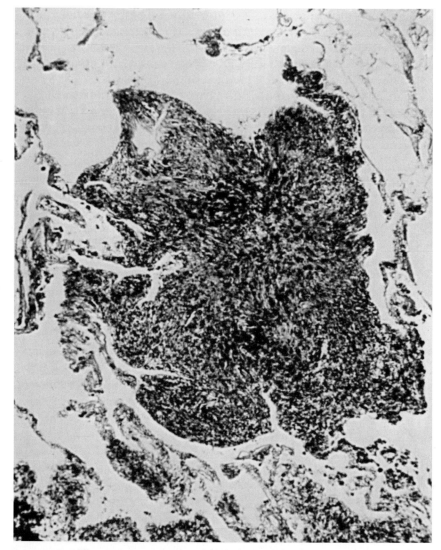

Figure 10-3 ▬— Histologic appearance of coal macule shows coal dust, dust-laden macrophages, and relatively small amounts of fibrous reaction. (From Morgan WKC and Seaton A: Occupational Lung Diseases. Philadelphia, WB Saunders Co., 1975.)

development of asbestosis is usually more than 10 to 20 years, although it may vary depending on the intensity of the exposure.

One theory of the pathogenesis of asbestosis suggests that asbestos fibers activate macrophages and induce the release of mediators that attract other inflammatory cells, including neutrophils, lymphocytes, and more alveolar macrophages. Unlike silica, asbestos is probably not cytotoxic to macrophages. That is, it does not seem to destroy or "kill" macrophages in the way that silica does. The mechanism of the often significant fibrotic reaction that occurs with asbestos may be related to the release of mediators from macrophages (e.g., fibronectin, insulin-like growth factor I, and platelet-derived growth factor) that can promote fibroblast recruitment and replication.

The earliest microscopic lesions appear around respiratory bronchioles, with an alveolitis that progresses to peribronchiolar fibrosis. The fibrosis subsequently becomes more generalized throughout the alveolar walls and can become quite marked. Areas of the lung that are heavily involved by the fibrotic process include the lung bases and the subpleural regions.

A characteristic finding of asbestos exposure is the *ferruginous body*, which is a rod-shaped body with clubbed ends (Fig. 10-4) that appears yellow-brown in stained tissue. These ferruginous bodies represent asbestos fibers that have been coated by macrophages with an iron-protein complex. Although it is common to see large numbers of these structures by light microscopy in patients with asbestosis, not all such coated fibers are asbestos, and ferruginous bodies may be seen even in the absence of parenchymal lung disease. Uncoated asbestos fibers, which are long and narrow, cannot be seen with light microscopy and require electron microscopy for their detection.

The chest radiograph in asbestosis shows a pattern of linear streaking that is generally most prominent at the lung bases (Fig. 10-5). In advanced cases the findings may be quite extensive and associated with cyst formation and honeycombing. Commonly, there is evidence of associated pleural disease, either in the form of diffuse pleural thickening or localized plaques (which may be calcified) or, much less frequently, in the form of pleural effusions. Because asbestos is a predisposing factor in the development of malignancies of the lung and pleura, either of these complications may also be seen on the chest radiograph.

The clinical, pathophysiologic, and diagnostic features of asbestosis usually follow the general description of interstitial lung disease given in Chapter 9. However, of the pneumoconioses already discussed, asbestosis is much more likely on physical examination to be associated with clubbing than is either silicosis or CWP.

Berylliosis

Berylliosis is a pneumoconiosis that is due to inhalation of the metal dust beryllium. The disease was initially described in individuals making fluorescent light bulbs, but more recent cases involve workers in the aerospace,

---

In asbestosis, microscopic examination of lung tissue often shows large numbers of ferruginous bodies.

Pulmonary complications of asbestos exposure are the following:
1. Interstitial lung disease (asbestosis)
2. Diffuse pleural thickening
3. Localized pleural plaques
4. Pleural effusions
5. Lung cancer
6. Pleural malignancy (mesothelioma)

Berylliosis, which resembles sarcoidosis in many respects, represents a cellular immune response to beryllium.

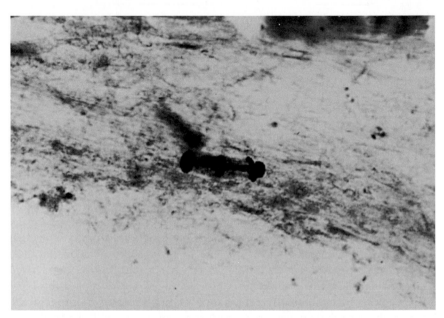

Figure 10-4 ▬▬ High-power photomicrograph of ferruginous body. Rod-shaped body with clubbed ends represents "coated" asbestos fiber. (Courtesy of Dr. Earl Kasdon.)

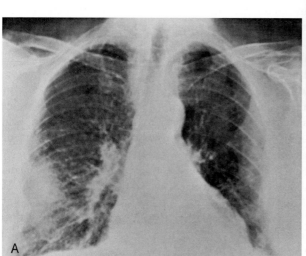
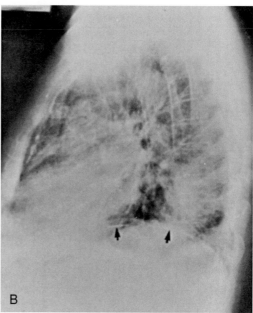

Figure 10-5 ━━ Chest radiograph of patient with parenchymal and pleural disease secondary to asbestos exposure. Interstitial markings are increased at lung bases, and there is extensive pleural thickening. Diaphragmatic calcification, which strongly suggests prior asbestos exposure, is highlighted by arrows. *A*, Posteroanterior and *B*, lateral views.

nuclear weapons, and electronics industries and in other industries in which beryllium is used. The histologic appearance of disease due to beryllium is quite different from that seen with the other pneumoconioses described earlier. Instead, the pathologic reaction within the lungs (and in hilar and mediastinal lymph nodes) involves formation of granulomas resembling those seen in sarcoidosis.

A great deal of research has been done to elucidate the pathogenesis of berylliosis, which is known to represent a cellular immune (delayed hypersensitivity) response to beryllium. Lymphocytes harvested from blood or from bronchoalveolar lavage fluid of patients with berylliosis demonstrate transformation (i.e., proliferation) when exposed to beryllium salts in vitro. Not only does this "beryllium lymphocyte transformation test" confirm the pathogenesis of the disease, but it also serves as a useful diagnostic test in individuals with a clinical picture consistent with berylliosis. In addition, sensitization to beryllium can be demonstrated in some workers before the onset of clinical disease, a finding that may be important for prevention or early intervention to arrest progression from subclinical to clinical disease.

Whether beryllium interacts directly with T lymphocytes or whether the metal first must bind to antigenic peptides is not known. Whatever the mechanism, the particular pattern of cytokine release by lymphocytes following exposure to beryllium suggests a response by the T_H1 class of helper (CD_4^+) lymphocytes. Studies also suggest that there may be a genetic susceptibility to development of the disease in response to exposure to beryllium. This susceptibility is identified by the presence of glutamate in position 69 of the human leukocyte antigen (HLA) DPB1 molecule.

Clinically and radiographically, the disease closely mimics sarcoidosis, which is described in Chapter 11. Specifically, patients with berylliosis demonstrate granulomatous inflammation in multiple organ systems, especially the pulmonary parenchyma and intrathoracic lymph nodes.

HYPERSENSITIVITY PNEUMONITIS

In *hypersensitivity pneumonitis*, immunologic phenomena directed against an antigen are responsible for the production of interstitial lung disease. This disorder is also sometimes referred to as *extrinsic allergic alveolitis*.

The antigens that induce the series of immunologic events are inhaled particulate or aerosol antigens from a variety of sources. Almost all the antigens are derived from microorganisms, plant proteins, and animal proteins, and exposure is generally related either to the patient's occupation or to some avocation. The first of the hypersensitivity pneumonitides to be described was *farmers' lung*, which is due to antigens from microorganisms (thermophilic actinomycetes) that may be present on moldy hay. The list of antigens and types of exposure has become quite extensive and includes such entities as air conditioner or humidifier lung (due to antigens from microorganisms contaminating a forced air system) and bird breeders' or fanciers' lung (due to bird proteins).

Interestingly, even when a large number of individuals are exposed to a given antigen by virtue of their occupation or avocation, disease develops in only a small percentage. Clearly, additional factors, perhaps genetic, determine who will contract the disease, but these factors have not yet been identified.

Pathogenetically, it is currently believed that a type IV immune reaction (cell-mediated or delayed hypersensitivity, mediated by T lymphocytes) causing a lymphocytic alveolitis is of prime importance in producing hypersensitivity pneumonitis, although a type III (immune-complex disease) mechanism may also have a contributory role. Evidence suggests that T lymphocytes in the lower respiratory tract become sensitized to the particular organic antigen. They may then release soluble cytokines that attract macrophages and possibly induce them to form granulomas in the lung. Antigen-antibody immune complexes may also be involved, with binding of complement and the resulting production of chemotactic factors and activation of macrophages.

Pathologic examination of the lung in hypersensitivity pneumonitis reveals an alveolitis composed primarily of lymphocytes (especially cytotoxic/suppressor CD8$^+$ cells) and macrophages, as well as the presence of granulomas. The granulomas are often poorly formed, unlike the well-defined granulomas characteristic of sarcoidosis (see Chapter 11). Often the pathologic changes have a peribronchiolar prominence, thus accounting for the frequent physiologic evidence for obstruction of small airways.

Clinically, hypersensitivity pneumonitis manifests in different ways—ranging from acute episodes of dyspnea, cough, fever, and infiltrates on chest radiograph, occurring approximately 4 to 6 hours after exposure to the offending antigen, to a chronic form of diffuse parenchymal lung disease. This latter presentation is a more insidious one, with the patient often reporting gradual onset of shortness of breath and cough, along with systemic symptoms of fatigue, loss of appetite, and weight loss. Antigen exposure is a more long-term problem in these circumstances, and unfortunately, because acute episodes are not necessarily an important feature, the patient does not associate the symptoms with any particular exposure.

Unlike its acute form, the chronic form of hypersensitivity pneumonitis behaves like other forms of interstitial lung disease. Unless the physician is attuned to the possibility that hypersensitivity to an antigen in the environment might be responsible for the patient's lung disease, this entity may easily be missed, and exposure to the antigen may continue.

Hypersensitivity pneumonitis represents an immunologic response to an inhaled organic antigen.

Hypersensitivity pneumonitis occurs either with acute episodes 4 to 6 hours after exposure to the offending antigen or with the more insidious course of chronic interstitial lung disease.

With an acute episode of hypersensitivity pneumonitis, the chest radiograph has patchy or diffuse infiltrates. As the disease becomes chronic, the abnormality may take on a more nodular quality, eventually appearing as the reticulonodular pattern characteristic of the other chronic interstitial lung diseases. In the chronic form of the disease, there is often an upper lobe predominance to the radiographic changes. High-resolution chest CT scanning may be particularly helpful in suggesting the diagnosis, often demonstrating a mosaic ground-glass pattern as illustrated in Figure 3-9.

The diagnosis is certainly more likely to be considered if the patient is able to give a history of acute episodes, either by themselves or punctuating a more chronic illness. Historic features concerning the patient's occupation and hobbies may provide valuable clues for detecting the responsible exposure. One of the standard diagnostic tests is a search for precipitating antibodies to the common organic antigens known to cause hypersensitivity pneumonitis. Unfortunately, false-positive and false-negative results for precipitins may cause diagnostic confusion. For instance, the finding of precipitins to thermophilic actinomycetes, the agent responsible for farmers' lung, is relatively common in healthy farmers without any evidence of the disease. In addition, making a diagnosis of hypersensitivity pneumonitis by the finding of precipitins obviously requires that the responsible antigen be included in the panel of antigens tested. If a lung biopsy is performed for diagnosis of interstitial lung disease, findings on microscopic examination may also suggest this entity.

The best treatment is avoidance of exposure. Unfortunately, the chronic form of the disease often leads to irreversible changes in the lung that persist even after exposure is terminated. Corticosteroids are sometimes administered to patients with persistent disease, but the results are variable.

DRUG-INDUCED PARENCHYMAL LUNG DISEASE

As the list of available pharmacologic agents expands every year, so does the list of potential complications. The lung is certainly one of the target organs for these side effects, and diffuse parenchymal lung disease is a particularly important (although not the only) manifestation of such drug toxicity. Each drug cannot be considered in detail here, nor can a complete list be included of the growing number of drugs that have been implicated. It is possible, however, to discuss briefly the general principles of drug-induced parenchymal lung disease and to mention the major agents that have been responsible.

The largest single category of drugs associated with disease of the alveolar wall includes the chemotherapeutic or cytotoxic agents, that is, those drugs designed primarily as antitumor agents. Individual drugs that have been commonly implicated in the development of lung disease are bleomycin, mitomycin, busulfan, cyclophosphamide, methotrexate, and the nitrosoureas, although several others have been described in smaller numbers of cases. In general, the risk of developing interstitial lung disease increases with higher cumulative doses of a particular agent. However, occasional cases are described with even a relatively low cumulative dose. In most cases, interstitial lung disease develops in a period ranging from a month to several years after use of the agent. Busulfan is particularly notable for the late development of complications, often several years after the onset of therapy.

The pathogenesis of chemotherapy-induced diffuse parenchymal lung disease often appears to involve either direct toxicity to normal lung

Chemotherapeutic and cytotoxic agents are the largest category of drugs associated with interstitial lung disease.

parenchymal cells or oxidant injury induced by generation of toxic oxygen radicals. One exception is methotrexate, for which hypersensitivity mechanisms may also play a role. When oxidant damage is involved, as with bleomycin, other agents that promote oxygen-free radical formation, such as radiation therapy or high concentrations of inhaled oxygen, can augment the injury due to the chemotherapeutic agent.

The pathologic appearance of interstitial lung disease caused by cytotoxic agents is frequently notable for the presence of atypical, bizarre-appearing type II alveolar epithelial cells with large hyperchromatic nuclei. When this feature is associated with the other usual findings of interstitial lung disease, the pathologist should suspect that a chemotherapeutic agent may be responsible. In conjunction with its presumed difference in pathogenesis, methotrexate does not produce the same degree of epithelial cell atypia as do the other cytotoxic agents; in contrast, granulomas, consistent with a hypersensitivity mechanism, are frequently seen.

> Cytotoxic drug-induced interstitial lung disease shows atypical, bizarre-appearing alveolar type II epithelial cells.

Clinically, fever is a common accompaniment to the respiratory symptoms associated with drug-induced interstitial lung disease. An increase in eosinophils in peripheral blood is also often noted in patients with methotrexate-induced lung disease.

For patients receiving these drugs in whom pulmonary infiltrates develop, often associated with fever, several diagnostic considerations routinely arise. In addition to the possibility of drug toxicity, there is concern about infection (because host defenses are generally impaired by the drug or by the underlying malignancy), dissemination of the malignancy through the lung, bleeding into the lung, and, in patients who have received radiation therapy, toxic effects from the irradiation. When the diagnosis is not clear, a lung biopsy is often performed, primarily to rule out an infectious process. If atypical epithelial cells but no infectious agents are found, a drug-induced process is suspected.

For patients who are believed to have a cytotoxic drug-related interstitial lung disease, the particular chemotherapeutic agent is generally discontinued. Steroids may be administered, but as with their use in other diffuse parenchymal diseases, the results are variable.

Several drugs that are not chemotherapeutic agents have also been implicated in the development of parenchymal lung disease. Nitrofurantoin, an antibiotic, has been associated with both acute and chronic reactions. The acute problem, which is presumably a hypersensitivity phenomenon, is often characterized by pulmonary infiltrates, pleural effusions, fever, and eosinophilia in peripheral blood. The chronic problem, which does not appear to be related to prior acute episodes, is characterized by a nonspecific interstitial pneumonitis and fibrosis akin to that of the other interstitial pneumonitides.

Therapy with injections of gold, which is used in rheumatoid arthritis, has also been associated with development of interstitial lung disease. The diagnosis here may be confusing, because the underlying disease (rheumatoid arthritis) can be associated with alveolitis and pulmonary fibrosis.

The antiarrhythmic agent amiodarone, which is now used quite commonly, has been associated with clinically significant parenchymal lung disease in approximately 5 to 10 percent of treated patients. In addition to nonspecific inflammation and fibrosis, the pathologic appearance of amiodarone-induced interstitial lung disease is notable for macrophages that appear foamy because of cytoplasmic phospholipid inclusions. However, similar foamy macrophages with cytoplasmic inclusions have been found in autopsy specimens of lung tissue from amiodarone-treated patients without interstitial inflammation and fibrosis. This finding suggests that the phospholipid inclusions may just be a marker of amiodarone use, and may not necessarily be directly responsible for the other pathologic and clinically important pulmonary consequences of amiodarone. Radiographically, patients with amiodarone-induced lung disease can develop either focal or diffuse infiltrates, and CT scanning commonly demonstrates a relatively high density of the infiltrates, resulting from a high iodine content within the amiodarone molecule.

A large number of drugs have also been linked with the development of an illness that resembles systemic lupus erythematosus, and patients with this "drug-induced lupus" may have parenchymal lung disease as one manifestation. In addition, a variety of drugs have been associated with pulmonary infiltrates and peripheral blood eosinophilia. This constellation of pulmonary infiltrates with eosinophilia, of which drugs are just one of several possible causes, is often abbreviated as the PIE syndrome.

RADIATION-INDUCED LUNG DISEASE

Interstitial lung disease is a potential complication of radiation therapy for tumors within or in close proximity to the thorax, particularly lymphoma (Hodgkin's disease) and carcinoma of the breast or lung. It has been estimated that signs and symptoms of clinically apparent injury will develop in 5 to 15 percent of patients whose radiation therapy includes exposure of portions of normal lung. However, radiographic changes in the absence of symptoms are even more frequent, occurring in 20 to 70 percent of exposed patients.

Radiation-induced pulmonary disease is generally divided into two phases, early pneumonitis and late fibrosis. The acute phase of radiation pneumonitis develops approximately 1 to 3 months after completion of a course of therapy, depending to a large extent upon the total dose and the volume of lung irradiated. The later stage of radiation fibrosis may directly follow earlier radiation-induced pneumonitis, may occur after a symptom-free latent interval, or occasionally may develop without any prior clinical evidence of acute pneumonitis. When fibrosis occurs, it does so generally 6 to 12 months after radiation has been completed.

> Radiation-induced lung disease includes an early period of radiation pneumonitis and a later period of radiation fibrosis.

Although the pathogenesis of radiation-induced lung disease is not entirely known, toxicity to capillary endothelial cells and, to a lesser extent, to type I alveolar epithelial cells is believed to be the primary mode of injury, perhaps mediated by oxygen-derived free radicals. In the period preceding chronic fibrosis, an alveolitis probably contributes directly to the development of the fibrotic changes. The possibility of hypersensitivity playing a role in the pathogenesis of the alveolitis has also been suggested by the finding of increased lymphocytes in bronchoalveolar fluid of the nonirradiated lung in patients with radiation-induced pneumonitis.

Early pathologic changes include swelling of endothelial cells, interstitial edema, mononuclear cell infiltrates, and atypical hyperplastic epithelial cells. Subsequent changes during the fibrotic stage consist of progressive fibrosis (indistinguishable from pulmonary fibrosis of other causes) and sclerosis of small vessels, with obliteration of a major portion of the capillary bed in the involved area.

Clinically, patients may have fever with the acute pneumonitis in conjunction with their respiratory symptoms. On chest radiograph, the acute pneumonitis is usually characterized by an infiltrate that conforms in shape

The interstitial pattern in radiation-induced lung disease conforms in distribution to the region of lung irradiated.

and location to the region of lung irradiated. Chest CT scanning may be particularly useful, both because it may detect subtle abnormalities earlier than they can be seen on chest radiograph, and because the cross-sectional views readily show the correspondence of the radiographic abnormalities to the radiation ports. However, for reasons that are still unclear, additional changes outside the field of radiation may develop in some patients. The pattern of chronic radiation fibrosis is an increase in interstitial markings, again generally corresponding in location to the irradiated region of lung, often with associated volume loss. The acute changes of the pneumonitis are potentially reversible, whereas the chronic fibrotic changes are generally permanent.

Diagnostic considerations are usually similar to the ones mentioned for drug-induced parenchymal lung disease. A history of recent irradiation occurring at the appropriate time is obviously crucial to the diagnosis. In addition, the finding of radiographic changes that conform to the radiation port, often with a relatively sharp cut-off, is strongly suggestive of the diagnosis.

Corticosteroids are frequently used to treat radiation-induced pneumonitis, often with reasonably good results. When the chronic changes of fibrosis have supervened, corticosteroids are much less effective.

References

Diseases Caused by Inhaled Inorganic Dusts

American Thoracic Society: Adverse effects of crystalline silica exposure. Am J Respir Crit Care Med 155:761-765, 1997.
Bateman ED and Benatar SR: Asbestos-induced diseases: clinical perspectives. Q J Med 62:183-194, 1987.
Castranova V and Vallyathan V: Silicosis and coal workers' pneumoconiosis. Environ Health Perspect 108 (Suppl):675-684, 2000.
Cohen R and Velho V: Update on respiratory disease from coal mine and silica dust. Clin Chest Med 23:811-826, 2002.
Davis GS: Pathogenesis of silicosis: current concepts and hypotheses. Lung 164:139-154, 1986.
Harvey B-G and Crystal RG: Pulmonary responses to chronic inorganic dust exposure. In Crystal RG, West JB, Weibel ER, and Barnes PJ (eds): The Lung: Scientific Foundations, 2nd ed. Philadelphia, Lippincott-Raven, 1997, pp 2339-2352.
Kamp DW and Weitzman SA: The molecular basis of asbestos-induced lung injury. Thorax 54:638-652, 1999.
Mapp CE (ed): Occupational lung disorders. Eur Respir Mon 4 (Monograph 11):1-355, 1999.
Morgan WKC and Seaton A: Occupational Lung Diseases, 2nd ed. Philadelphia, WB Saunders Co., 1984.
Mossman BT and Churg A: Mechanisms in the pathogenesis of asbestosis and silicosis. Am J Respir Crit Care Med 157:1666-1680, 1998.
Mossman BT and Gee JBL: Asbestos-related diseases. N Engl J Med 320:1721-1730, 1989.
Newman LS: Immunology, genetics, and epidemiology of beryllium disease. Chest 109:40S-43S, 1996.
Rom WN, Travis WD, and Brody AR: Cellular and molecular basis of the asbestos-related diseases. Am Rev Respir Dis 143:408-422, 1991.
Saltini C and Amicosante M: Beryllium disease. Am J Med Sci 321:89-98, 2001.

Hypersensitivity Pneumonitis

Bertorelli G, Bocchino V, and Olivieri D: Hypersensitivity pneumonitis. Eur Respir Mon 5 (Monograph 14):120-136, 2000.
Fink JN: Clinical features of hypersensitivity pneumonitis. Chest 89:193S-195S, 1986.
Fink JN et al: Interstitial lung disease due to contamination of forced air systems. Ann Intern Med 84:406-413, 1976.
Pepys J: Clinical and therapeutic significance of patterns of allergic reactions of the lungs to extrinsic agents. Am Rev Respir Dis 116:573-588, 1977.
Reynolds HY: Hypersensitivity pneumonitis. Clin Chest Med 3:503-519, 1982.
Roberts RC and Moore VL: Immunopathogenesis of hypersensitivity pneumonitis. Am Rev Respir Dis 116:1075-1090, 1977.
Rose C and King TE Jr: Controversies in hypersensitivity pneumonitis. Am Rev Respir Dis 145:1-2, 1992.
Salvaggio JE and deShazo RD: Pathogenesis of hypersensitivity pneumonitis. Chest 190S-193S, 1986.

Trentin L, Facco M, and Semenzato G: Hypersensitivity pneumonitis. Eur Respir Mon 4 (Monograph 11):301-319, 1999.

Drug-Induced Parenchymal Lung Disease

Batist G and Andrews JL Jr: Pulmonary toxicity of antineoplastic drugs. JAMA 246:1449-1453, 1981.
Cooper JAD Jr, White DA, and Matthay RA: Drug-induced pulmonary disease. Am Rev Respir Dis 133:321-340, 488-505, 1986.
Dunn M and Glassroth J: Pulmonary complications of amiodarone toxicity. Prog Cardiovasc Dis 31:447-453, 1989.
Foucher P et al: Drugs that may injure the respiratory system. Eur Respir J 10:265-279, 1997.
Ginsberg SJ and Comis RL: The pulmonary toxicity of antineoplastic agents. Semin Oncol 9:34-51, 1982.
Imokawa S, Colby TV, Leslie KO, and Helmers RA: Methotrexate pneumonitis: review of the literature and histopathological findings in nine patients. Eur Respir J 15:373-381, 2000.
Renz CL: Drug-induced pulmonary diseases. *In* Leff AR (ed): Pulmonary and Critical Care Pharmacology and Therapeutics. New York, McGraw-Hill, 1996, pp 707-719.
Sleijfer S: Bleomycin-induced pneumonitis. Chest 120:617-624, 2001.

Radiation-Induced Lung Disease

Cameron EH and Crystal RG: Radiation-induced lung injury. *In* Crystal RG, West JB, Weibel ER, and Barnes PJ (eds): The Lung: Scientific Foundations, 2nd ed. Philadelphia, Lippincott-Raven, 1997, pp 2647-2651.
Gibson PG et al: Radiation-induced lung injury: a hypersensitivity pneumonitis? Ann Intern Med 109:288-291, 1988.
Gross NJ: Pulmonary effects of radiation therapy. Ann Intern Med 86:81-92, 1977.
Movsas B et al: Pulmonary radiation injury. Chest 111:1061-1076, 1997.
Rosiello RA and Merrill WW: Radiation-induced lung injury. Clin Chest Med 11:65-71, 1990.

Diffuse Parenchymal Lung Diseases of Unknown Etiology

Approximately 65 percent of patients with diffuse parenchymal lung disease are victims of a process for which no etiologic agent has been identified, even though a specific name may be attached to the disease entity. Included in this category of disease are idiopathic pulmonary fibrosis, pulmonary fibrosis associated with connective tissue disease, sarcoidosis, and pulmonary Langerhans'-cell histiocytosis, as well as a variety of other disorders. Because many general aspects of these problems were discussed in Chapter 9, the focus here is on the specific diseases and their particular characteristics.

IDIOPATHIC PULMONARY FIBROSIS

Although the name *idiopathic pulmonary fibrosis* (IPF) has often been used nonspecifically to describe fibrotic interstitial lung disease without an identifiable diagnosis, most clinicians and investigators believe that IPF represents a specific disease entity. This chapter adopts that assumption and considers pulmonary fibrosis associated with an underlying connective tissue disease as a separate entity. Other names that have been used interchangeably with IPF include cryptogenic fibrosing alveolitis and usual interstitial pneumonia. However, the latter term is now generally used as a description of the pathologic pattern associated with IPF, a pattern that can also occasionally be seen in other clinical settings besides IPF.

As implied by the name, IPF does not yet have a recognizable inciting agent. Whether the primary agent, if one exists, reaches the lung via the airways or the blood stream has also not been settled. Over the past several years, the theory behind the pathogenesis of IPF has changed considerably. For many years it was thought that exposure to an unknown agent (perhaps an antigen leading to formation of antigen-antibody complexes) led to alveolar inflammation, which was perpetuated by release of chemotactic factors from inflammatory cells. The ongoing inflammation was believed to be responsible for the subsequent development of fibrosis.

Over the past several years, however, a newer conceptual framework has emerged, in which alveolar inflammation does not play a critical role in the eventual development of fibrosis. Rather, fibrosis is believed to result directly from alveolar epithelial injury and is thought to be a manifestation of abnormal wound healing within the lung parenchyma. According to this newer theory, injury to alveolar epithelial cells (still from an unidentified source or agent) is the primary initiating event. Whereas injury to type I alveolar epithelial cells would normally be followed by a repair process that includes proliferation of type II cells and differentiation into type I cells, this repair process is impaired, at least in part because of disruption of the basement membrane, which is normally important for the re-epithelialization process. At the same time, alveolar epithelial cells express a variety of profibrotic cytokines and growth factors, including platelet-derived growth factor (PDGF) and transforming growth factor-β1 (TGF–β1), which enhance fibroblast migration and proliferation. Fibroblastic foci develop in sites of alveolar injury, and appear to be responsible for increased extracellular matrix deposition. This process is summarized in Figure 11-1.

Clinically, the most common age at presentation of patients with IPF is between 50 and 70 years, and the onset of the disease is generally insidious. The symptoms are similar to those of other interstitial lung diseases, with dyspnea being the most prominent complaint. In addition to the classic finding of dry crackles or rales on physical examination, patients frequently have evidence of clubbing of the digits.

The chest radiograph shows an interstitial (reticular or reticulonodular) pattern that is generally bilateral and relatively diffuse, though typically more prominent at the bases of the lungs (see Fig. 3-6). Neither pleural effusions

> Idiopathic pulmonary fibrosis is thought to represent a dysregulated pattern of fibrosis in response to alveolar epithelial injury.

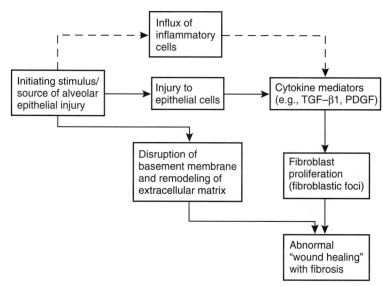

Figure 11-1 ◾— Proposed pathogenetic sequence in IPF. The dotted lines indicate that, although there is an influx of inflammatory cells, this is not thought to be a primary component of the pathogenesis. TGF–β1 = transforming growth factor-beta1; PDGF = platelet-derived growth factor.

The chest radiograph in IPF demonstrates a diffuse interstitial pattern without pleural disease or hilar enlargement.

nor hilar enlargement is found on the radiograph. High-resolution computed tomographic (HRCT) scanning often has a characteristic appearance, showing interstitial densities that are patchy, peripheral, subpleural, and associated with small cystic spaces (Fig. 11-2). Many patients have serologic abnormalities, such as a positive test result for antinuclear antibodies, that are generally found in patients with autoimmune or connective tissue disease. However, in the absence of other suggestive clinical features, these abnormalities are thought to be nonspecific and not indicative of an underlying rheumatologic disease.

The diagnosis is often made via lung biopsy, but only in the appropriate clinical setting when other etiologic factors for interstitial lung disease cannot be identified. As mentioned earlier, the histologic expression of IPF is in the form of UIP (see Fig. 9-3), and patients who have a pathologic pattern more compatible with DIP or NSIP (see Chapter 9 as well as the next section of this chapter) should not be considered to have IPF. Additionally, granulomas are not seen on a biopsy specimen. If they are found, they indicate the presence of another disorder.

From the time of clinical presentation, patients have a relatively poor prognosis, with mean survival in the range of 2 to 5 years. Corticosteroids are frequently used to treat patients with IPF; cytotoxic and other immunosuppressive agents, especially azathioprine or cyclophosphamide, have also been used in conjunction with steroids in many cases. Unfortunately, the response of IPF to both steroids and to other immunosuppressive agents has generally been poor, with relatively few patients demonstrating significant improvement. As a result, interest has shifted away from suppressing the inflammatory response, and clinical investigators are focusing on identifying and testing agents that suppress fibrosis or interfere with mediators involved in the fibrotic process. In some patients with severe IPF, especially those who are younger, lung transplantation is used as the only therapeutic alternative to progressive respiratory failure and death.

Prognosis and response to corticosteroid or other immunosuppressive therapy in IPF is generally poor.

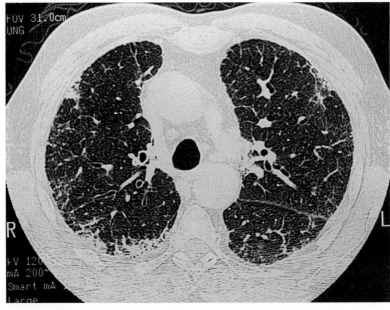

Figure 11-2 ■— High-resolution CT scan of IPF shows scattered interstitial densities, especially in the subpleural regions.

OTHER IDIOPATHIC INTERSTITIAL PNEUMONIAS

Several other disorders besides IPF fall under the category of the idiopathic interstitial pneumonias, and have often been confused with IPF. Although these are uncommon disorders, we will briefly describe some of them here, largely to clarify how their pathologic features differ from UIP and their clinical features differ from IPF. They are also mentioned in Chapter 9 as part of the discussion of the pathology of the interstitial pneumonias.

Desquamative interstitial pneumonia (DIP) occurs largely in smokers and generally has a subacute rather than chronic onset. Imaging studies with chest radiography and high-resolution CT scanning often show a ground-glass (hazy) pattern, and lung biopsy shows a uniform accumulation of intra-alveolar macrophages with little or no fibrosis. The prognosis is much better than in IPF, with patients often improving after cessation of smoking and, when necessary, responding to corticosteroids.

Nonspecific interstitial pneumonia (NSIP) also differs from UIP in its radiographic pattern, its histologic appearance, and its prognosis and response to treatment. As with DIP, imaging studies often show a ground-glass pattern that reflects inflammation rather than fibrosis, and lung biopsy shows a predominantly inflammatory response in the alveolar walls, with relatively little fibrosis. Although NSIP is often idiopathic and not associated with any underlying disease or inciting agent, it can represent the histologic appearance of parenchymal lung disease associated with one of the connective tissue diseases or with drug-induced pulmonary toxicity. Based on the prominence of inflammation rather than fibrosis, the prognosis is much better than in IPF, and patients often respond to treatment with corticosteroids.

Acute interstitial pneumonia (AIP) is a more acute or fulminant type of pulmonary parenchymal disease that begins with the clinical picture of acute respiratory distress syndrome (ARDS, see Chapter 28), but without any of the usual inciting events associated with development of ARDS. Imaging studies of AIP typically show features of ARDS, including areas of ground-glass opacification and alveolar filling (as opposed to a purely interstitial pattern). The histologic pattern is that of diffuse alveolar damage (DAD), often showing some organization and fibrosis. Although the mortality is high overall, some patients do well, with clinical resolution of the disease and without long-term sequelae.

One confusing aspect of the nomenclature of the idiopathic interstitial pneumonias is the relationship underlying AIP, UIP (or IPF), and a disorder called *Hamman-Rich syndrome.* More than 65 years ago Hamman and Rich described a number of cases of parenchymal lung disease that were subsequently thought to represent the first-described cases of IPF, and the term Hamman-Rich syndrome was for many years used synonymously with IPF. However, it is now believed that the cases described by Hamman and Rich were actually cases of AIP rather than IPF, and it is more appropriate that Hamman-Rich syndrome be considered synonymous with AIP rather than with either UIP or IPF.

PULMONARY PARENCHYMAL INVOLVEMENT COMPLICATING CONNECTIVE TISSUE DISEASE

The connective tissue diseases, also commonly called either collagen vascular diseases or systemic rheumatic diseases, include rheumatoid arthritis, systemic lupus erythematosus, progressive systemic sclerosis (scleroderma), polymyositis-dermatomyositis, Sjögren's syndrome, and some overlap syndromes that have features of more than one of these disorders. Although they form a diverse group, all are multisystem, inflammatory diseases that are mediated immunologically. The organ systems that are likely to be involved vary with each disease and are mentioned briefly in the following discussion of each entity.

Each disease is complicated and has been the focus of an extensive amount of research into etiology and pathogenesis. However, because none of them primarily affects the lung, they are not considered in detail here. Rather, a brief discussion will note how they affect the respiratory system, particularly with regard to development of parenchymal lung disease. Some clinicians include additional disorders among connective tissue diseases, but this discussion is limited to those in the preceding paragraph, each of which has the potential for pulmonary involvement.

Four assertions are true of each of these disorders. First, although the patients generally have evidence of the underlying connective tissue disease before pulmonary manifestations develop, some patients have lung disease as the presenting problem, occasionally predating other manifestations of their illness by several years. Second, detailed histologic or physiologic evaluation of patients with these diseases shows that pulmonary involvement is much more common than is clinically suspected. Third, the histopathology of interstitial lung disease associated with connective tissue disorders is generally that of UIP and is therefore indistinguishable from the pattern seen in IPF. However, in some cases, the histopathology demonstrates NSIP rather than UIP. Fourth, the interstitial lung disease that may develop with each of these entities preferentially affects the lower rather than the upper lung zones. This fact is usually apparent on examination of the chest radiograph.

Rheumatoid arthritis is a disorder whose primary manifestations consist of inflammatory joint disease. The most common site of involvement within the thorax is the pleura. This involvement takes the form of pleurisy, pleural effusions, or both. The lung parenchyma may become involved, with one or multiple nodules or with development of interstitial lung disease. The latter is usually relatively mild, although severe cases are occasionally seen. Occasionally, patients with rheumatoid arthritis develop airway complications in the form of bronchiolitis (an inflammatory process involving small airways) or bronchiectasis.

Systemic lupus erythematosus is a multisystem disease that primarily affects joints and skin but often has more serious involvement of several organ systems, including kidneys, lungs, nervous system, and heart. Its most frequent presentation within the chest is in the form of pleural disease, specifically pleuritic chest pain or pleural effusion, or both. The lung parenchyma may be involved by an acute pneumonitis, in which infiltrates often involve the alveolar spaces as well as the alveolar walls, or less frequently by chronic interstitial lung disease. In the latter, extensive fibrosis is usually not a prominent feature of the histology.

Progressive systemic sclerosis or *scleroderma* is a disease whose most obvious manifestations are in the skin and the small blood vessels. Other organ systems, including the gastrointestinal tract, lungs, kidneys, and heart, are involved relatively frequently. Of all the connective tissue diseases, scleroderma is the one in which pulmonary involvement tends to be most severe and most likely associated with significant scarring of the pulmonary parenchyma. Pulmonary fibrosis complicating scleroderma appears to be strongly associated with the presence of a particular serologic marker, an

---

Histologic and physiologic changes suggest that pulmonary involvement in most connective tissue diseases is common, often with a histologic pattern of UIP or NSIP.

In rheumatoid arthritis and lupus, pleural disease is more common than is clinically evident interstitial lung disease.

Scleroderma lung disease is notable for interstitial fibrosis; disease of the small pulmonary vessels may be independent of the interstitial process.

autoantibody to topoisomerase I (antitopoisomerase I, also called Scl 70). Another potential pulmonary manifestation of scleroderma is disease of the small pulmonary blood vessels, which is discussed in Chapter 14. This involvement appears to be independent of the fibrotic process affecting the alveolar walls.

In *polymyositis-dermatomyositis,* muscles and skin are the primary sites of the inflammatory process. The interstitial lung disease of polymyositis-dermatomyositis is relatively infrequent and has no particular distinguishing features. Patients may also have respiratory problems as a result of their muscle disease, with weakness of the diaphragm or other inspiratory muscles. In addition, difficulty in swallowing may lead to recurrent episodes of aspiration pneumonia.

In *Sjögren's syndrome,* a lymphocytic infiltration affects salivary and lacrimal glands and is associated with dry mouth and dry eyes (keratoconjunctivitis sicca). When patients with Sjögren's syndrome have pulmonary parenchymal involvement, the histologic appearance is most commonly that of a lymphocytic infiltrate within the alveolar walls (called *lymphocytic interstitial pneumonia*) rather than either UIP or NSIP. Other lymphocytic complications of the lung can also develop in patients with Sjögren's syndrome, specifically either a localized, mass-like lesion called a pseudolymphoma, or an actual lymphoma.

Finally, a number of overlap syndromes, often also called *undifferentiated connective tissue disease,* have features of several of these disorders, particularly scleroderma, lupus, and polymyositis. Such patients may develop any of the complications noted with the more classic individual disorders, including interstitial lung disease, pleural disease, and pulmonary vascular disease.

SARCOIDOSIS

Sarcoidosis is defined as a systemic disorder in which granulomas, typically described as noncaseating, can be found in affected tissues or organ systems. An important qualification is that these granulomas occur in the absence of any exogenous (infectious or environmental) agents known to be associated with granulomatous inflammation. The lung is the most frequently involved organ, with potential manifestations including parenchymal lung disease, enlargement of hilar and mediastinal lymph nodes, or both.

Sarcoidosis is a systemic granulomatous disease that most commonly affects the lungs, the hilar and mediastinal lymph nodes, or both.

Sarcoidosis is a relatively common disorder that particularly affects young adults between 20 and 40 years of age. It is slightly more common in women than in men, and in the United States is more common in blacks than in whites. However, this racial predilection is not seen throughout the world, as the disease is notably prevalent in the white population of Scandinavia. Although a common stereotype in the United States is that the disease is primarily one of young black women, a substantial number of men and individuals of other ethnic and age groups are also affected. Of all the disorders of unknown cause affecting the alveolar wall, it is clearly the most prevalent.

Despite increasing knowledge about the cells involved in the inflammatory and granulomatous response in sarcoidosis, and despite the identification of multiple cytokines and chemokines that appear to be involved in the pathogenesis of the disease, the fundamental etiology of sarcoidosis remains as mysterious as it was when the disease was first described more than a century ago. It has been hypothesized that sarcoidosis represents an immunologic response to an exogenous agent in a genetically susceptible individual, but neither an exogenous agent nor a specific genetic susceptibility has been convincingly demonstrated. Interest has focused on a wide range of potential exogenous inciting agents, especially microorganisms such as viruses, mycobacteria, and other bacteria (e.g., *Propionibacterium acnes*). However, the identity of an infectious agent as a trigger for sarcoidosis remains elusive, and we do not at present even know if such an infectious agent exists.

On the other hand, we do have substantial information about cells and mediators that appear to be important in the inflammatory and granulomatous tissue reaction in sarcoidosis (see Figure 11-3). The critical cells are macrophages and T lymphocytes; the presumption is that processing of the responsible antigen by alveolar macrophages results in recruitment of helper T lymphocytes (CD4$^+$ cells) with a Th1 profile. A host of pro-inflammatory cytokines and chemokines, such as interleukin-2 (IL-2), interferon-γ (IFN-γ), tumor necrosis factor-α (TNF-α), and interleukin-12 (IL-12), appear to be important in recruiting and activating inflammatory cells, perpetuating the inflammatory response, and inducing the formation of granulomas. Profibrotic cytokines such as transforming growth factor-β (TGF-β), platelet-derived growth factor (PDGF), and insulin-like growth factor-1 (IGF-1) may subsequently result in fibrosis as a complication of the initial inflammatory reaction.

The accumulation of CD4$^+$ lymphocytes at the sites of active disease appears to result in secondary immunologic phenomena that are well recognized in sarcoidosis. First, presumably because of this concentration of activated lymphocytes in affected tissues, there is a relative depletion of CD4$^+$ cells in peripheral blood, leading to an apparent depression of cell-mediated immunity, at least as measured by cutaneous delayed hypersensitivity (skin testing). However, patients with sarcoidosis are not unduly susceptible to opportunistic infections that characteristically affect the immunosuppressed host with impaired cellular immunity. Second, T lymphocytes in sarcoidosis

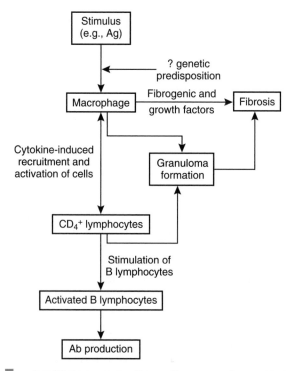

Figure 11-3 ■— Simplified proposed pathogenetic sequence in sarcoidosis.

nonspecifically activate B lymphocytes and the humoral immune system, leading to production of a variety of immunoglobulins and the common finding of hyperglobulinemia.

The characteristic histopathologic feature of sarcoidosis is the non-caseating granuloma (see Fig. 9-2). This discrete collection of tissue macrophages (also called epithelioid histiocytes) composing the granuloma does not show evidence of frank necrosis or caseation, as would appear in such disorders as tuberculosis or histoplasmosis. In addition to granulomas, in which multinucleated giant cells are frequently seen (see Fig. 9-2), there is often an alveolitis. The alveolitis is composed of mononuclear cells, including macrophages and lymphocytes, with the latter presumed to be of particular importance in the pathogenesis of the disease.

Patients with sarcoidosis seek consultation most frequently either as a result of abnormalities detected on an incidental chest radiograph or because of respiratory symptoms, mainly dyspnea or a nonproductive cough. Because many other organ systems may be involved with noncaseating granulomas, other manifestations occur but are less common. Eye involvement (e.g., anterior uveitis [inflammation in the anterior chamber of the eye]) and skin involvement (e.g., skin papules or plaques) are particularly common extrathoracic manifestations of sarcoidosis, but there may also be cardiac, neuromuscular, hematologic, hepatic, endocrine, and peripheral lymph node findings. Although symptoms are often insidious in onset, some patients with sarcoidosis have a more acute presentation called *Löfgren's syndrome*, in which the chest radiographic finding of bilateral hilar lymphadenopathy is accompanied by erythema nodosum (painful red nodules, typically on the anterior surface of the lower legs) and often fever and arthralgias.

The chest radiograph in sarcoidosis generally shows one of the following patterns: (1) enlargement of lymph nodes, most commonly bilateral hilar lymphadenopathy, with or without paratracheal node enlargement (Fig. 11-4); (2) parenchymal lung disease (in the form of interstitial disease, nodules, or alveolar infiltrates); or (3) both adenopathy and parenchymal disease (Fig. 11-5). High-resolution CT scanning, although not generally necessary, is more sensitive than plain chest radiography in detecting parenchymal lung disease, and it may show a particularly characteristic pattern of small nodules preferentially distributed along bronchovascular bundles (Fig. 11-6). In addition, HRCT often demonstrates mediastinal lymphadenopathy that cannot be seen on plain chest radiography.

The course of the radiographic findings in sarcoidosis is quite variable. Over time, both the adenopathy and the interstitial lung disease may regress spontaneously. At the other extreme, the interstitial disease may progress to a condition of extensive scarring and end-stage lung disease, at which time the patient has severe respiratory compromise.

As mentioned earlier, patients often display abnormalities in the immune system. Clinically, these patients may have anergy, i.e., failure to respond to skin tests requiring intact delayed hypersensitivity; they may also have hyperglobulinemia—evidence of a hyperactive humoral immune system. Calcium metabolism may be abnormal in sarcoidosis, occurring as a result of increased formation of the active form of vitamin D ($1,25$-dihydroxy-D_3) by activated macrophages in granulomas. Increased amounts of the active form of vitamin D lead to enhanced calcium absorption from the gastrointestinal tract, potentially causing hypercalciuria or, less frequently, hypercalcemia.

The diagnosis of sarcoidosis can be made in several ways. When the clinical diagnosis strongly suggests sarcoidosis, tissue confirmation is sometimes

The characteristic pathologic feature of sarcoidosis is the noncaseating granuloma; an alveolitis composed primarily of mononuclear cells may also occur.

The chest radiograph in sarcoidosis shows symmetrically enlarged hilar lymph nodes or interstitial lung disease, or both.

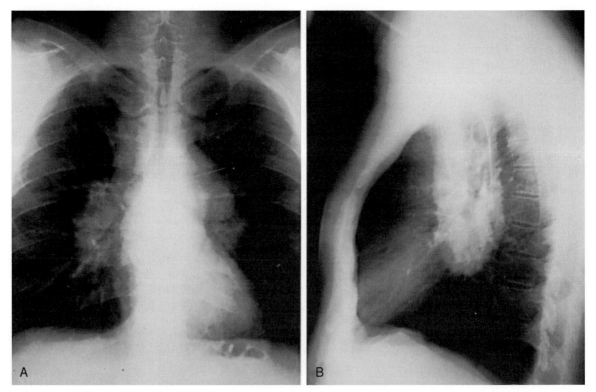

Figure 11-4 ◼— Radiographic appearance of stage I sarcoidosis shows bilateral hilar and paratracheal adenopathy. Enlarged nodes can be seen on (*A*) posteroanterior and (*B*) lateral views.

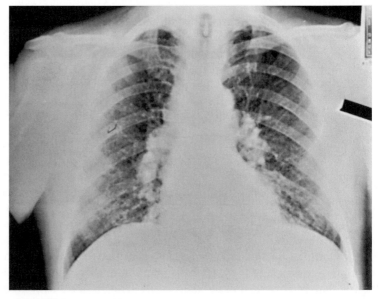

Figure 11-5 ◼— Chest radiograph shows characteristic features of stage II sarcoidosis: bilateral hilar adenopathy and diffuse interstitial lung disease. In stage III sarcoidosis (not shown), patients have diffuse interstitial lung disease without hilar adenopathy.

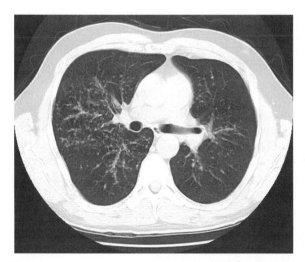

Figure 11-6 ▪— Chest CT scan demonstrates a micronodular pattern in a patient with sarcoidosis.

unnecessary. An example of such a presentation would be bilateral hilar lymphadenopathy found on an incidental chest radiograph in a symptom-free young black woman. On the other hand, when the patient has symptoms or when there is a question about the diagnosis, tissue sampling is usually undertaken to look for noncaseating granulomas and to rule out other causes. The lung is generally the most appropriate source of tissue, samples of which are frequently obtained with a transbronchial biopsy through a fiberoptic bronchoscope. Interestingly, even when the chest radiograph shows only hilar adenopathy without obvious parenchymal lung disease, the alveolar walls usually are studded with granulomas that may be seen on transbronchial lung biopsy. Other ways of obtaining tissue include performing a biopsy of a lymph node in the mediastinum (via mediastinoscopy) or a thoracoscopic lung biopsy. In addition, biopsy specimens can be obtained easily from involved areas of skin (when skin involvement is suspected on physical examination), or they are occasionally obtained from a variety of other involved tissues or organs, such as peripheral lymph nodes, conjunctiva, minor salivary glands, or liver.

> In sarcoidosis, transbronchial lung biopsy through a fiberoptic bronchoscope usually demonstrates granulomas in the lung parenchyma, even when the chest radiograph does not show interstitial lung disease.

Serum levels of angiotensin-converting enzyme have been found to be elevated in a large percentage of patients with sarcoidosis. This enzyme, which is normally synthesized by vascular endothelial cells, appears to be produced in the granulomas of sarcoidosis, suggesting it may be useful for diagnosing or following the disease. However, because it is not specific for sarcoidosis and often is normal in the presence of relatively inactive disease, its routine use has generally fallen out of favor.

The natural history of sarcoidosis is quite variable. In some patients, all clinical and radiographic manifestations are resolved within 1 to 2 years. Other patients have persistent radiographic changes, either with or without persisting symptoms. A minority of patients show continued progression of their radiographic abnormalities, with or without additional extrathoracic disease, and may have debilitating respiratory symptoms. In addition to pulmonary function tests, which are most useful for quantitating functional impairment, it has been suggested that assessing the alveolitis of the disease would be clinically useful. However, techniques such as gallium scanning and bronchoalveolar lavage have not received widespread acceptance for clinical use in evaluating the "activity" of the disease.

The initial treatment decision confronting the clinician is whether or not to institute therapy for the patient with sarcoidosis. Many patients do not need to be treated, especially when the disease is causing neither significant symptoms nor significant functional organ involvement. The fact that the disease may improve or resolve spontaneously also complicates decisions about instituting therapy. When treatment is indicated because of symptoms and significant tissue involvement affecting organ function, the drug of choice is usually systemic corticosteroids. In patients with refractory disease, a variety of other agents, especially immunosuppressive drugs, have also been used, either with or instead of corticosteroids.

> The variable natural history of sarcoidosis often makes decisions about use of corticosteroids difficult.

MISCELLANEOUS DISORDERS INVOLVING THE PULMONARY PARENCHYMA

An exhaustive description of all the remaining diseases of unknown etiology affecting the pulmonary parenchyma obviously cannot be presented here. Instead, a brief description of several additional diseases will acquaint the reader with their major features. These include (1) pulmonary Langerhans'-cell histiocytosis, (2) lymphangioleiomyomatosis, (3) Goodpasture's syndrome, (4) Wegener's granulomatosis, (5) chronic eosinophilic pneumonia, (6) bronchiolitis obliterans with organizing pneumonia, and (7) pulmonary alveolar proteinosis. For each of these relatively uncommon disorders, certain pathologic, clinical, or radiographic features distinguish them from the diffuse parenchymal lung diseases described earlier in this chapter. However, the defining feature for each of these disorders is a relatively specific pathologic appearance involving various components of the pulmonary parenchyma.

Pulmonary Langerhans'-Cell Histiocytosis

Pulmonary Langerhans'-cell histiocytosis, also called either *eosinophilic granuloma of the lung* or *pulmonary histiocytosis X,* is thought to represent part of a spectrum of disorders involving histiocytic infiltration of one or more organ systems. Whereas multisystem involvement in *Langerhans'-cell histiocytosis* or *histiocytosis X* is typically seen with the childhood disorders called Letterer-Siwe disease or Hand-Schüller-Christian disease (which are not discussed here), isolated or predominant pulmonary involvement in pulmonary Langerhans'-cell histiocytosis occurs mainly in young to middle-aged adults.

The responsible histiocytic cell appears to be a type of antigen-presenting dendritic or phagocytic cell called a Langerhans' cell. An interesting ultrastructural feature of these cells is the presence of cytoplasmic rod-like structures called X bodies (hence the name histiocytosis X) or Birbeck's granules, which can be seen by electron microscopy. Light-microscopic examination of the lung, in addition to demonstrating these histiocytes, reveals infiltration by eosinophils, lymphocytes, macrophages, and plasma cells. Although the disease occurs almost exclusively in smokers, the role of smoking in causing the disease or contributing to its pathogenesis has not yet been well defined.

The clinical presentation of pulmonary Langerhans'-cell histiocytosis typically features a pattern of nodular or reticulonodular disease on chest radiograph, often accompanied by respiratory symptoms of dyspnea, cough, or

> Pulmonary Langerhans'-cell histiocytosis (also called eosinophilic granuloma of the lung or histiocytosis X) enters into the differential diagnosis of unexplained interstitial disease, particularly in the young or middle-aged adult.

both. Occasionally, patients have a spontaneous pneumothorax, which may be the presenting feature of the disease. The radiographic findings tend to be more prominent in the upper lung zones, with high-resolution CT scans showing small cysts in addition to the nodular or reticulonodular changes. In some cases, progression leads to a pattern of extensive cystic disease and honeycombing. Unlike the typical restrictive pattern in most of the diffuse parenchymal lung diseases, pulmonary function testing in pulmonary Langerhans'-cell histiocytosis may show restrictive changes, obstructive changes, or both, accompanied by unusually normal or large lung volumes on chest radiography.

The natural history of the disease is variable. In some patients the disease is self-limited, and the radiographic and functional changes may stabilize over time, especially with cessation of smoking. In others, extensive disease and significant functional impairment follow. There is no clearly effective treatment for the disease, although corticosteroids are often tried if smoking cessation alone is ineffective.

Lymphangioleiomyomatosis

Lymphangioleiomyomatosis (LAM) is a rare pulmonary disease characterized by proliferation of atypical smooth muscle cells around lymphatics, blood vessels, and airways, accompanied by the presence of numerous small cysts throughout the pulmonary parenchyma. It occurs almost exclusively in women of childbearing age, suggesting that hormonal influences play a role in development of the disease. In addition, recent studies suggest that mutations in a gene on chromosome 16 (tuberous sclerosis complex 2, or TSC2) may also be important in the pathogenesis of the disease.

The clinical manifestations of LAM follow from the presence of cysts and from the involvement of lymphatics, blood vessels, and airways. The overall pathologic process in the pulmonary parenchyma may lead to dyspnea and cough, while vascular involvement may result in hemoptysis, lymphatic obstruction may produce chylous (milky-appearing) pleural effusions, and airway involvement may produce airflow obstruction. Rupture of subpleural cysts can lead to development of a spontaneous pneumothorax.

The chest radiograph typically shows a reticular pattern, and cystic changes can sometimes also be seen. High-resolution CT scanning is much better than plain chest radiography for demonstrating the cystic disease throughout the pulmonary parenchyma. As is true for pulmonary Langerhans'-cell histiocytosis, pulmonary function testing is not typical of most diffuse parenchymal diseases, as patients may demonstrate obstructive disease, restrictive disease, or both, and lung volumes on chest radiograph appear normal or increased rather than decreased.

Because of the hormonal dependence of the disease, treatment has focused on hormonal manipulation, most commonly with either oophorectomy or administration of progesterone.

Goodpasture's Syndrome

Goodpasture's syndrome is a disease that has become well known not because of its incidence, which is extremely low, but because of its interesting pathogenetic and immunologic features. In this syndrome two organ systems are involved: the lungs and the kidneys. In the lungs, patients have episodes of pulmonary hemorrhage, and pulmonary fibrosis may develop, presumably as a consequence of the recurrent episodes of bleeding. In the

Lymphangioleiomyomatosis is characterized by proliferation of atypical smooth muscle cells within the lung.

kidneys, patients have a glomerulonephritis characterized by linear deposits of antibody along the glomerular basement membrane. Studies on peripheral blood have demonstrated that these patients have circulating antibodies against a component of type IV collagen in their own glomerular basement membrane, often abbreviated anti-GBM antibodies. It is believed that these antibodies cross-react with the basement membrane of the alveolar wall and that their deposition in the kidney and lung is responsible for the clinical manifestations of the disease.

Why these true autoantibodies develop in patients with Goodpasture's syndrome is not entirely clear. In some patients, onset of the disease appears to follow influenza infection or exposure to a toxic hydrocarbon. Presumably, injury to basement membranes and release of previously unexposed antigenic determinants are involved, or there may be incidental formation of antibodies (against an unrelated antigen) that happen to cross-react with alveolar and glomerular basement membranes.

Therapy for Goodpasture's syndrome is based on decreasing the burden of anti-GBM antibodies presented to the lung and kidney. Plasmapheresis is capable of directly removing anti-GBM antibodies from the circulation. Immunosuppressive therapy (e.g., prednisone plus cyclophosphamide), aimed at decreasing the formation of anti-GBM antibodies, is usually given in conjunction with plasmapheresis.

> In Goodpasture's syndrome, autoantibodies directed against the glomerular basement membrane may cross-react with the basement membrane of alveolar walls.

Wegener's Granulomatosis

A group of disorders termed the *granulomatous vasculitides* may affect the alveolar wall as part of a more generalized disease. The most well known of these disorders is *Wegener's granulomatosis,* a disease characterized primarily but not exclusively by involvement of the upper respiratory tract, the lungs, and the kidneys. The pathologic process in the lungs and the upper respiratory tract consists of a necrotizing, granulomatous vasculitis, and a focal glomerulonephritis is present in the kidney. On chest radiograph, patients commonly have one or several nodules (often large) or infiltrates, often with associated cavitation of the lesion(s) (Fig. 11-7). Unlike most of the other disorders of the pulmonary parenchyma discussed in Chapter 10 and this chapter, diffuse interstitial lung disease is not the characteristic radiographic finding in this entity.

Patients with Wegener's granulomatosis typically have antibodies in their serum directed against proteinase 3, a serine protease that is present in the azurophil granules found in the cytoplasm of neutrophils. Immunofluorescent techniques allow detection of these antibodies by demonstration of a coarse, diffuse cytoplasmic pattern of staining when the patient's serum is incubated with normal neutrophils. The presence of antineutrophil cytoplasmic antibodies (ANCA), specifically with a cytoplasmic staining pattern (c-ANCA), has become an important component of the diagnostic evaluation for Wegener's granulomatosis, although the sensitivity of the test has varied considerably in different series. It has also been proposed that these antibodies might have a pathogenetic role in development of the disease.

Although Wegener's granulomatosis was once considered an aggressive and fatal disease, its prognosis has dramatically improved since cytotoxic agents, specifically cyclophosphamide, have been used in its treatment. Prednisone is also generally added for the initial period of therapy. Whereas the mean survival time without treatment was 5 months, patients are achieving complete and long-term remissions with institution of appropriate therapy.

> Wegener's granulomatosis is characterized pathologically by granulomatous vasculitis of the lung and upper respiratory tract and by glomerulonephritis; the clinical corollary is pulmonary, upper respiratory tract, and renal disease.

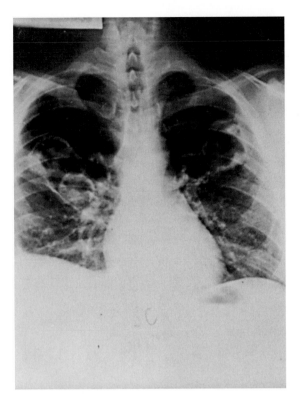

Figure 11-7 — Chest radiograph shows multiple cavitary pulmonary nodules in patient with Wegener's granulomatosis.

Reports on the combination antibiotic trimethoprim-sulfamethoxazole, either for treatment of selected patients or for prevention of relapse following successful immunosuppressive therapy, are also intriguing. What this finding means in terms of pathogenesis of the disease is unclear, as is the place of this less toxic therapy in the overall strategy for management.

Chronic Eosinophilic Pneumonia

Chronic eosinophilic pneumonia is a disorder in which the pulmonary interstitium and alveolar spaces are infiltrated primarily by eosinophils and, to a lesser extent, by macrophages. The clinical presentation typically occurs over weeks to months, with systemic symptoms such as fever and weight loss accompanying dyspnea and a nonproductive cough. The clues suggesting this diagnosis are often found on the chest radiograph and the routine white blood cell differential count. The radiograph frequently shows pulmonary infiltrates with a peripheral distribution and a pattern more suggestive of alveolar filling than of interstitial disease (Fig. 11-8). Because the typical radiographic pattern of pulmonary edema with congestive heart failure has central pulmonary infiltrates with sparing of the lung periphery, the prominent peripheral pattern often seen in chronic eosinophilic pneumonia has been described as the "photographic negative of pulmonary edema." The majority of patients also have increased numbers of eosinophils in peripheral blood, although this finding is not uniformly present and therefore not critical for the diagnosis.

Treatment is gratifying to patient and physician alike, because chronic eosinophilic pneumonia characteristically shows a dramatic response to corticosteroid therapy. Clinical improvement and radiographic resolution

Chronic eosinophilic pneumonia is often suggested on chest radiograph by a pattern of peripheral pulmonary infiltrates.

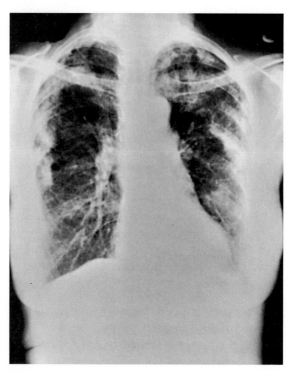

Figure 11-8 ■— Chest radiograph shows pattern of peripheral pulmonary infiltrates characteristic of chronic eosinophilic pneumonia.

generally occur within days to weeks, although therapy often needs to be prolonged for months to prevent recurrence.

Bronchiolitis Obliterans with Organizing Pneumonia

Bronchiolitis obliterans with organizing pneumonia (BOOP) is a disorder characterized by connective tissue plugs in small airways (hence the term *bronchiolitis obliterans*) accompanied by a mononuclear cell infiltration of the surrounding pulmonary parenchyma (organizing pneumonia). Although this histologic picture can sometimes be associated with connective tissue disease, toxic fume inhalation, or infection, the large majority of cases have no identifiable cause and are considered idiopathic. When no cause for BOOP is found, the term *cryptogenic organizing pneumonia* has often been used.

Like chronic eosinophilic pneumonia, BOOP often has a subacute presentation (over weeks to months) with systemic (constitutional) as well as respiratory symptoms. The chest radiograph shows patchy infiltrates, generally with an alveolar rather than an interstitial pattern, often mimicking a community-acquired pneumonia (Fig. 11-9). Also like chronic eosinophilic pneumonia, the response to corticosteroids is often dramatic and occurs over days to weeks. Therapy is usually prolonged for months to prevent relapse.

> On chest radiograph, bronchiolitis obliterans with organizing pneumonia (BOOP) often mimics a pneumonia, with one or more alveolar infiltrates.

Pulmonary Alveolar Proteinosis

Pulmonary alveolar proteinosis is a parenchymal lung disease in which the primary pathologic process affects the alveolar spaces, not the alveolar walls. Alveolar spaces are filled with a proteinaceous phospholipid material that represents components of pulmonary surfactant. Alveolar macrophages, in the

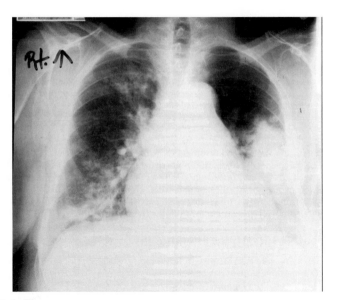

Figure 11-9 ■— Chest radiograph demonstrating patchy alveolar opacities in a patient with bronchiolitis obliterans with organizing pneumonia (BOOP). The enlarged cardiac silhouette is due to an unrelated cardiomyopathy.

process of phagocytosing this intra-alveolar material, become "overfed" and develop secondary functional abnormalities, including inability to handle certain microorganisms.

Although the mechanism of abnormal accumulation of surfactant-like material in alveolar spaces is not known with certainty, current theories center around abnormal clearance of the material. According to one hypothesis, alveolar type II cells, which are responsible not only for production but also for re-uptake of surfactant (essentially a "recycling" process), are deficient in carrying out this normal re-uptake process, thus overwhelming an additional clearance mechanism for surfactant provided by alveolar macrophages. Alternatively, a more recent theory is based on an animal model for alveolar proteinosis, in which mice lacking granulocyte-macrophage colony stimulating factor (GM-CSF) or the receptor for GM-CSF develop a pulmonary process that closely mimics human pulmonary alveolar proteinosis. According to this theory, the human disease might be related to a relative deficiency or loss of responsiveness to GM-CSF, which appears necessary for the effective clearance of surfactant by alveolar macrophages.

An animal model suggests that defective uptake of surfactant by alveolar macrophages, due to a decreased amount or effect of GM-CSF, may underlie the pathogenesis of pulmonary alveolar proteinosis.

Patients with alveolar proteinosis present primarily with dyspnea and cough accompanying a chest radiographic picture notable for bilateral alveolar infiltrates. HRCT generally shows a distinctive pattern that suggests the diagnosis, called a "crazy paving" pattern (produced by thickening of interlobular septa accompanied by ground-glass alveolar filling). Because of macrophage functional defects, patients are susceptible to certain types of superimposed respiratory infections, especially with the organism *Nocardia*.

Alveolar proteinosis is generally treated by a procedure called whole lung lavage, done while the patient is under general anesthesia, which involves "washing out" the material filling the alveolar spaces. The prognosis of this disease is generally relatively good, although patients may require additional treatments with whole lung lavage.

References

Idiopathic Pulmonary Fibrosis

American Thoracic Society and European Respiratory Society: Idiopathic pulmonary fibrosis: diagnosis and treatment. Am J Respir Crit Care Med 161:646-664, 2000.

British Thoracic Society: The diagnosis, assessment and treatment of diffuse parenchymal lung disease in adults. Thorax 54 (Suppl):S1-S30, 1999.

Costabel U and King TE: International consensus statement on idiopathic pulmonary fibrosis. Eur Respir J 17:163-167, 2001.

Freudenberger T and Raghu G: Idiopathic pulmonary fibrosis: an evolving approach to diagnosis and treatment. Eur Respir Mon 5 (Monograph 14):79-95, 2000.

Gross TJ and Hunninghake GW: Idiopathic pulmonary fibrosis. N Engl J Med 345:517-525, 2001.

Michaelson JE, Aguayo SM, and Roman J: Idiopathic pulmonary fibrosis: a practical approach for diagnosis and management. Chest 118:788-794, 2000.

Selman M, King TE Jr, and Pardo A: Idiopathic pulmonary fibrosis: prevailing and evolving hypotheses about its pathogenesis and implications for therapy. Ann Intern Med 134:136-151, 2001.

Other Idiopathic Interstitial Pneumonias

American Thoracic Society and European Respiratory Society: American Thoracic Society/European Respiratory Society international multidisciplinary consensus classification of the idiopathic interstitial pneumonias. Am J Respir Crit Care Med 165:277-304, 2002.

Bouros D, Nicholson AC, Polychronopoulos V, and du Bois RM: Acute interstitial pneumonia. Eur Respir J 15:412-418, 2000.

Collard HR and King TE Jr: Demystifying idiopathic interstitial pneumonia. Arch Intern Med 163:17-29, 2003.

Young DA, Cherniack RM, King TE, and Schwarz MI: Acute interstitial pneumonitis. Case series and review of the literature. Medicine 79:369-378, 2000.

Pulmonary Parenchymal Involvement Complicating Connective Tissue Disease

Eisenberg H: The interstitial lung diseases associated with collagen-vascular disorders. Clin Chest Med 3:565-578, 1982.

Gochuico BR: Potential pathogenesis and clinical aspects of pulmonary fibrosis associated with rheumatoid arthritis. Am J Med Sci 321:83-88, 2001.

Hunninghake GW and Fauci AS: Pulmonary involvement in the collagen vascular diseases. Am Rev Respir Dis 119:471-503, 1979.

Keane MP and Lynch JP: Pleuropulmonary manifestations of systemic lupus erythematosus. Thorax 55:159-166, 2000.

Lynch JP III and Hunninghake GW: Pulmonary complications of collagen vascular disease. Annu Rev Med 43:17-35, 1992.

Minai OA, Dweik RA, and Arroliga AC: Manifestations of scleroderma pulmonary disease. Clin Chest Med 19:713-731, 1998.

Mortenson RL and Corbridge T: Connective tissue disorders involving the lung—etiology, pathogenesis, and diagnosis. In Leff AR (ed): Pulmonary and Critical Care Pharmacology and Therapeutics. New York, McGraw-Hill, 1996, pp 1073-1084.

Schwarz MI: The lung in polymyositis. Clin Chest Med 19:701-712, 1998.

Sarcoidosis

American Thoracic Society: Statement on sarcoidosis. Am J Respir Crit Care Med 160:736-755, 1999.

DeRemee RA: Sarcoidosis. Mayo Clin Proc 70:177-181, 1995.

Eklund A and Grunewald J: Sarcoidosis. Eur Respir Mon 5 (Monograph 14):96-119, 2000.

Gibson GJ: Sarcoidosis: old and new treatments. Thorax 56:336-339, 2001.

Johns CJ and Michele TM: The clinical management of sarcoidosis. A 50-year experience at the Johns Hopkins Hospital. Medicine 78:65-111, 1999.

Mitchell DN and Scadding JG: Sarcoidosis. Am Rev Respir Dis 110:774-802, 1974.

Newman LS, Rose CS, and Maier LA: Sarcoidosis. N Engl J Med 336:1224-1234, 1997.

Paramothayan S and Jones PW: Corticosteroid therapy in pulmonary sarcoidosis. A systematic review. JAMA 287:1301-1307, 2002.

Miscellaneous Disorders Involving the Pulmonary Parenchyma

Alasaly K et al: Cryptogenic organizing pneumonia. Medicine 74:201-211, 1995.

Allen JN and Davis WB: Eosinophilic lung diseases. Am J Respir Crit Care Med 150:1423-1438, 1994.

Ball JA and Young KR: Pulmonary manifestations of Goodpasture's syndrome. Antiglomerular basement membrane disease and related disorders. Clin Chest Med 19:777-791, 1998.

Carsillo T, Astrinidis A, and Henske EP: Mutations in the tuberous sclerosis complex gene TSC2 are a cause of sporadic pulmonary lymphangioleiomyomatosis. PNAS 97:6085-6090, 2000.

Cordier J-F: Organising pneumonia. Thorax 55:318-328, 2000.

Costabel U and Guzman J: Alveolar proteinosis. Eur Respir Mon 5 (Monograph 14):194-205, 2000.

Epler GR: Bronchiolitis obliterans organizing pneumonia. Arch Intern Med 161:158-164, 2001.

Hoffman GS et al: Wegener's granulomatosis: an analysis of 158 patients. Ann Intern Med 116:488-498, 1992.

Jederlinic PJ, Sicilian L, and Gaensler EA: Chronic eosinophilic pneumonia. Medicine 67:154-162, 1988.

Johnson S: Lymphangioleiomyomatosis: clinical features, management and basic mechanisms. Thorax 54:254-264, 1999.

Langford CA and Hoffman GS: Wegener's granulomatosis. Thorax 54:629-637, 1999.

Langford CA and Sneller MC: Update on the diagnosis and treatment of Wegener's granulomatosis. Adv Intern Med 46:177-206, 2001.

Leatherman JW: Immune alveolar hemorrhage. Chest 91:891-897, 1987.

Leatherman JW, Davies SF, and Hoidal JR: Alveolar hemorrhage syndromes: diffuse microvascular lung hemorrhage in immune and idiopathic disorders. Medicine 63:343-361, 1984.

Rao JK et al: The role of antineutrophil cytoplasmic antibody (c-ANCA) testing in the diagnosis of Wegener granulomatosis. Ann Intern Med 123:925-932, 1995.

Shah PL et al: Pulmonary alveolar proteinosis: clinical aspects and current concepts on pathogenesis. Thorax 55:67-77, 2000.

Sneller MC: Wegener's granulomatosis. JAMA 273:1288-1291, 1995.

Stegman CA et al: Trimethoprim-sulfamethoxazole (co-trimoxazole) for the prevention of relapses of Wegener's granulomatosis. N Engl J Med 335:16-20, 1996.

Strizheva GD et al: The spectrum of mutations in TSC1 and TSC2 in women with tuberous sclerosis and lymphangioleiomyomatosis. Am J Respir Crit Care Med 163:253-258, 2001.

Sullivan EJ: Lymphangioleiomyomatosis. A review. Chest 114:1689-1703, 1998.

Tazi A, Soler P, and Hance AJ: Adult pulmonary Langerhans' cell histiocytosis. Thorax 55:405-416, 2000.

Vassallo R et al: Pulmonary Langerhans'-cell histiocytosis. N Engl J Med 342:1969-1978, 2000.

Vassallo R et al: Clinical outcomes of pulmonary Langerhans'-cell histiocytosis in adults. N Engl J Med 346:484-490, 2002.

Anatomic and Physiologic Aspects of the Pulmonary Vasculature

ANATOMY

PHYSIOLOGY
    Pulmonary Vascular Resistance
    Distribution of Pulmonary Blood
    Flow

Pulmonary Vascular Response to
    Hypoxia
Other Aspects of Pulmonary
    Vascular Physiology

The pulmonary vasculature is responsible for transporting desaturated blood to the lungs and then carrying freshly oxygenated blood back to the left atrium and ventricle for pumping to peripheral tissues. Although the pulmonary circulation is often called the "lesser circulation," the lungs are the only organ system that receives the entire cardiac output. This extensive system of pulmonary vessels is susceptible to a variety of disease processes, ranging from those that primarily affect the vasculature to those that are either secondary to airway or pulmonary parenchymal disease or due to transport of material that is foreign to the pulmonary vessels, including blood clots.

Before diseases of the pulmonary vasculature are considered in Chapters 13 and 14, a few of the general anatomic and physiologic aspects of the pulmonary vessels are discussed in this chapter. Included in the discussion on physiology are several topics relating to hemodynamics of the pulmonary circulation as well as a brief consideration of some nonrespiratory, metabolic functions of the pulmonary circulation.

ANATOMY

In contrast to the systemic arteries, which carry blood from the left ventricle to the rest of the body, the pulmonary arteries are relatively thin-walled vessels that normally do not need to withstand particularly high pressures. The pulmonary trunk, which carries the outflow from the right ventricle, divides almost immediately into the right and left main pulmonary arteries, which subsequently divide into smaller branches. Throughout these progressive divisions, the pulmonary arteries and their branches travel with companion airways, following closely the course of the progressively dividing bronchial tree. By the time the vessels are considered arterioles, the outer diameter is less than approximately 0.1 mm. An important feature of the smaller pulmonary arteries is the presence of smooth muscle within the walls, which is responsible for the vasoconstrictive response to various stimuli, particularly hypoxia.

The pulmonary capillaries form an extensive network of communicating channels coursing through alveolar walls. Rather than being described as a series of separate vessels, the capillary system has been described as a continuous meshwork or sheet bounded by alveolar walls on each side and interrupted by "posts" of connective tissue, akin to the appearance of an underground parking garage. The capillaries are in close proximity to alveolar gas, separated only by alveolar epithelial cells and a small amount of interstitium present in some regions of the alveolar wall (see Figs. 8-1 and 8-2). The design of this capillary system is extraordinarily well suited to the requirements of gas-exchange, inasmuch as it contains an enormous effective surface area of contact between pulmonary capillaries and alveolar gas. The pulmonary veins, responsible for transporting oxygenated blood from the pulmonary capillaries to the left atrium, progressively combine into larger vessels until four major pulmonary veins enter the left atrium. Unlike the pulmonary arteries and their branches, the pulmonary venous system does not follow the course of the corresponding bronchial structures.

The bronchial arteries, which are part of the systemic circulation, provide nutrient blood flow to a variety of nonalveolar structures, such as the bronchi and the visceral pleural surface. Generally, a single bronchial artery of variable origin (upper right intercostal, right subclavian, or internal mammary artery) supplies the right lung. Two bronchial arteries, usually arising from the thoracic aorta, supply the left lung. Venous blood from the large, extrapulmonary airways drains via bronchial veins into the azygos vein and eventually into the right atrium. In contrast, venous blood from intrapulmonary airways drains into the pulmonary venous system, thus eventually providing a small amount of anatomic shunting of desaturated blood to the systemic arterial circulation.

An extensive network of lymphatic channels is also located primarily within the connective tissue sheaths around small vessels and airways. Although these channels do not generally course through the interstitial tissue of the alveolar walls, they are in close enough proximity to be effective at removing liquid and some solutes that constantly pass into the interstitium of the alveolar wall.

PHYSIOLOGY

Pulmonary Vascular Resistance

Although the pulmonary circulation handles the same cardiac output from the right ventricle as the systemic circulation handles from the left, the former operates under much lower pressures and has substantially less resistance to flow than does the latter. The systolic and diastolic pressures in the pulmonary artery are normally approximately 25 and 10 mm Hg, respectively, in contrast to 120 and 80 mm Hg in the systemic arteries. The pulmonary resistance can be calculated according to the following formula:

$$R = \text{change in pressure/flow}$$

The change or drop in pressure across the pulmonary circuit is the mean pulmonary artery pressure minus the mean left atrial pressure. Left atrial pressure is difficult to measure directly, but a reasonably accurate indirect assessment can be made by measuring the "back pressure" in the pulmonary artery when forward flow has been occluded. A special catheter designed for this purpose, called a *pulmonary artery balloon occlusion catheter,* or *Swan-Ganz catheter,* has had wide clinical application for such pressure measurements.

Assuming mean pulmonary artery (PA) and left atrial (LA) pressures of 15 and 6 mm Hg, respectively, along with a cardiac output of 6 L/min, the pulmonary resistance is (15-6)/6 mm Hg/L/min, or 1.5 mm Hg/L/min. This resistance is approximately one-tenth that found in the systemic circulation.

When cardiac output increases (e.g., during exercise), the pulmonary circulation is able to decrease its resistance and to handle the extra flow with only a minimal increase in pulmonary artery pressure. Two mechanisms appear to be responsible: recruitment of new vessels and, to a lesser extent, distention of previously perfused vessels. In normal resting conditions, some of the pulmonary vessels receive no blood flow but are capable of carrying part of the pulmonary blood flow should the pressure increase. In addition, because pulmonary vessels have relatively thin walls, they are distensible and can enlarge their diameter under increased pressure to accommodate additional blood flow. With a means for increasing the total cross-sectional area of the pulmonary vasculature on demand, the pulmonary circulation is capable of lowering its resistance when the need for increased flow arises.

Another factor that affects pulmonary vascular resistance is lung volume. In discussing the nature of this effect, it is useful to distinguish two categories of pulmonary vessels on the basis of their size and location. One category, called *alveolar vessels,* includes the capillary network coursing through alveolar walls. When alveoli are expanded and lung volume is raised, these vessels are compressed in the stretched alveolar walls, and their contribution to pulmonary vascular resistance is increased. In contrast, when alveoli are emptied and lung volume is lowered, the resistance of these alveolar vessels is diminished. The other category consists of the larger vessels, called *extra-alveolar vessels;* they are not compressed by air-filled alveoli. The supporting structure that surrounds the walls of these vessels has attachments to alveolar walls, and the elastic recoil of the alveolar walls provides radial traction to keep these vessels open. This concept is similar to the one discussed in Chapter 6 concerning the effect of alveolar wall attachments on airway diameter (see Fig. 6-6). When lung volume is increased, elastic recoil of the alveolar walls is increased, and the extra-alveolar vessels become larger. When lung volume is decreased, the resistance of the extra-alveolar vessels increases. This differential effect of lung volume on the resistance of alveolar versus extra-alveolar vessels is shown in Figure 12-1. The total pulmonary vascular resistance is least at the normal resting expiratory position of the lung, i.e., at functional residual capacity.

Distribution of Pulmonary Blood Flow

The relatively low pressures in the pulmonary artery have important implications for the way blood flow is distributed in the lung. When a person is in the upright position, blood going to the upper zones of the lung is flowing against gravity and must be under sufficient pressure in the pulmonary artery to make this antigravitational journey. Because the top of the lung is approximately 15 cm above the level of the main pulmonary arteries, a pressure of 15 cm H_2O is required to achieve perfusion of the apices. The mean pulmonary artery pressure of 15 mm Hg (approximately 19 cm H_2O) is normally just sufficient to achieve flow to this region. In contrast, flow to the lower lung

Pulmonary vascular resistance = (mean PA pressure − mean LA pressure)/cardiac output; LA pressure is indirectly determined from occluded PA pressure.

When cardiac output increases, recruitment and distention of pulmonary vessels prevent a significant increase in pulmonary artery pressure.

The distribution of blood flow within the lung is strongly influenced by gravity.

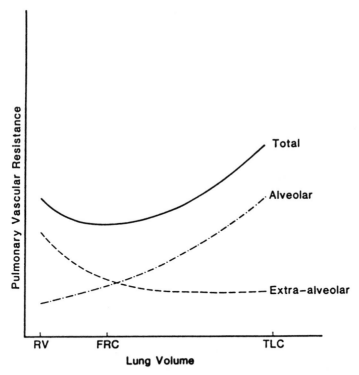

Figure 12-1 ■— Effect of lung volume on total pulmonary vascular resistance (solid line), alveolar vessel resistance (dashed-dotted line), and extra-alveolar vessel resistance (dashed line). Note that total resistance is least at functional residual capacity (FRC). TLC = total lung capacity; RV = residual volume. (From Taylor AE, Rehder K, Hyatt RE, and Parker JC: Clinical Respiratory Physiology, p. 75. Philadelphia, WB Saunders Co., 1989.)

zones—that is, below the level of the main pulmonary arteries—is assisted by gravity. Therefore, in the upright individual, gravity provides a normal gradient of blood flow from the apex to the base of the lung, with the base receiving substantially greater flow than the apex (see Fig. 1-4). As discussed in Chapter 1, this distribution of blood flow in the lung has major implications for the manner in which ventilation and perfusion are matched.

The three-zone model presented in Chapter 1 for describing the determinants of pulmonary blood flow is actually more complicated, as a zone 4 has been recognized. In this zone, which occupies the base of the lung, blood flow progressively diminishes as the most dependent region of the lung is approached. In order to explain why a zone 4 exists, we must return to the concept of extra-alveolar pulmonary vessels. At the lung bases, the weight of the lung results in decreased alveolar volume, accompanied by distortion and compression of extra-alveolar vessels. As a result, the resistance of the extra-alveolar vessels increases considerably, the total vascular resistance in this zone increases, and blood flow diminishes.

The distribution of blood flow in the lung can be measured conveniently with radioactive isotopes. A particularly useful technique involves intravenous injection of labeled particles, specifically macroaggregates of albumin, that are of sufficient size to lodge in the pulmonary capillaries. An external counter over the lung can then sense the distribution of lodged particles and hence the distribution of blood flow to the lung. This technique, when performed in the upright individual, not only confirms the expected gradient of blood flow in the lung but also detects regions of decreased or absent perfusion in disease states, as discussed in Chapter 3.

Pulmonary Vascular Response to Hypoxia

An important physiologic feature of the pulmonary circulation is its response to hypoxia. When alveoli in an area of lung contain gas with a low P_{O_2}, generally less than 60 to 70 torr, the vessels supplying that region of lung undergo vasoconstriction. This response occurs primarily at the level of the small arteries or arterioles and serves as a protective mechanism for decreasing perfusion to poorly ventilated alveoli. Hence, ventilation-perfusion mismatch is decreased, and areas of low ventilation-perfusion ratio, which contribute hypoxemic blood, are minimized. When there are localized regions of lung with a low P_{O_2}, then the vasoconstrictive response is also localized. In these circumstances the overall pulmonary vascular resistance does not increase significantly. However, with a generalized decrease in P_{O_2}, as in many forms of lung disease or in persons exposed to high altitude, pulmonary vasoconstriction is generalized. In this circumstance, pulmonary vascular resistance and pulmonary artery pressure are both increased. What would be a protective response in the case of localized disease is thus detrimental in the case of generalized disease and widespread alveolar hypoxia.

There is one setting in which such generalized pulmonary vasoconstriction in response to alveolar hypoxia is most beneficial: the fetus. In utero, the alveoli receive no aeration, making the entire lung hypoxic. As a result there is marked pulmonary vasoconstriction, accompanied by very high pulmonary vascular resistance and diversion of blood away from the lung. Instead, blood preferentially goes through the ductus arteriosus from the pulmonary artery to the aorta, and through the foramen ovale from the right to the left atrium.

At birth, when the first few breaths are taken, oxygen flows into the alveoli, and the pulmonary vasoconstriction is reversed. As a result of this pulmonary vasodilation (as well as constriction of the ductus arteriosus), right ventricular output passes through the lungs, where the blood is oxygenated. Interestingly, the hypoxic vasoconstriction that persists throughout adult life is probably directly related to this important fetal response.

The mechanism of hypoxic vasoconstriction remains unknown. One theory suggests that alveolar hypoxia acts on pulmonary vascular smooth muscle cells by inhibiting a membrane potassium ion channel, which leads to membrane depolarization and subsequent influx of calcium ions. The increase in intracellular calcium is then responsible for inducing pulmonary vascular smooth muscle cell contraction. Alternatively, hypoxia may alter release of vasoactive mediators; popular candidates have included mediators released from vascular endothelial cells, such as the vasodilating factor nitric oxide (previously called endothelial-derived relaxing factor) and the constricting factor known as endothelin. Nitric oxide, which is produced by vascular endothelial cells, acts via increasing cyclic GMP to produce vascular smooth muscle relaxation. Although the overall role of nitric oxide in regulating the pulmonary circulation, either in normal circumstances or in the setting of disease or alveolar hypoxia, is unclear, there is ongoing interest in its potential usefulness as a therapeutic agent in disorders associated with pulmonary hypertension.

Pulmonary vasoconstriction occurs in response to alveolar hypoxia; this protective mechanism reduces blood flow to poorly ventilated alveoli, minimizing ventilation-perfusion mismatch.

Other Aspects of Pulmonary Vascular Physiology

An additional stimulus for pulmonary vasoconstriction is a low blood pH value. Although this effect is less important than the effect of hypoxia, the two stimuli do appear to have a synergistic effect on increasing pulmonary vascular resistance. Any effect of PCO_2 on the pulmonary vasculature appears to be small; although hypercapnia may increase pulmonary vascular resistance, the effect is apparently mediated by changes in blood pH.

A low pH value in blood is an additional stimulus for pulmonary vasoconstriction.

A variety of other factors that influence pulmonary vascular tone are being increasingly recognized. Autonomic innervation of the pulmonary arterial system is present although not extensive. Sympathetic and parasympathetic stimulation have the expected opposing effects, causing vasoconstriction and vasodilation, respectively. Humoral stimuli altering vascular tone are numerous; examples include histamine and the prostaglandin products of arachidonic acid metabolism. Most recently, interest has focused on two molecules mentioned earlier in the discussion of hypoxic vasoconstriction, each of which is known to have important effects on the pulmonary vasculature: nitric oxide (a potent vasodilator) and endothelin (a potent vasoconstrictor). In addition to a possible role that these compounds may have in the pathophysiology of disease states involving the pulmonary vasculature, there may be a therapeutic benefit for agents that affect the production or effect of these vasoactive molecules.

Another important aspect of pulmonary vascular physiology relates to fluid movement from pulmonary capillaries into the interstitium of the alveolar wall. Because of the importance of abnormalities in fluid transport across the capillaries in acute respiratory distress syndrome and respiratory failure, this topic is discussed specifically in Chapter 28.

Finally, although transport of blood between the heart and the lungs is the most obvious function of the pulmonary vasculature, these vessels have additional nonrespiratory, metabolic functions. A substantial amount of evidence shows that the pulmonary circulation has an important role in the inactivation of certain circulating bioactive chemicals. For example, serotonin (5-hydroxytryptamine) and bradykinin are primarily inactivated in the lung, probably at the level of the vascular endothelium. In addition, angiotensin I, an inactive decapeptide, is converted to the active octapeptide angiotensin II by angiotensin-converting enzyme, which is produced by pulmonary vascular endothelial cells. Although the metabolic functions of the pulmonary vasculature are certainly important in modifying the effects of these substances, it is not known whether derangements in these functions are important consequences of diseases affecting the vasculature.

References

Archer SL, Weir EK, Reeve HL, and Michelakis E: Molecular identification of O_2 sensors and O_2-sensitive potassium channels in the pulmonary circulation. Adv Exp Med Biol 475:219-240, 2000.

Barnes PJ and Liu SF: Regulation of pulmonary vascular tone. Pharmacol Rev 47:87-131, 1995.

Brij SO and Peacock AJ: Cellular responses to hypoxia in the pulmonary circulation. Thorax 53:1075-1079, 1998.

Chen YF and Oparil S: Endothelial dysfunction in the pulmonary vascular bed. Am J Med Sci 320:223-232, 2000.

Coppock EA, Martens JR, and Tamkun MM: Molecular basis of hypoxia-induced pulmonary vasoconstriction: role of voltage-gated K^+ channels. Am J Physiol Lung Cell Mol Physiol 281:L1-L12, 2001.

Cutaia M and Rounds S: Hypoxic pulmonary vasoconstriction: physiologic significance, mechanism, and clinical relevance. Chest 97:706-718, 1990.

Keith IM: The role of endogenous lung neuropeptides in regulation of the pulmonary circulation. Physiol Rev 49:519-537, 2000.

Leff AR and Schumacker PT: Respiratory Physiology: Basics and Applications. Philadelphia, WB Saunders Co., 1993.

Vender RL: Chronic hypoxic pulmonary hypertension: cell biology to pathophysiology. Chest 106:236-243, 1994.

Weibel ER: The Pathway for Oxygen: Structure and Function in the Mammalian Respiratory System. Cambridge, MA, Harvard University Press, 1984.

West JB: Respiratory Physiology—The Essentials, 6th ed. Baltimore, Lippincott Williams & Wilkins, 2000.

Zapol WM et al: Nitric oxide and the lung. Am J Respir Crit Care Med 149:1375-1380, 1994.

chapter 13

Pulmonary Embolism

ETIOLOGY AND PATHOGENESIS
PATHOLOGY
PATHOPHYSIOLOGY
CLINICAL FEATURES
DIAGNOSTIC EVALUATION
TREATMENT

Pulmonary embolism is one of the most important disorders that affect the pulmonary vasculature. Not only is it found in more than 60 percent of autopsies in which careful search is made but it is also widely misdiagnosed, in terms of both "overdiagnosis" when not present and "underdiagnosis" when present.

The term *pulmonary embolism,* or more precisely, *pulmonary thromboembolism,* refers to the movement of a blood clot from a systemic vein through the right side of the heart to the pulmonary circulation, where it lodges in one or more branches of the pulmonary artery. The clinical consequences of this common problem are quite variable, ranging from none to sudden death, depending on the size of the embolus and the medical condition of the patient. Although pulmonary embolism is intimately associated with the development of a thrombus elsewhere in the circulation, the focus in this chapter is on the pulmonary manifestations of thromboembolic disease, not on the clinical effects or diagnosis of the clot at the site of formation.

ETIOLOGY AND PATHOGENESIS

A thrombus—blood clot—is the material that travels to the pulmonary circulation in pulmonary thromboembolic disease. Other material can also travel via the vasculature to the pulmonary arteries, including tumor cells or fragments, fat, amniotic fluid, and a variety of foreign materials that can be introduced into the circulation. This text does not consider these additional, much less common, types of embolism, which have quite different clinical presentations than do thromboemboli.

In the majority of cases, the lower extremities are the source of thrombi that embolize to the lungs. Although these thrombi frequently originate in the veins of the calf, propagation of the clots to the veins of the thigh is necessary to produce sufficiently large thrombi for clinically important embolism. Rarely do pulmonary emboli originate in the arms, pelvis, or right-sided chambers of the heart; these sources combined probably account for less than 10 percent of all pulmonary emboli. However, not all thrombi resulting in embolic disease are clinically apparent. In fact, only about 50 percent of

Thrombi in the deep veins of the lower extremities are the usual source of pulmonary emboli.

181

patients with pulmonary emboli have previous clinical evidence of venous thrombosis in the lower extremities or elsewhere.

It is commonly said that the following three factors potentially contribute to the genesis of venous thrombosis: (1) alteration in the mechanism of blood coagulation, i.e., hypercoagulability, (2) damage to the endothelium of the vessel wall, and (3) stasis or stagnation of blood flow. In practice, many specific risk factors for thromboemboli have been identified, including immobilization (e.g., bed rest, prolonged sitting during travel, immobilization of an extremity after fracture), the postoperative state, congestive heart failure, obesity, underlying carcinoma, pregnancy and the postpartum state, use of oral contraceptives, and chronic deep venous insufficiency. Patients at particularly high risk are those who have had trauma or surgery related to the pelvis or lower extremities, especially hip fracture or either hip or knee replacement.

A number of genetic predispositions to hypercoagulability have been recognized. These include deficiency of proteins with antithrombotic activity (antithrombin III, protein C, protein S) or the presence of abnormal variants of some of the clotting factors that are part of the coagulation cascade, especially factor V and prothrombin (factor II). In the genetic defect called factor V Leiden, which is usually due to a single base pair substitution leading to replacement of an arginine residue by glutamine, the factor V protein becomes resistant to the action of activated protein C. Individuals who are heterozygous for factor V Leiden have a 3- to 5-fold increased risk of venous thrombosis, and the much less common homozygous state confers a significantly higher risk. In the genetic variant of prothrombin that is often called the *prothrombin gene mutation*, there is also a single base pair deletion which, by an unknown mechanism, leads to increased plasma levels of prothrombin and predisposes to venous thrombosis. Whereas deficiencies of the antithrombotic proteins are rare, factor V Leiden may have a prevalence of up to 5 percent, and the fact that it is found in about 20 percent of patients with a first episode of venous thromboembolism suggests it is an important risk factor. Both factor V Leiden and the prothrombin gene mutation are relatively common in the white population but rare among blacks and Asians.

PATHOLOGY

The pathologic changes that result from occlusion of a pulmonary artery depend to a large extent on the location of the occlusion and the presence of other disorders that compromise O_2 supply to the pulmonary parenchyma. There are two major consequences of vascular occlusion in the lung parenchyma distal to the site of occlusion. First, if minimal or no other O_2 supply reaches the parenchyma, either from the airways or from the bronchial arterial circulation, then frank necrosis of lung tissue (pulmonary infarction) will result. According to one estimate, only 10 to 15 percent of all pulmonary emboli result in pulmonary infarction. It has sometimes been said that compromise of two of the three O_2 sources to the lung—pulmonary artery, bronchial artery, and alveolar gas—is necessary before infarction results. Second, when the integrity of the parenchyma is maintained and infarction does not result, hemorrhage and edema often occur in lung tissue supplied by the occluded pulmonary artery. The name *congestive atelectasis* has sometimes been applied to this process of parenchymal hemorrhage and edema without infarction.

Embolic occlusion of a vessel may lead to infarction or congestive atelectasis of the lung parenchyma.

With either pulmonary infarction or congestive atelectasis, the pathologic process generally extends to the visceral pleural surface, and corresponding radiographic changes are therefore often pleura-based. In some cases, pleural effusion may also result. As part of the natural history of infarction, there is generally contraction of the infarcted parenchyma and eventual formation of a scar. With congestive atelectasis but no infarction, resolution of the process and resorption of the blood may leave few or no pathologic sequelae.

In many cases, neither of these pathologic changes occurs, and relatively little alteration of the distal lung parenchyma is found, presumably because of incomplete occlusion or sufficient nutrient O_2 from other sources. Frequently, the thrombus quickly fragments or undergoes a process of lysis, with smaller fragments moving progressively distally in the pulmonary arterial circulation. Whether this rapid process of clot dissolution occurs is also important in determining the pathologic consequences of pulmonary embolism.

With clots that do not fragment or lyse, there is generally a slower process of organization in the vessel wall and eventual recanalization. Webs may form within the arterial lumen and may sometimes be detected on a pulmonary arteriogram or on postmortem examination as the only evidence for prior embolic disease.

PATHOPHYSIOLOGY

When a thrombus migrates to and lodges within a pulmonary vessel, a variety of consequences ensue. These relate not only to mechanical obstruction of one or more vessels but also to the secondary effects of various mediators released from the thrombus. The effects of mechanical occlusion of the vessels are discussed first, followed by a consideration of how chemical mediators contribute to the clinical effects.

When a vessel is occluded by an embolus and forward blood flow through the vessel stops, perfusion of pulmonary capillaries normally supplied by that vessel ceases. If ventilation to the corresponding alveoli continues, then the ventilation is wasted, and the region of lung serves as dead space. As discussed in Chapter 1, assuming that minute ventilation remains constant, increasing the dead space automatically decreases alveolar ventilation and hence CO_2 excretion. However, despite the potential for CO_2 retention in pulmonary embolic disease, hypercapnia is an unusual consequence of pulmonary embolus, mainly because patients routinely increase their minute ventilation after an embolus occurs and more than compensate for the increase in dead space. In fact, the usual consequence of a pulmonary embolus is hyperventilation and hypocapnia, not hypercapnia. However, if minute ventilation is fixed—for example, in an unconscious or anesthetized patient whose ventilation is controlled by a mechanical ventilator—then a rise in P_{CO_2} may result from a relatively large pulmonary embolus.

Pulmonary emboli are typically associated with hypocapnia, resulting from an increase in overall minute ventilation.

In addition to creating an area of dead space, another potential consequence of mechanical occlusion of one or more vessels is an increase in pulmonary vascular resistance. As discussed in Chapter 12, the pulmonary vascular bed is capable of recruitment and distention of vessels. It is therefore not surprising that experimental evidence indicates no increase in resistance or pressure in the pulmonary vasculature until about 50 to 70 percent of the vascular bed is occluded. The experimental model is somewhat different from the clinical setting, however, because release of chemical mediators may cause vasoconstriction and additional compromise of the pulmonary vasculature.

When there has been even further limitation of the vascular bed by the combination of mechanical occlusion and the effects of chemical mediators, the pulmonary vascular resistance and pulmonary artery pressure may rise so high that the right ventricle cannot cope with the acute increase in workload. As a result, the forward output of the right ventricle may diminish, blood pressure may fall, and the individual may have a syncopal (fainting) episode or go into hypotensive shock. In addition, "backward" failure of the right ventricle may occur, which manifests acutely with elevation of systemic venous pressure and appears on physical examination as distention of jugular veins.

The hemodynamic consequences of an acute pulmonary embolus depend to a large extent on the presence of preexisting emboli or pulmonary vascular disease. When there have been prior emboli, the right ventricular wall has already thickened (hypertrophied), and higher pressures can be maintained. On the other hand, an additional embolus in an already compromised pulmonary vascular bed may act as "the straw that broke the camel's back" and induce decompensation of the right ventricle.

In addition to the direct mechanical effects of vessel occlusion, thrombi appear to release chemical mediators that have secondary effects on both airways and blood vessels of the lung. The exact source and nature of the chemical mediators are not entirely clear. Platelets that adhere to the thrombus are presumably an important source of such mediators as histamine, serotonin, and prostaglandins. Bronchoconstriction, largely at the level of small airways, appears to be an important effect of mediator release and is thought to be an explanation for the hypoxemia that so commonly accompanies pulmonary embolism. Constriction of small airways in regions of lung that are uninvolved with emboli and have maintained blood flow leads to regions of ventilation-perfusion mismatch (low ventilation-perfusion ratio) and to hypoxemia. Whether this is the primary explanation for the hypoxemia of pulmonary embolism is unknown; however, it is a contributing factor.

> Bronchoconstriction of small airways, induced by chemical mediators released from the thrombus, may be an important mechanism of hypoxemia in pulmonary embolism.

As mentioned earlier, the chemical mediators also affect the pulmonary vasculature. Vasoconstriction of pulmonary arteries and arterioles compounds the loss of vascular bed by clot and adds to the likelihood of major vascular compromise.

Three additional features of the pathophysiology of pulmonary embolism are worth mentioning. First, as a result of vascular compromise to one or more regions of lung, synthesis of the surface-active material surfactant by alveoli in the affected region is compromised. Consequently, alveoli may be more likely to collapse, and liquid may more likely leak into alveolar spaces. Second, hypocapnia appears to have the effect of inducing secondary bronchoconstriction of small airways. With the hypocapnia that occurs in pulmonary embolus, and particularly with the low alveolar P_{CO_2} in dead space regions of lung, secondary bronchoconstriction results. Both of these mechanisms, along with the small airway constriction induced by chemical mediators, may contribute to the volume loss or atelectasis that is frequently observed in chest radiographs of patients with pulmonary embolism.

Finally, as mentioned in Chapter 12, a variety of bioactive substances are inactivated in the lung. Whether pulmonary embolism disturbs some of these nonrespiratory, metabolic functions of the lung is not clear, and whether clinical consequences might ensue from such a potential disturbance is totally unknown.

CLINICAL FEATURES

Most frequently, pulmonary embolism develops in the setting of one of the risk factors previously mentioned. Commonly, the embolus does not produce any significant symptoms, and the entire episode goes unnoticed by the patient and the physician. When the patient does have symptoms, acute onset of dyspnea is the most frequent complaint. Less common is pleuritic chest pain or hemoptysis. Syncope is an occasional presentation, particularly in the setting of a massive embolus, defined as the obstruction of two or more lobes (or their equivalent).

Symptoms of pulmonary embolism are the following:
1. Dyspnea
2. Pleuritic chest pain
3. Hemoptysis
4. Syncope

On physical examination, the most common findings are tachycardia and tachypnea. Results of chest examination may be entirely normal or may show a variety of nonspecific findings, such as decreased air entry, localized rales, or wheezing. With pulmonary infarction extending to the pleura, a pleural friction rub may be heard, as may findings of a pleural effusion. Cardiac examination may show evidence of acute right ventricular overload, i.e., acute cor pulmonale, in which case the pulmonic component of the second heart sound (P_2) is increased, a right-sided S_4 is heard, and a right ventricular heave may be present. If the right ventricle fails, a right-sided S_3 may be heard, and jugular veins may also be distended. Examination of the lower extremities may reveal changes suggesting a thrombus, including tenderness, swelling, or a cord (palpable clot within a vessel). However, as only approximately 50 percent of patients with emboli arising from leg veins have clinical evidence of deep venous thrombosis, absence of these findings should not be surprising.

DIAGNOSTIC EVALUATION

The initial diagnostic evaluation of the patient with suspected pulmonary embolism generally includes a chest radiograph and measurement of arterial blood gases. The radiographic findings in acute pulmonary embolism are quite variable. Most frequently, the radiographic findings are normal. When they are not, the abnormalities are often nonspecific, including areas of atelectasis or elevation of a hemidiaphragm, indicating volume loss. This volume loss may be related to decreased ventilation to the involved area as a result of small airways constriction and possibly loss of surfactant. In addition, if pleuritic chest pain is present, the patient may try to avoid pain by breathing more shallowly, which also contributes to atelectasis.

Occasionally, there is a localized area of decreased perfusion on the chest radiograph, corresponding to the region in which the vessel has been occluded. This finding is called *Westermark's sign* but is often difficult to read unless prior radiographs are available for comparison. With a large proximal embolus, occasionally there may be enlargement of a pulmonary artery near the hilum as a result of distention of the vessel by the clot itself. There may also be an apparent abrupt termination of the vessel, although this condition is usually difficult to see on a plain chest radiograph.

Both congestive atelectasis and infarction may appear as an opacified region on the radiograph. Classically, the density is shaped like a truncated cone, fanning out toward and reaching the pleural surface. This finding, called a *Hampton's hump*, is also relatively infrequent. Finally, pleural disease, in the form of an effusion, may also be seen as an accompaniment of pulmonary embolic disease.

Characteristic arterial blood gas values in pulmonary embolic disease are the following:

1. Decreased P_{O_2}
2. Decreased P_{CO_2}
3. Increased pH

Arterial blood gas values characteristically show hypoxemia and a respiratory alkalosis, i.e., hypocapnia. Because the P_{CO_2} is decreased, the arterial P_{O_2} appears higher than it would if hyperventilation were not present. However, if the alveolar-arterial O_2 difference (AaD_{O_2}) is calculated, it is found to be increased. Occasionally, the P_{O_2} is normal, so that the presence of a normal P_{O_2} does not exclude the diagnosis of pulmonary embolism.

Traditionally, the major screening test for pulmonary embolism has been the perfusion lung scan, described in Chapter 3. However, the diagnostic evaluation of suspected pulmonary embolism is currently in a state of transition, as contrast CT angiography is increasingly being used either instead of, or in addition to, perfusion lung scanning. Evaluation of the large veins in the lower extremities, typically using ultrasound techniques, is also a commonly used diagnostic strategy, since identification of a clot in a vein above the popliteal fossa warrants the same treatment as a documented pulmonary embolus, and often obviates the need for further evaluation.

When blood flow is obstructed by a clot within the pulmonary arterial system, perfusion lung scanning demonstrates absence of perfusion to the region of lung supplied by the occluded vessel (Fig. 13-1). If results of the scan are normal, pulmonary embolism is, for all practical purposes, excluded. Abnormalities, however, do not automatically indicate the presence of embolic disease. False-positive lung scans are common because local decreases in blood flow may result from primary disease of the parenchyma or the airways. A ventilation scan, involving inhalation of a xenon radioisotope, is often added, because if regions of decreased blood flow are secondary to airways disease, there should be corresponding abnormalities on the ventilation scan. If parenchymal disease, such as a pneumonia, is the cause of a perfusion

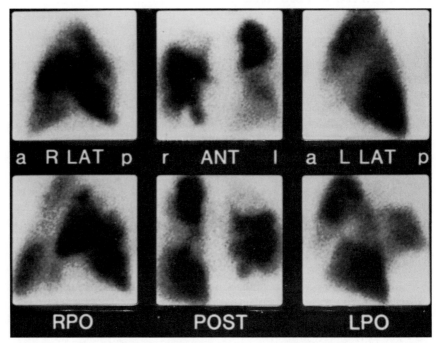

Figure 13-1 ▬— Positive results of perfusion scan shows multiple perfusion defects in patient with pulmonary emboli. Six views of complete scan are shown: right lateral (R LAT); anterior (ANT); left lateral (L LAT); right posterior oblique (RPO); posterior (POST); and left posterior oblique (LPO). a = anterior; p = posterior; r = right; l = left. Compare with normal scan results in Figure 3-11. (Courtesy of Dr. Henry Royal.)

defect, then there should be a corresponding abnormality on the chest radiograph.

Interpretation of the perfusion lung scan is a complicated process and depends on the clinical setting, the results of the chest radiograph, and frequently the findings on a ventilation lung scan. Because the perfusion scan is often not definitive, a probability is placed on the likelihood of pulmonary embolism, taking into account the size and number of defects and the presence or absence of corresponding abnormalities on the radiograph and the ventilation lung scan. The scan results are then analyzed in conjunction with the *pretest probability* of pulmonary embolism, a term that is used to represent the clinician's assessment of the likelihood of pulmonary embolism based on the patient's clinical presentation.

When the lung scan is not conclusive, it is critical that additional diagnostic evaluation be performed. As mentioned, there are different options for further work-up, focusing either on the veins of the lower extremities or on the pulmonary vasculature itself. However, because lower extremity studies are often negative even in the presence of documented pulmonary embolism, a negative lower extremity study does not preclude the need for further evaluation of the pulmonary arteries if there is a reasonably high suspicion of pulmonary thromboembolism.

Major techniques for diagnosis of pulmonary emboli include ventilation-perfusion lung scanning, pulmonary angiography, and CT angiography.

Evaluation of the pulmonary arterial system to identify intraluminal thrombus can be done somewhat invasively, using a more traditional procedure that is called pulmonary angiography and is discussed in Chapter 3. Although angiography is generally considered the "gold standard" for diagnosis of embolic disease, it also has pitfalls in interpretation and is not entirely without risk. Nevertheless, it is frequently useful, and the finding of a filling defect within a vessel or an abrupt cut-off is considered diagnostic of a pulmonary embolus (Fig. 13-2). The more recent technique of CT angiography,

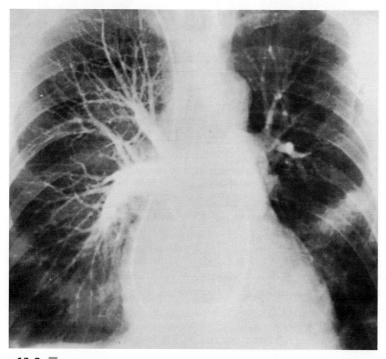

Figure 13-2 ■— Positive results of pulmonary angiogram show occlusion of vessel supplying left lower lobe. Area of density in left midlung probably represents pulmonary infarct. (Courtesy of Dr. Morris Simon.)

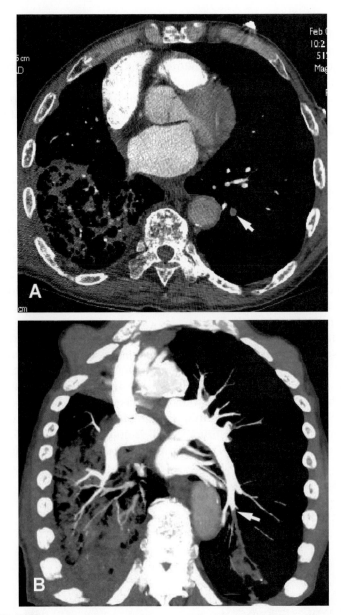

Figure 13-3 ■— Chest CT angiography demonstrating a pulmonary embolus in a midsized vessel in the left lung. *A*, Standard cross-sectional view showing a blood vessel (seen on end) filled by clot rather than radiopaque contrast dye (arrow). *B*, An image displayed in a reformatted oblique view shows the same vessel in its longitudinal course. The arrow shows the absence of radiopaque dye in the vessel at the edge of the clot. (Courtesy of Dr. Phillip Boiselle.)

also discussed in Chapter 3, is a less invasive, more conveniently performed procedure, although it is not as sensitive as traditional pulmonary angiography in detecting thrombus in smaller vessels. Nevertheless, as CT technology is continuing to improve, CT angiography is rapidly becoming a standard procedure, and is now often used in lieu of perfusion lung scanning as part of the initial diagnostic evaluation for suspected pulmonary embolism (Fig. 13-3).

An additional test that is used in some centers as part of the diagnostic strategy for venous thromboembolic disease is measurement of plasma levels of D-dimer, a degradation product of cross-linked fibrin. Plasma levels of D-dimer increase in the setting of venous thrombosis, but the test is nonspecific and the results are dependent upon the particular assay used. When D-dimer measurement is used in clinical practice, normal levels found with a sensitive assay (such as the enzyme-linked immunosorbent assay, or ELISA) are considered strong evidence against thromboembolic disease, but elevated levels are considered nonspecific and therefore nondiagnostic.

TREATMENT

The standard treatment for a pulmonary embolus involves anticoagulant therapy, initially intravenous heparin and then an oral coumarin derivative (warfarin), the latter usually given for at least 3 to 6 months. Recently, low-molecular-weight fractions of heparin, administered subcutaneously, are being used more frequently in lieu of standard, unfractionated heparin. Low-molecular-weight heparin has a number of potential advantages over unfractionated heparin, including less risk of heparin-induced thrombocytopenia. In addition, it does not need laboratory monitoring of coagulation tests to guide dosage adjustment, and it can be given subcutaneously in one or two daily doses, avoiding the need for continuous intravenous infusion.

> Options for therapy of pulmonary embolism are the following:
> 1. Anticoagulation (heparin, warfarin)
> 2. Thrombolysis (streptokinase, urokinase, t-PA)
> 3. Inferior vena caval filter

However, the rationale for the use of all anticoagulants is to prevent formation of new thrombi or propagation of old ones (in the legs), not to dissolve clots that have already embolized to the lungs. As a result, there has been a great deal of interest for years in the use of thrombolytic agents—streptokinase, urokinase, and tissue plasminogen activator (t-PA)—for treatment of pulmonary emboli. These agents, which may actually lyse recent blood clots, ideally are given within the first several days of the embolic event, but may be effective even up to two weeks following the embolus. Although the overall mortality rate is comparable whether thrombolytic agents or heparin is used for initial therapy, there may be specific subgroups of patients most likely to benefit from thrombolytic therapy, namely those patients with massive pulmonary embolus and those with hemodynamic compromise as a result of vascular occlusion. When one of these agents is used, the initial intravenous infusion of the thrombolytic agent is followed by standard anticoagulant therapy.

In some circumstances, treatment of pulmonary embolism involves placement of a filtering device into the inferior vena cava, with the goal of trapping thrombi from the lower extremities en route to the pulmonary circulation. This type of device is used most frequently if there are contraindications to anticoagulant therapy, such as bleeding problems, or if the patient already has such limited pulmonary vascular reserve that an additional clot to the lungs would be fatal.

Finally, no discussion of the treatment of pulmonary embolism is complete without a consideration of prophylactic methods used in the high-risk patient to prevent deep venous thrombosis. The most common forms of prophylaxis have traditionally been (1) external compression of the lower extremities with an intermittently inflating pneumatic device and (2) heparin administered subcutaneously in low dosage. Low-molecular-weight heparin now appears to be at least as effective and safe as low-dose unfractionated heparin. One or another method of prophylaxis is now generally used in patients about to undergo thoracic or abdominal surgery and in a variety of other high-risk patients who are at bed rest in the hospital. In the highest risk patients—those with hip fracture or hip or knee replacement surgery—either low-molecular-weight heparin or warfarin is more effective for prophylaxis than low-dose subcutaneous standard heparin.

References

General Reviews

American Thoracic Society. The diagnostic approach to acute venous thromboembolism. Clinical practice guideline. Am J Respir Crit Care Med 160:1043-1066, 1999.
Dalen JE: Pulmonary embolism: what have we learned since Virchow? Chest 122:1440-1456 and 1801-1817, 2002.
Goldhaber SZ: Pulmonary embolism. New Engl J Med 339:93-104, 1998.
Hyers TM: Venous thromboembolism. Am J Respir Crit Care Med 159:1-14, 1999.

Specific Aspects

Aguilar D and Goldhaber SZ: Clinical uses of low-molecular-weight heparins. Chest 115:1418-1423, 1999.
Arcasoy SM and Kreit JW: Thrombolytic therapy of pulmonary embolism: a comprehensive review of current evidence. Chest 115:1695-1707, 1999.
Bell WR, Simon TL, and DeMets DL: The clinical features of submassive and massive pulmonary emboli. Am J Med 62:355-360, 1977.
Dalen JE: The uncertain role of thrombolytic therapy in the treatment of pulmonary embolism. Arch Intern Med 162:2521-2523, 2002.
Elliott CG: Pulmonary physiology during pulmonary embolism. Chest 101:163S-171S, 1992.
Geerts WH et al: Prevention of venous thromboembolism. Chest 119 (Suppl):132S-175S, 2001.
Ginsberg JS: Management of venous thromboembolism. N Engl J Med 335:1816-1828, 1996.
Goldhaber SZ: Thrombolytic therapy in venous thromboembolism: clinical trials and current indications. Clin Chest Med 16:307-320, 1995.
Hillarp A, Zoller B, and Dahlback B: Activated protein C resistance as a basis for venous thrombosis. Am J Med 101:534-540, 1996.
Hirsh J and Bates SM: Clinical trials that have influenced the treatment of venous thromboembolism: a historical perspective. Ann Intern Med 134:409-417, 2001.
Hyers TM et al: Antithrombotic therapy for venous thromboembolic disease. Chest 119 (Suppl):176S-193S, 2001.
Indik JH and Alpert JS: Detection of pulmonary embolism by D-dimer assay, spiral computed tomography, and magnetic resonance imaging. Prog Cardiovasc Dis 42:261-272, 2000.
PIOPED Investigators: Value of the ventilation/perfusion scan in acute pulmonary embolism: results of the Prospective Investigation of Pulmonary Embolism Diagnosis (PIOPED). JAMA 263:2753-2759, 1990.
Rathbun SW, Raskob GE, and Whitsett TL: Sensitivity and specificity of helical computed tomography in the diagnosis of pulmonary embolism: a systematic review. Ann Intern Med 132:227-232, 2000.
Robin ED: Overdiagnosis and overtreatment of pulmonary embolism: the emperor may have no clothes. Ann Intern Med 87:775-781, 1977.
Ryu JH, Swensen SJ, Olson EJ, and Pellikka PA: Diagnosis of pulmonary embolism with use of computed tomographic angiography. Mayo Clin Proc 76:59-65, 2001.
Seligsohn U and Lubetsky A: Genetic susceptibility to venous thrombosis. N Engl J Med 344:1222-1231, 2001.

chapter **14**

Pulmonary Hypertension

Elevation of intravascular pressure within the pulmonary circulation is the hallmark of pulmonary hypertension. In this chapter, the specific reference is to elevated pulmonary arterial pressure (often defined as either a pulmonary artery systolic pressure above 40 torr, or a mean pressure above 25 torr at rest or 30 torr with exercise), although in some cases an elevation in pulmonary venous pressure is an important forerunner of pulmonary arterial hypertension. Because pulmonary hypertension has a number of causes that presumably act by several different mechanisms, this chapter begins with a consideration of features relevant to pulmonary hypertension in general and follows with a discussion of a few of the important specific causes of pulmonary hypertension.

First, clarification of two points is pertinent. As already mentioned, pulmonary hypertension merely refers to the elevation of pulmonary vascular pressure; such elevation in pressure may be acute or chronic, depending on the causative factors. In some cases, chronic pulmonary hypertension is punctuated by further acute elevations in pressure, often as a result of exacerbations of the underlying disease. Second, the development of right ventricular hypertrophy is the consequence of pulmonary hypertension, whatever the primary cause of the latter. When pulmonary hypertension is due to disorders of any part of the respiratory apparatus (airways, parenchyma and blood vessels, chest wall, respiratory musculature, or the central nervous system controller), the term *cor pulmonale* is used to refer to the resulting right ventricular hypertrophy. This term is not used to describe the right ventricular changes occurring as a consequence of primary cardiac disease or of increased flow to the pulmonary vascular bed.

PATHOGENESIS

A number of factors contribute to the pathogenesis of pulmonary arterial hypertension, both acutely and chronically. First, as mentioned in Chapter 13, occlusion of a sufficient cross-sectional area of the pulmonary arteries by material within the vessels, such as pulmonary emboli, is obviously an important factor. In acute conditions, with massive pulmonary emboli occluding more than one-half to two-thirds of the vasculature, pulmonary arterial pressure is elevated. The right ventricle may dilate as a response to its acutely increased workload, because there is insufficient time for hypertrophy. In chronic conditions, in contrast, multiple and recurrent pulmonary emboli may elevate pulmonary arterial pressures during a period sufficient for right ventricular hypertrophy to occur.

Second, diminution of cross-sectional area as a consequence of primary disease of the pulmonary arterial walls is another potential factor. Disorders acting by this mechanism are characterized by intimal and medial changes (see discussion of Pathology) leading to thickening of the arterial and arteriolar walls, and to narrowing or obliteration of the lumen. This group of disorders with primary pulmonary arterial pathology includes *primary pulmonary hypertension,* which is usually sporadic but occasionally may be familial, and pulmonary hypertension associated with other diseases (scleroderma, portal hypertension, HIV infection) or exogenous agents (drugs and toxins). Compromise of the pulmonary vasculature and increased resistance to flow may be so pronounced in these primary disorders of the vessel wall that the level of pulmonary hypertension is quite severe.

Third, the total cross-sectional area of the pulmonary vascular bed is compromised by primary parenchymal disease, with loss of blood vessels from either a scarring or a destructive process affecting the alveolar walls. Interstitial lung disease and emphysema can affect the pulmonary vasculature via this mechanism, although obviously the underlying disorder in the parenchyma appears quite different. With these diseases, it is common for pulmonary arterial pressure to be relatively normal at rest but elevated with exercise because of insufficient recruitment or distention of vessels to handle the increase in cardiac output.

A fourth and most important mechanism of pulmonary hypertension is vasoconstriction in response to hypoxia and, to a lesser extent, to acidosis. The importance of this mechanism is related to its potential reversibility when a normal PO_2 and pH value are achieved. In several causes of cor pulmonale, particularly chronic obstructive lung disease with type B physiology, hypoxia is the single most important factor leading to pulmonary hypertension and is also potentially the most treatable. As mentioned in Chapter 12, acidosis, either respiratory or metabolic, causes pulmonary vasoconstriction and, although it is less important than hypoxia, may augment the vasoconstrictive response to hypoxia.

When flow through the pulmonary vascular bed is increased, as in patients with congenital intracardiac (left-to-right) shunts, the vasculature is initially able to handle the augmented flow without any anatomic changes in the arteries or arterioles. However, over a prolonged period, there is thickening of the vessel walls, and pulmonary arterial resistance increases. Eventually, as a result of the high pulmonary vascular resistance, right-sided cardiac pressures may become so elevated that the intracardiac shunt reverses in direction. This conversion to a right-to-left shunt is commonly called *Eisenmenger's syndrome,* and it is a potentially important consequence of an atrial or ventricular septal defect or a patent ductus arteriosus.

Factors contributing to pulmonary arterial hypertension are the following:

1. Occlusion of vessels by emboli
2. Primary thickening of arterial walls
3. Loss of vessels by scarring or destruction of alveolar walls
4. Pulmonary vasoconstriction (from hypoxia, acidosis)
5. Increased pulmonary vascular flow (left-to-right shunt)
6. Elevated left atrial pressure

A final and very common mechanism of pulmonary arterial hypertension is elevation of pressure distally, in either the left atrium or the left ventricle, and progressive elevation of the "back-pressure," first in the pulmonary capillaries and then in the pulmonary arterioles and arteries. As is the case with pulmonary hypertension eventually induced by increased flow in the pulmonary vasculature, here too the initial elevation in pressure is not accompanied by anatomic changes in the pulmonary arteries. Eventually, however, structural changes are seen, and measured pulmonary vascular resistance may be substantially increased. The major disorders that result in pulmonary hypertension by this final mechanism are mitral stenosis and chronic left ventricular failure.

PATHOLOGY

In many ways the pathologic findings in the pulmonary vessels of patients with pulmonary hypertension are similar, regardless of the underlying cause. This section specifically focuses on these general changes.

The most prominent abnormalities are frequently seen in vessels of the pulmonary arterial tree whose diameter is less than 1 mm, namely the small muscular arteries (0.1 to 1 mm) and the arterioles (less than 0.1 mm). The muscular arteries show hypertrophy of the media, composed of smooth muscle, and hyperplasia of the intimal layer lining the vessel lumen. In the arterioles, a significant muscular component to the vessel wall is normally not present, but with pulmonary hypertension these vessels undergo "muscularization" of their walls (Fig. 14-1A). In addition, the arteriolar intima proliferates. As a result of these changes, the luminal diameter is significantly decreased, and the pulmonary vascular resistance is elevated. Ultimately, the lumen may be completely obliterated, and the overall number of small vessels is greatly diminished. In some cases, particularly when the pulmonary hypertension is due to primary pulmonary vascular disease or is secondary to congenital intracardiac shunts, the small arterioles may demonstrate so-called *plexiform changes,* appearing as a plexus of small slit-like vascular channels.

When pulmonary hypertension becomes marked, additional changes are commonly seen in the larger (elastic) pulmonary arteries (Fig. 14-1B). These vessels, which normally have much thinner walls than do vessels of comparable size in the systemic circulation, develop thickening of the wall, particularly in the media. They also develop the types of atherosclerotic plaques that are generally seen only in the higher pressure systemic circulation.

A secondary problem that may develop in patients with pulmonary hypertension of any cause is in situ thrombosis in the pulmonary vasculature. Presumably, endothelial damage and sluggish flow in some of the pulmonary arterial vessels can contribute to thrombus formation. The development of in situ thrombosis can worsen the degree of pulmonary hypertension by further compromising the pulmonary vascular bed.

The cardiac consequences of pulmonary hypertension are manifest pathologically as changes in the right ventricular wall. The magnitude of the changes depends primarily on the severity and chronicity of the pulmonary hypertension rather than on the nature of the underlying disorder. The major finding is concentric hypertrophy of the right ventricular wall. If the right ventricle fails as a result of the chronic increase in workload, then dilation of the right ventricle is also observed.

Pathologic features of pulmonary hypertension are the following:

1. Intimal hyperplasia and medial hypertrophy of small arteries and arterioles
2. Eventual obliteration of the lumen of small arteries and arterioles
3. Thickening of the wall of larger (elastic) pulmonary arteries
4. Right ventricular hypertrophy (with or without dilatation)

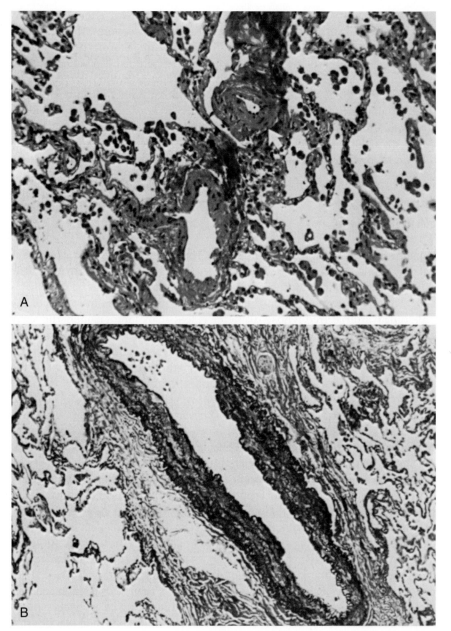

Figure 14-1 ◼— Histologic changes in pulmonary hypertension. *A*, Moderate-power photomicrograph shows thickened wall of pulmonary arteriole (*arrow*). *B*, Low-power photomicrograph (elastic tissue stain) shows thickened wall of branch of pulmonary artery. (Courtesy of Dr. Earl Kasdon.)

PATHOPHYSIOLOGY

The pathophysiologic hallmark of pulmonary hypertension is by definition an increase in pressure within the pulmonary circulation. If the primary component of the vascular change occurs at the level of the pulmonary arteries or arterioles, as is true of cor pulmonale, then the pulmonary arterial pressures (both systolic and diastolic) rise, whereas the pulmonary capillary pressure remains normal. If, on the other hand, the pulmonary arterial hypertension is secondary to pulmonary venous and pulmonary capillary hypertension, as is the case with mitral stenosis or left ventricular failure, then the pulmonary capillary pressure is obviously also elevated above its normal level.

As pulmonary hypertension progresses, the right ventricular systolic pressure rises in conjunction with the increase in pulmonary arterial systolic pressure. The cardiac output usually remains normal early in the course of the process. When the right ventricle fails, the right ventricular end-diastolic pressure rises, and the cardiac output may decrease as well. The right atrial pressure also rises, which may be apparent on physical examination of the neck veins by an elevation in the jugular venous pressure.

CLINICAL FEATURES

Although the overall constellation of symptoms in patients with pulmonary hypertension depends on the underlying disease, certain characteristic complaints can be attributed to the pulmonary hypertension itself. Dyspnea, especially on exertion, is frequently observed in all forms of pulmonary hypertension. However, in patients with pulmonary hypertension secondary to underlying lung disease, it is often difficult to know how much the pulmonary hypertension, as opposed to the underlying lung disease, is responsible for the symptom. Patients may have substernal chest pain that is difficult, if not impossible, to distinguish from classic angina pectoris, particularly because the pain is frequently precipitated by exertion. It has been presumed that the chest pain is related to the increased workload of the right ventricle and to right ventricular ischemia, as opposed to the more frequent ischemia of the left ventricle associated with coronary artery disease. In many cases, as a result of an inability to increase cardiac output with exercise, patients may experience exertional fatigue or even syncope.

Physical examination shows several features that are more related to the cardiac consequences of pulmonary hypertension than to the actual disease of the pulmonary vessels. Pulmonary hypertension itself does not cause any changes on examination of the lungs, although patients with underlying lung disease obviously often have findings related to their primary disease. On cardiac examination, patients frequently exhibit an accentuation of the component of the second heart sound due to pulmonic valve closure (P_2), which is attributable to high pressure in the pulmonary artery. With right ventricular hypertrophy, there is often a prominent lift or heave of the region immediately to the left of the lower sternum, corresponding to a prominent right ventricular impulse during systole. As the right atrium contracts and empties its contents into the poorly compliant, hypertrophied right ventricle, a presystolic gallop (S_4) originating from the right ventricle may be heard. When the right ventricle fails, a mid-diastolic gallop (S_3) in the parasternal region is frequently heard, the jugular veins become distended, and peripheral edema may develop. Occasionally, murmurs of pulmonic or tricuspid valve insufficiency may be heard.

Clinical features of pulmonary hypertension are the following:

1. Symptoms: dyspnea, substernal chest pain, fatigue, syncope
2. Physical signs: loud P_2, prominent parasternal (right ventricular) impulse, right-sided S_4; also, right-sided S_3, jugular venous distention, peripheral edema in case of right ventricular failure

DIAGNOSTIC FEATURES

Most often the status of the pulmonary vessels is initially assessed by chest radiography. With mild pulmonary hypertension originating at the arterial or arteriolar level, frequently no abnormalities are seen. As the pulmonary arterial hypertension becomes more significant, the central (hilar) pulmonary arteries increase in size, and the vessels often rapidly taper off, so that the distal vasculature appears attenuated (Fig. 14-2). With hypertrophy of the right ventricle, the cardiac silhouette may enlarge. This feature is most apparent on the lateral radiograph, which shows bulging of the anterior cardiac border.

When pulmonary hypertension is a consequence of either increased flow to the pulmonary vasculature (as in congenital heart disease with initial left-to-right shunting) or increased back-pressure from the pulmonary veins and pulmonary capillaries (as in mitral stenosis or left ventricular failure), the findings are significantly altered. In the case of congenital heart disease with left-to-right shunting, pulmonary blood flow is prominent until there is reversal of the left-to-right shunt. When there is elevation of pulmonary venous pressure from mitral stenosis or left ventricular failure, the chest radiograph often shows redistribution of blood flow from lower to upper lung zones, accompanied by evidence of interstitial or alveolar edema.

Perfusion lung scanning is frequently a valuable adjunct in the assessment of patients with pulmonary hypertension. In particular, focal perfusion defects may suggest recurrent pulmonary emboli as a likely cause for the elevation in pulmonary arterial pressure. Angiography, performed either as CT angiography or as traditional pulmonary angiography, may also be useful either instead of, or in addition to perfusion scanning, with precautions taken to avoid complications that have been reported following administration of intravenous contrast agents to patients with severe pulmonary hypertension.

Pulmonary function tests in evaluating the patient with pulmonary hypertension are useful primarily for detecting underlying airflow obstruction (from chronic obstructive lung disease) or restricted lung volumes (from inter-

Pulmonary function tests may demonstrate underlying restrictive or obstructive disease; tests may also show decrease in diffusing capacity from loss of the pulmonary vascular bed.

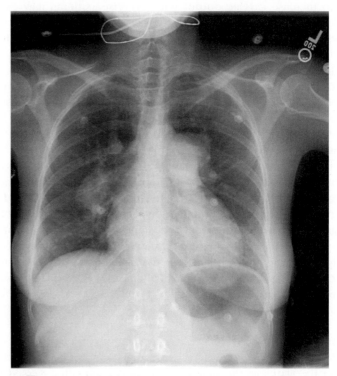

Figure 14-2 ▬— Chest radiograph of patient with pulmonary hypertension due to recurrent thromboemboli. Central pulmonary arteries are large bilaterally, but there is rapid tapering of vessels distally.

stitial lung disease). As a result of the pulmonary hypertension itself and loss of the pulmonary vascular bed, the diffusing capacity may be decreased and is often the only additional abnormality noted.

Arterial blood gas analysis is highly useful for determining whether hypoxemia or acidosis plays a role in the pathogenesis of the pulmonary hypertension. Arterial PO_2 may also be mildly decreased as a result of the pulmonary vascular disease, apparently because of nonuniform distribution of disease and ventilation-perfusion mismatch.

Echocardiography and electrocardiography may aid in the diagnosis of pulmonary hypertension by demonstrating right ventricular hypertrophy, and more sophisticated echocardiographic techniques allow estimation of pulmonary arterial pressure. Description of the specific findings is beyond the scope of this chapter but may be found in standard textbooks of cardiology.

Definitive quantitation of the degree of pulmonary hypertension is made by cardiac catheterization. In many circumstances, such evaluation is not deemed necessary. However, in circumstances such as evaluation of suspected primary pulmonary hypertension, measurements of right ventricular, pulmonary artery, and pulmonary capillary pressures are important in making the diagnosis, determining the severity of the disease, and assessing the response to acute vasodilator testing as a guide to the patient's subsequent management.

SPECIFIC DISORDERS ASSOCIATED WITH PULMONARY HYPERTENSION

Primary Pulmonary Arterial Disease: Primary Pulmonary Hypertension and Related Disorders

For purposes of our discussion here, the term primary pulmonary arterial disease can be subdivided to include two types of processes: (1) a disorder called primary pulmonary hypertension, a disease of unknown cause found most commonly in women from 20 to 40 years of age, and (2) a group of disorders with a pathologic appearance and clinical presentation similar to those of primary pulmonary hypertension, but with an accompanying process or etiologic agent known to be associated with this disease pattern. Such underlying processes or agents include connective tissue disease (particularly scleroderma), portal hypertension accompanying cirrhosis, infection with the human immunodeficiency virus (HIV), and exposure to certain drugs or toxins. In particular, several appetite suppressants have been associated with pulmonary hypertension, including aminorex (withdrawn from the market many years ago) and the drugs fenfluramine and dexfenfluramine (withdrawn from the market in 1997). It is also well recognized that chronic and recurrent pulmonary embolization can closely mimic primary pulmonary hypertension. Consequently, the diagnosis of primary pulmonary hypertension cannot be made until the presence of chronic thromboemboli has been excluded.

Primary pulmonary hypertension usually occurs as a sporadic (i.e., nonfamilial) disorder in young women, although the disease has a familial basis in approximately 6 to 10 percent of cases. Several theories have arisen about the pathogenesis of primary pulmonary hypertension, but the relative roles of each and their possible interrelationships have yet to be elucidated. One theory focuses on the importance of an imbalance between vasoconstrictor

Often, primary pulmonary hypertension appears in young women, is associated with Raynaud's syndrome, and has a poor prognosis.

and vasodilator influences on the pulmonary vasculature. According to this theory, there is an increase in such vasoconstrictors as endothelin-1 and thromboxane and/or a decrease in the vasodilators prostacyclin and nitric oxide. Interestingly, because the vasoconstrictors also act as growth factors and the vasodilators act as anti-growth factors, these mediators may be important in the vascular remodeling, i.e., the structural changes, seen in primary pulmonary hypertension. Another theory attributes importance to abnormalities in the membrane potassium channel of smooth muscle cells, subsequently leading to increased calcium influx and vasoconstriction.

Recent information about the genetic basis of familial primary pulmonary hypertension may also have relevance to the pathogenesis of the sporadic, nonfamilial cases of primary pulmonary hypertension. In familial primary pulmonary hypertension, there is a mutation in the gene for the bone morphogenetic protein receptor II (BMPR2), which acts as a receptor for transforming growth factor-β (TGF-β). It has been proposed that, under the proper conditions, the presence of the mutant BMPR2 leads to partial loss of an inhibitory effect of BMPR2 on vascular smooth muscle cell growth. The smooth muscle cell changes may then lead indirectly to endothelial cell injury and proliferation. Because some patients with nonfamilial primary pulmonary hypertension have also been reported with a mutation in BMPR2, it is reasonable to presume that this and perhaps other genetic factors may also play a role in the development of sporadic, nonfamilial primary pulmonary hypertension.

The prognosis in primary pulmonary hypertension is generally considered poor; patients frequently die within several years of diagnosis. Treatment has focused on the use of vasodilators in an attempt to reduce pulmonary arterial pressure, but the results have been inconsistent, presumably because the pathology of the disease involves structural remodeling of the vessels in addition to vasoconstriction. Unfortunately, even when there is some vasodilation of pulmonary vessels, use of these agents may be limited by dilation of systemic blood vessels and subsequent systemic arterial hypotension. Typically, before a particular vasodilator regimen is initiated, patients undergo acute vasodilator testing in the setting of a pulmonary artery catheterization, so that the effect of one or more vasodilators on pulmonary arterial pressures, cardiac output, and systemic blood pressure can be evaluated in a controlled setting.

Among the vasodilators that have been used therapeutically are the calcium channel blockers, such as nifedipine or diltiazem, which are given orally. More recently, there has been therapeutic success with continuous intravenous infusion of prostacyclin (PGI_2, also called epoprostenol), which has been associated with clinical and hemodynamic improvement as well as improved survival. In fact, the long-term effect of prostacyclin suggests that it may reverse some of the vascular remodeling and proliferative changes in the pulmonary arterial system in addition to its vasodilator effect. However, the drug is extremely expensive, and the need for continuous intravenous infusion makes it inconvenient and more logistically difficult to administer than an oral agent. Early results with an oral endothelin receptor antagonist—bosentan—have also been encouraging, but further experience is needed to assess its overall value and longer term effectiveness.

There has also been significant interest in the development of vasodilators that are selective for the pulmonary circulation, without any corresponding effect on the systemic vasculature. Inhaled nitric oxide is such an agent. It is thought to have a selective effect by virtue of reaching smooth muscle cells of pulmonary arterioles through diffusion across the alveolar-capillary membrane; subsequent binding of nitric oxide to hemoglobin leads to inactivation of the nitric oxide, thus preventing a systemic vasodilator effect. Its limitation is that it is administered by inhalation, so that it is used primarily for acute vasodilator testing or for short-term therapy, as its longer term use is impractical.

Patients with primary pulmonary hypertension are also usually placed on long-term anticoagulation therapy with warfarin. The rationale is to decrease in situ thrombosis in the pulmonary arterial system, and objective data suggest that anticoagulation may improve survival in these patients.

For some patients with debilitating disease and a poor response to therapy, combined heart-lung transplantation or lung transplantation alone has been done successfully. However, this form of therapy has very limited availability and is not a realistic option for most patients.

Chronic Pulmonary Thromboembolism

The typical presentation of chronic pulmonary thromboembolism is with symptoms and findings related to chronic pulmonary hypertension rather than with a history suggesting one or more acute episodes of pulmonary embolism. In some cases the thromboemboli are large and proximal and presumably have been occurring over months to years. In these patients, surgical removal of the proximal thrombi (thromboendarterectomy) may be a feasible therapeutic option. In other cases there is extensive thromboembolic occlusion of smaller vessels. Although it has generally been assumed that this type of small vessel occlusion is a result of multiple small pulmonary emboli, it has also been suggested that primary thrombosis of the microvasculature, perhaps secondary to endothelial damage, may be playing a role. For the small vessel or microvascular form of chronic pulmonary thromboembolism, therapy involves anticoagulation and sometimes vasodilators.

Pulmonary Hypertension Secondary to Airway or Parenchymal Lung Disease

The most common causes of cor pulmonale appear to be chronic obstructive lung disease and interstitial lung disease. In the former category, patients with type B physiology—i.e., those with a prominent component of chronic bronchitis who are considered "blue bloaters"—are particularly susceptible to development of pulmonary hypertension. Hypoxia is the single most important etiologic factor in these patients. Additional contributory factors include respiratory acidosis, which may worsen vasoconstriction; secondary polycythemia, a consequence of chronic hypoxemia, which further increases pulmonary artery pressures as a result of increased blood viscosity; and loss of pulmonary vascular bed caused by coexistent emphysema.

Any of the interstitial lung diseases, when relatively severe, may also be associated with cor pulmonale. In these patients the major contributing factors appear to be loss of vascular bed, as a result of the scarring process in the alveolar walls, and hypoxia.

In obstructive and interstitial disease, important therapy can be offered, namely correction of alveolar hypoxia and hypoxemia by administration of supplemental O_2. In these patients the goal is to maintain arterial Po_2 at a level greater than approximately 60 torr, above which hypoxic vasoconstriction is largely eliminated. Other forms of therapy aimed more specifically at the underlying disease are discussed in Chapters 6, 10, and 11.

> Obstructive disease, interstitial disease, and a variety of neural, muscular, and chest wall diseases may produce pulmonary hypertension and cor pulmonale.

In addition to these two categories of lung disease, other disorders of the respiratory apparatus associated with hypoxemia and hypercapnia may be complicated by development of cor pulmonale. Specifically, disorders of control of breathing, of the chest bellows, and of the neural apparatus controlling the chest bellows may be complicated by cor pulmonale. These disorders are discussed in more detail in Chapters 18 and 19.

Pulmonary Arterial Hypertension Associated with Pulmonary Venous Hypertension

Mitral stenosis and chronic left ventricular failure are the two disorders most frequently associated with pulmonary venous, and subsequently pulmonary arterial, hypertension. The resulting right ventricular hypertrophy is not included in the category of cor pulmonale, because the underlying problem resulting in pulmonary hypertension is clearly of cardiac, not pulmonary, origin.

With pulmonary venous hypertension, the pathologic and many of the clinical and diagnostic features are different in a relatively predictable way. Pathologically, dilated and tortuous capillaries and small veins may result from high pressures in the pulmonary veins and capillaries, along with chronic extravasation of red blood cells into the pulmonary parenchyma. In the process of handling the interstitial and alveolar hemoglobin, macrophages may become loaded with hemosiderin, a breakdown product of hemoglobin. These macrophages can be detected by appropriate staining of sputum for iron. Not infrequently, the alveolar walls have a fibrotic response, presumably secondary to the long-standing extravasation of blood, so that a component of interstitial lung disease with fibrosis may be seen.

> Long-standing pulmonary venous hypertension is associated with extravasation of erythrocytes into the pulmonary parenchyma, hemosiderin-laden macrophages, and a fibrotic interstitial response.

As mentioned earlier in the discussion of radiographic abnormalities, the presence of pulmonary venous hypertension adds several features to the chest radiograph, including redistribution of blood flow to the upper lobes and interstitial and alveolar edema. In addition, there are frequently Kerley's B lines, small horizontal lines extending to the pleura at both lung bases, which reflect thickening of or fluid in lymphatic vessels in interlobular septa, a consequence of interstitial edema.

> Radiographic evidence of pulmonary venous hypertension includes the following:
> 1. Redistribution of the blood flow to upper zones
> 2. Interstitial and alveolar edema
> 3. Kerley's B lines

Treatment of these disorders certainly revolves around attempts to "correct" the cardiac disease, or at least to decrease pulmonary venous and capillary pressures. The potential reversibility of the pulmonary arterial hypertension depends on the chronicity of the disease and the degree to which the venous hypertension can be alleviated.

References

General Reviews

Chatterjee K, DeMarco T, and Alpert JS: Pulmonary hypertension. Hemodynamic diagnosis and treatment. Arch Intern Med 162:1925-1933, 2002.

Fishman AP et al: Mechanisms of proliferative and obliterative vascular diseases. Insights from the pulmonary and systemic circulations. Am J Respir Crit Care Med 158:670-674, 1998.

Gaine S: Pulmonary hypertension. JAMA 284:3160-3168, 2000.

Hoeper MM, Galiè N, Simonneau G, and Rubin LJ: New treatments for pulmonary arterial hypertension. Am J Respir Crit Care Med 165:1209-1216, 2002.

Rubin LJ: Approach to the diagnosis and treatment of pulmonary hypertension. Chest 96:659-664, 1989.

Voelkel NF and Tuder RM: Cellular and molecular mechanisms in the pathogenesis of severe pulmonary hypertension. Eur Respir J 8:2129-2138, 1995.

Voelkel NF and Tuder RM: Severe pulmonary hypertensive diseases: a perspective. Eur Respir J 14:1246-1250, 1999.

Primary Pulmonary Hypertension and Related Disorders

Abenhaim L et al: Appetite-suppressant drugs and the risk of primary pulmonary hypertension. N Engl J Med 335:609-616, 1996.

Barst RJ et al: A comparison of continuous intravenous epoprostenol (prostacyclin) with conventional therapy for primary pulmonary hypertension. N Engl J Med 334:296-301, 1996.

Eddahibi S, et al: Pathobiology of pulmonary arterial hypertension. Eur Respir J 20:1559-1572, 2002.

Fishman AP: Epoprostenol (prostacyclin) and pulmonary hypertension. Ann Intern Med 132:500-502, 2000.

Gaine SP and Rubin LJ: Primary pulmonary hypertension. Lancet 352:719-725, 1998.

Hoeper MM: Pulmonary hypertension in collagen vascular disease. Eur Respir J 19:571-576, 2002.

Hughes JD and Rubin LJ: Primary pulmonary hypertension: an analysis of 28 cases and a review of the literature. Medicine 65:56-72, 1986.

Kuo PC et al: Distinctive clinical features of portopulmonary hypertension. Chest 112:980-986, 1997.

Loscalzo J: Genetic clues to the cause of primary pulmonary hypertension. N Engl J Med 345:367-371, 2001.

Peacock AJ: Primary pulmonary hypertension. Thorax 54:1107-1118, 1999.

Pepke-Zaba J et al: Inhaled nitric oxide as a cause of selective pulmonary vasodilatation in pulmonary hypertension. Lancet 338:1173-1174, 1991.

Rich S: Executive summary of the World Symposium on PPH. 1999. Available at: http://www.who.int/ncd/cvd/pph.html.

Rich S et al: Primary pulmonary hypertension: a national prospective study. Ann Intern Med 107:216-223, 1987.

Rubin LJ: Primary pulmonary hypertension. N Engl J Med 336:111-117, 1997.

Rubin LJ et al: Bosentan therapy for pulmonary arterial hypertension. N Engl J Med 346:896-903, 2002.

Rudarakanchana N, Trembath RC, and Morrell NW: New insights into the pathogenesis and treatment of primary pulmonary hypertension. Thorax 56:888-890, 2001.

Speich R et al: Primary pulmonary hypertension in HIV infection. 100:1268-1271, 1991.

Voelkel NF, Clarke WR, and Higenbottam T: Obesity, dexfenfluramine, and pulmonary hypertension. Am J Respir Crit Care Med 155:786-788, 1997.

Chronic Pulmonary Thromboembolism

Fedullo PF et al: Chronic thromboembolic pulmonary hypertension. Clin Chest Med 16:353-374, 1995.

Fedullo PF, Auger WR, Kerr KM, and Rubin LJ: Chronic thromboembolic pulmonary hypertension. N Engl J Med 345:1465-1472, 2001.

Rich S, Levitsky S, and Brundage BH: Pulmonary hypertension from chronic pulmonary thromboembolism. Ann Intern Med 108:425-434, 1988.

Pulmonary Hypertension Associated with Cardiac Disease

Cortese DA: Pulmonary function in mitral stenosis. Mayo Clin Proc 53:321-326, 1978.

Dalen JE et al: Early reduction of pulmonary vascular resistance after mitral-valve replacement. N Engl J Med 277:387-394, 1967.

Dexter L: Pulmonary vascular disease in acquired and congenital heart disease. Arch Intern Med 139:922-928, 1979.

Cor Pulmonale

Fishman AP: Chronic cor pulmonale. Am Rev Respir Dis 114:775-794, 1976.

MacNee W: Pathophysiology of cor pulmonale in chronic obstructive pulmonary disease. Am J Respir Crit Care Med 150:833-852 and 1158-1168, 1994.

Palevsky HI and Fishman AP: Chronic cor pulmonale: etiology and management. JAMA 263:2347-2353, 1990.

Pleural Disease

In moving from the lung to other structures that are part of the process of respiration, the adjacent pleura is considered next. In clinical medicine, the pleura is important not only because diseases of the lung commonly cause secondary abnormalities in the pleura, but also because it is a major site of disease in its own right. Not infrequently, pleural disease is a manifestation of a multisystem process that is inflammatory, immune, or malignant.

In this chapter, a discussion of the anatomy of the pleura is followed, first, by presentation of a few physiologic principles concerning fluid formation and absorption by the pleura and, second, by discussion of two types of abnormalities that affect the pleura: liquid in the pleural space (pleural effusion) and air in the pleural space (pneumothorax). A comprehensive treatment of all the disorders that affect the pleura is beyond the scope of this text. Rather, the purpose is to cover the major categories and to give the reader an understanding of the way in which different factors interact in the production of pleural disease. The primary malignancy of the pleura, called *mesothelioma,* is discussed in Chapter 21, which deals with neoplastic disease.

ANATOMY

The term *pleura* refers to the thin lining layer on the outer surface of the lung (*visceral pleura*), the corresponding lining layer on the inner surface of the chest wall (*parietal pleura*), and the space between them (the *pleural space*) (Fig. 15-1). Because the visceral and parietal pleural surfaces normally touch each other, the space between them is only a potential space; it contains a thin layer of serous fluid coating the apposing surfaces. When air or a larger amount of fluid accumulates in the pleural space, the visceral and parietal pleural surfaces are separated, and the fact that there is a space between the lung and the chest wall becomes more apparent.

The pleura lines not only those surfaces of the lung that are in direct contact with the chest wall, but also the diaphragmatic and mediastinal borders of the lung. These surfaces are called the *diaphragmatic* and

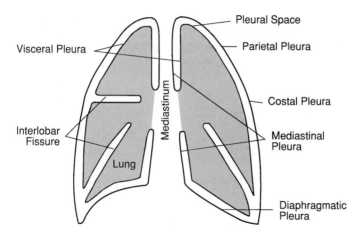

Figure 15-1 ■— Anatomic features of pleura. Pleural space is located between visceral and parietal pleural surfaces. Pleura lines surfaces of lung in contact with chest wall (costal pleura) and mediastinal and diaphragmatic borders (mediastinal and diaphragmatic pleura, respectively). (From Lowell JR: Pleural Effusions: A Comprehensive Review. Baltimore, University Park Press, 1977, p 7.)

mediastinal pleura, respectively (see Fig. 15-1). Visceral pleura also separates the lobes of the lung from each other; therefore, the major and minor fissures are defined by two apposing visceral pleural surfaces.

Each of the two pleural surfaces, visceral and parietal, is a thin membrane, the surface of which consists of specific lining cells called *mesothelial cells.* Beneath the mesothelial cell layer is a thin layer of connective tissue. Blood vessels and lymphatic vessels course throughout the connective tissue and are important in the dynamics of liquid formation and resorption in the pleural space. On the parietal but not on the visceral pleural surface, openings called *stomas* are located between the mesothelial cells. These stomas lead to lymphatic channels, allowing a passageway for liquid from the pleural space to the lymphatic system. There are also some sensory nerve endings in the parietal and diaphragmatic pleura that are apparently responsible for the characteristic "pleuritic chest pain" arising from the pleura.

The blood vessels supplying the parietal pleural surface originate from the systemic arterial circulation, primarily the intercostal arteries. Venous blood from the parietal pleura drains to the systemic venous system. The visceral pleura is also supplied primarily by systemic arteries, specifically branches of the bronchial arterial circulation. However, unlike the parietal pleura, the visceral pleura has its venous drainage into the pulmonary venous system. Depending on their location, the lymphatic vessels that drain the pleural surfaces transport their fluid contents to different lymph nodes. Ultimately, any liquid transported by the lymphatic channels finds its way to the right lymphatic or thoracic ducts, which empty into the systemic venous circulation.

PHYSIOLOGY

The pleural space normally contains only a small quantity of liquid, approximately 10 mL or so, which lubricates the apposing surfaces of the visceral and parietal pleurae. According to the current concept of pleural fluid formation and resorption, there is ongoing formation of fluid primarily from the parietal pleural surface, and fluid is resorbed through the stomas into the lymphatic channels of the parietal pleura (Fig. 15-2). The normal rates of formation and resorption of fluid, which must be equal if the quantity of fluid within the pleural space is not changing, are believed to be approximately 15 to 20 mL/d.

The normally occurring liquid in the pleural space is an ultrafiltrate from the pleural capillaries. Several different forces either promote or oppose fluid filtration, and the net movement of fluid from the pleural capillaries to the pleural space depends on the magnitude of these counterbalancing forces. For capillaries adjacent to a pericapillary space, the hydrostatic pressure in the capillary promotes movement of fluid out of the vessel and into the pericapillary space, whereas the colloid osmotic pressure (the osmotic pressure exerted by protein drawing in fluid) hinders movement of liquid out of the capillary. Likewise, hydrostatic and colloid osmotic pressures in the pericapillary space comprise the opposing forces that act on liquid within the pericapillary region.

The effect of these forces is summarized in the Starling equation, which describes the movement of fluid between vascular and extravascular compartments of any part of the body, not just the pleura.

$$\text{Fluid movement} = K[(P_c - P_{is}) - \sigma(COP_c - COP_{is})]$$

where K = filtration coefficient (a function of the permeability of the pleural surface), P = hydrostatic pressure, COP = colloid osmotic pressure, σ is a

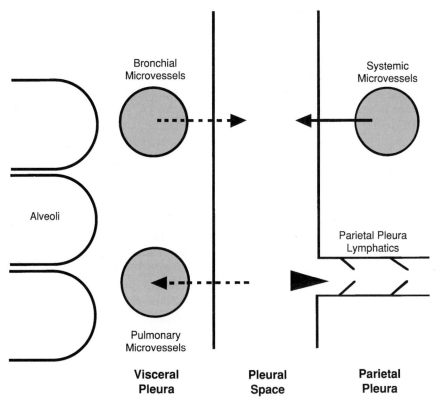

Figure 15-2 ■— Schematic diagram of normal filtration and resorption of fluid in pleural space. Solid arrow shows filtration of fluid from parietal pleural microvessels into pleural space. Arrowhead indicates removal of fluid through stomas and into parietal pleural lymphatics. Dashed arrows indicate a minor role for filtration and resorption of fluid by visceral pleural microvessels. (Adapted from Pistolesi M, Miniati M, and Giuntini C: Am Rev Respir Dis 140:825-847, 1989.)

measure of capillary permeability to protein (called the reflection coefficient), and the subscripts "c" and "is" refer to the capillary and the pericapillary interstitial space, respectively. In this case the pericapillary interstitial space is essentially the pleural space, and P_{is} and COP_{is} therefore refer to intrapleural pressure and the colloid osmotic pressure of pleural fluid, respectively. The intrapleural pressure—that is, the hydrostatic pressure within the pleural space—is negative, reflecting the outward elastic recoil of the chest wall and the inward elastic recoil of the lung.

When values obtained by direct measurement or by estimation are put into the Starling equation, it is found that there is a net pressure of approximately 9 cm H_2O favoring movement of fluid from the parietal pleura to the pleural space. The critical factor responsible for the forces favoring formation of pleural fluid is the difference between the positive hydrostatic pressure in the pleural capillaries and the negative hydrostatic pressure in the pleural space.

Applying the same equation to fluid filtration from the visceral pleura is more difficult. The visceral pleural capillaries are supplied by the systemic arterial circulation but are drained into the pulmonary venous rather than the systemic venous circulation. Although currently unknown, the hydrostatic pressure in the visceral pleural capillaries is estimated to be less than in the parietal pleural capillaries. As a result the driving pressure for the formation of pleural fluid is normally greater at the parietal than at the visceral pleural surface, and most of the small amount of normal pleural fluid is thought to originate from filtration through capillaries of the parietal pleura.

Resorption of pleural fluid, including protein and cells in the fluid, occurs through the stomas between mesothelial cells on the parietal pleural surface. The fluid enters lymphatic channels, and valves within these channels ensure unidirectional flow. Movement of fluid through the valved lymphatics is believed to be aided by respiratory motion. When pleural fluid formation is increased, as occurs in many of the pathologic states to be discussed, the parietal pleural lymphatics are capable of increasing their flow substantially to accommodate at least some of the excess fluid formed.

> The Starling equation can be applied to the parietal pleura:
>
> P_c = 30 cm H_2O
> P_{is} (mean intrapleural pressure) = −5 cm H_2O
> COP_c = 32 cm H_2O
> COP_{is} = 6 cm H_2O
> σ = 1, K = 1

> Fluid movement at parietal pleura = [30 − (−5)] − 1(32 − 6) = 9 cm H_2O

> Pleural fluid is filtered from the parietal pleura into the pleural space and reabsorbed through stomas into the parietal pleural lymphatics.

PLEURAL EFFUSION

In the normal individual, resorption of pleural fluid maintains pace with pleural fluid formation so that fluid does not accumulate. However, a variety of diseases affect the forces governing pleural fluid filtration and resorption, resulting in fluid formation exceeding fluid removal, that is, development of pleural effusion. The pathogenesis (dynamics) of fluid accumulation is discussed first, followed by a consideration of some of the etiologic factors, clinical features, and diagnostic approaches to pleural effusions.

Pathogenesis of Pleural Fluid Accumulation

In theory, a change in the magnitude of any of the factors in the Starling equation can cause sufficient imbalance of pleural fluid dynamics to result in pleural fluid accumulation. In practice, it is easiest to divide these changes into the following two categories: (1) alteration of the permeability of the pleural surface, i.e., changes in the filtration coefficient (K) and the reflection coefficient (σ) so that the pleura is more permeable to fluid and to larger molecular-weight components of blood; and (2) alteration in the driving pressure, encompassing a change in hydrostatic or colloid osmotic pressures of the parietal or visceral pleura, without any change in pleural permeability.

The most common types of disease causing a change in the filtration and reflection coefficients are inflammatory or neoplastic diseases involving the pleura. In these circumstances the pleural surface is more permeable to proteins, so that the accumulated fluid has a relatively high protein content. This type of fluid, because of a change in permeability and its association with a relatively high protein content, is termed an *exudate*.

In contrast, an increase in hydrostatic pressure within pleural capillaries (e.g., as might be seen in congestive heart failure) or a decrease in plasma colloid osmotic pressure (as in hypoproteinemia) results in accumulation of fluid with a low protein content, because the pleural barrier is still relatively impermeable to proteins. This type of fluid, because of a change in the driving pressure (without increased permeability) and the presence of a low protein content, is termed a *transudate*.

Another general mechanism accounting for some pleural effusions reflects neither altered permeability nor altered driving pressure. Rather, the fluid originates in the peritoneum as ascitic fluid and travels to the pleural space primarily via small diaphragmatic defects and perhaps also by diaphragmatic lymphatics. Considering that intrapleural pressure is more negative than intraperitoneal pressure, it is not surprising that fluid moves from the peritoneum to the pleural space when such defects exist.

Finally, interference with the resorptive process for pleural fluid can contribute to the development of effusions. This is seen primarily with blockage of the lymphatic drainage from the pleural space, as may occur when tumor cells invade the lymphatic channels or the draining lymph nodes.

Increased permeability of the pleural surface is associated with exudative pleural fluid; changes in pleural hydrostatic or colloid osmotic pressures are associated with transudative pleural fluid.

Etiology of Pleural Effusion

The numerous causes of pleural fluid accumulation are best divided into transudative and exudative categories (Table 15-1). As will be discussed, this distinction is generally easy to make and is most important in guiding the physician along the best route for further evaluation. Transudative fluid usually implies that the pathologic process is not one primarily involving the pleural surfaces, whereas exudative fluid often suggests that the pleura is affected by the disease process causing the effusion.

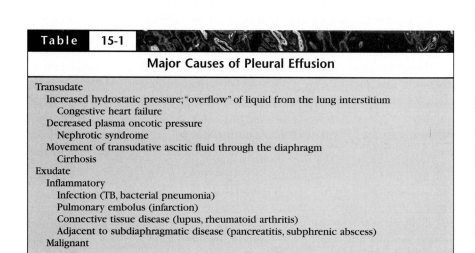

Table 15-1
Major Causes of Pleural Effusion

Transudate
  Increased hydrostatic pressure; "overflow" of liquid from the lung interstitium
    Congestive heart failure
  Decreased plasma oncotic pressure
    Nephrotic syndrome
  Movement of transudative ascitic fluid through the diaphragm
    Cirrhosis
Exudate
  Inflammatory
    Infection (TB, bacterial pneumonia)
    Pulmonary embolus (infarction)
    Connective tissue disease (lupus, rheumatoid arthritis)
    Adjacent to subdiaphragmatic disease (pancreatitis, subphrenic abscess)
  Malignant

Transudative Pleural Fluid

Most frequently, transudative pleural fluid is associated with congestive heart failure. Although the traditional explanation had been that an elevation of hydrostatic pressure in the pleural capillaries was responsible for increased flux of fluid from these vessels into the pleural space, recent data suggest an alternative explanation. The source of pleural fluid in congestive heart failure appears primarily to be liquid accumulating in the lung interstitium, which then leaks across the visceral pleura and into the pleural space, akin to leakage of fluid from the surface of a wet sponge. On the basis of clinical studies, pulmonary venous hypertension (with left-sided heart failure) appears to be a more important factor contributing to effusions than is systemic venous hypertension (with right-sided failure). Pleural effusion is particularly likely to occur when both ventricles have failed and pulmonary and systemic venous hypertension coexist.

Patients with hypoproteinemia have decreased plasma colloid osmotic pressure, and pleural fluid may develop because hydrostatic pressure in pleural capillaries is now less opposed by the osmotic pressure provided by plasma proteins. The most common circumstance resulting in hypoproteinemia and pleural effusion is nephrotic syndrome, with excessive renal losses of protein.

Movement of transudative ascitic fluid through diaphragmatic defects and into the pleural space appears to be the most important mechanism for the pleural effusions sometimes seen in liver disease, especially cirrhosis. Although these patients may also have decreased hepatic synthesis of protein, hypoproteinemia has only a minor role in the pathogenesis of these effusions.

> Ascitic fluid may travel through diaphragmatic defects into the pleural space.

Exudative Pleural Fluid

Exudative pleural fluid generally implies an increase in the permeability of the pleural surfaces, so that protein and fluid more readily enter the pleural space. Although a wide variety of processes can result in exudative pleural effusions, the two main etiologic categories are inflammatory and neoplastic disease. The inflammatory processes often originate within the lung but extend to the visceral pleural surface. Infection (especially bacterial pneumonia and tuberculosis) and pulmonary embolus (often with infarction) are two common examples. In the case of pneumonia extending to the pleural surface, an associated pleural effusion is called a *parapneumonic effusion.* When the effusion itself harbors organisms or when it has the appearance of pus (as a result of an exuberant inflammatory response with many thousands of neutrophils), then the effusion is called an *empyema.* Although infection within the pleural space is commonly secondary to a pneumonia, empyema may also result from infection introduced through the chest wall, as in trauma or surgery involving the thorax.

In tuberculosis there may be rupture of a subpleural focus of infection into the pleural space, after which an inflammatory response of the pleura ensues (with or without growth of the tubercle bacilli within the pleural space). In some cases the pulmonary focus is not apparent, and pleural involvement is the major manifestation of tuberculosis within the thorax.

Other forms of inflammatory disease affecting the pleura primarily involve the pleural surface as opposed to the lung. Several of the connective tissue diseases, particularly systemic lupus erythematosus and rheumatoid arthritis, are associated with pleural involvement that is independent of changes within the pulmonary parenchyma. Inflammatory processes below the diaphragm, such as pancreatitis and subphrenic abscess, are often accompanied by "sympathetic" pleural inflammation and development of an exudative pleural effusion.

With these disorders, inflammation of the diaphragm itself may lead to increased permeability of vessels in the diaphragmatic pleura and leakage of fluid into the pleural space. When ascites is present, as is common in pancreatitis, transport of fluid from the abdomen through defects in the diaphragm may also contribute to pleural fluid accumulation.

Malignancy may cause pleural effusion by several mechanisms, but the resulting fluid is generally exudative in nature. Commonly, malignant cells are found on the pleural surface, arriving there either by direct extension from an intrapulmonary malignancy or by hematogenous (blood-stream) dissemination from a distant source. In other cases, lymphatic channels or lymph nodes are blocked by foci of tumor so that the normal lymphatic clearance mechanism for protein and fluid from the pleural space is impaired. In these latter cases, malignant cells are generally not found on examination of the pleural fluid.

A host of other disorders may have pleural effusion as a clinical manifestation. The list includes such varied processes as hypothyroidism, benign ovarian tumors (Meigs' syndrome), asbestos exposure, and primary disorders of the lymphatic channels. Detailed discussion of the various disorders with potential for pleural fluid accumulation may be found in references listed at the end of this chapter.

Clinical Features

A patient with pleural fluid may or may not have symptoms caused by the pleural disease. Whether symptoms are present depends on the size of the effusion(s) and the nature of the underlying process. The inflammatory processes affecting the pleura frequently result in pleuritic chest pain, i.e., a sharp pain aggravated by respiration. When an effusion is quite large, patients may experience dyspnea resulting from compromise of the underlying lung. With small or moderate-sized effusions, a patient with otherwise normal lungs generally does not have dyspnea just from the presence of fluid in the pleural space. When the pleural fluid has an inflammatory nature or is frankly infected, fever is also commonly present.

Common clinical features with pleural effusion(s) are the following:
Symptoms: pleuritic chest pain, dyspnea
Physical signs: dullness, decreased breath sounds, egophony at upper level, pleural friction rub

On physical examination of the chest, the region overlying the effusion is dull to percussion. Breath sounds are also usually decreased in this region as a result of decreased transmission of sound through the fluid medium in the pleura. At the upper level of the effusion, egophony may sometimes be heard as a manifestation of increased transmission of sound resulting from compression (atelectasis) of the underlying lung parenchyma. A scratchy, pleural friction rub may be present, particularly with an inflammatory process involving the pleural surfaces.

Diagnostic Approach

The posteroanterior and lateral chest radiographs are clearly most important in the initial evaluation of the patient with suspected pleural effusion (Fig. 15-3). With a small effusion, blunting of the normally sharp angle between the diaphragm and the chest wall (costophrenic angle) is seen. Often this blunting is first apparent on inspection of the posterior costophrenic angle on the lateral radiograph, because this is the most dependent area of the pleural space. With a larger effusion, a homogeneous opacity of liquid density appears and is most obvious at the lung base(s) when the patient is upright. The fluid may also track along the lateral chest wall, forming a meniscus.

When certain inflammatory effusions persist for a time, fluid may no longer be free-flowing within the pleural space, as fibrous bands of tissue

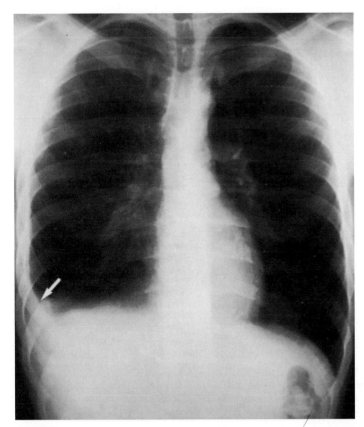

Figure 15-3 ■ Chest radiograph shows small right pleural effusion. Right costophrenic angle is blunted by the effusion (*arrow*). Curvature of lateral rib overlies meniscus of pleural fluid.

(loculations) form within the pleura. In such circumstances, fluid is not necessarily positioned as one would expect from the effects of gravity, and atypical appearances may be found. To detect whether fluid is free-flowing or whether small costophrenic angle densities represent pleural fluid, a lateral decubitus chest radiograph may be extremely useful. In this view, the patient lies on a side, and free-flowing fluid shifts position to line the most dependent part of the pleural space (Fig. 15-4).

Another technique frequently used to evaluate the presence and location of pleural fluid is ultrasonography. When pleural fluid is present, a characteristic echo-free space can be detected between the chest wall and lung. Ultrasonography is particularly useful in locating a small effusion not apparent on physical examination and in guiding the physician to a suitable site for thoracentesis.

When pleural fluid is present and the etiologic diagnosis is uncertain, sampling the fluid by thoracentesis (withdrawal of fluid by a needle or catheter) allows determination of the cellular and chemical characteristics of the fluid. These features define whether it is transudative or exudative and frequently give other clues about the cause. Although different criteria have been used, the most common criteria include the levels of protein and of the enzyme lactic dehydrogenase (LDH) within the fluid, both in absolute numbers and relative to the corresponding values in serum. Exudative fluid has high levels of protein or LDH, or both, whereas transudative fluid is associated with low levels of both.

An exudative effusion is defined by one or more of the following:

1. Pleural fluid/serum protein ratio >0.5
2. Pleural fluid/serum LDH ratio >0.6
3. Pleural fluid LDH >$\frac{2}{3}$ × upper limit of normal serum LDH

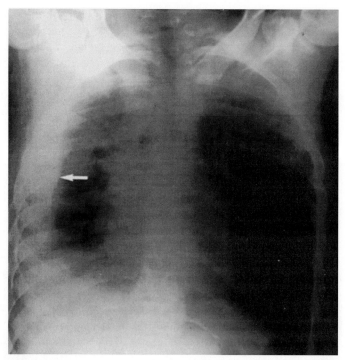

Figure 15-4 ■— Right lateral decubitus chest radiograph of patient in Figure 15-3. With the patient lying on right side, pleural fluid (*arrow*) flows freely to dependent part of pleural space adjacent to right lateral chest wall. Film is shown upright for convenience of comparison with Figure 15-3.

Pleural fluid obtained by thoracentesis is also routinely analyzed for absolute numbers and types of cellular constituents, for bacteria (by stains and cultures), and for glucose level. In many cases, amylase level and pH value of the pleural fluid are also measured. Special slides are prepared for cytologic examination, and a search for malignant cells is made. Detailed discussions of the findings in different disorders are in the references at the end of this chapter.

In some cases, pleural tissue is sampled by pleural biopsy, generally performed with a relatively large cutting needle inserted through the skin of the chest wall. Histologic examination of this tissue is useful for demonstrating granulomas of tuberculosis or implants of tumor cells from a malignant process. Pleural tissue may also be obtained under direct vision with the aid of a thoracoscope passed through the chest wall and into the pleural space.

Pulmonary function tests are generally not part of the routine evaluation of patients with pleural effusion. However, a significant effusion may impair lung expansion sufficiently to cause a restrictive pattern (with decreased lung volumes) on pulmonary function testing.

Treatment

The treatment of pleural effusion depends entirely on the nature of the underlying process and is usually directed at this process rather than at the effusion itself. In cases in which there is a high likelihood that the effusion will eventuate in extensive fibrosis or loculation of the pleural space—for example, with an empyema or a hemothorax (blood in the pleural space, often secondary to trauma)—the fluid is drained with a catheter or a relatively large-bore tube inserted into the pleural space. If loculation has already occurred, then thoracoscopy or an open surgical approach may be necessary to break up fibrous adhesions and allow effective drainage of the fluid.

In other cases in which there are recurrent large effusions, especially those caused by malignancy, the fluid is initially drained with a tube that is passed into the pleural space, and an irritating agent (e.g., talc or a tetracycline derivative) is instilled via the tube into the pleural space to induce inflammation and to cause the visceral and parietal pleural surfaces to become adherent. This process of sclerosis (also called *pleurodesis*) eliminates the pleural space and, if effective, prevents recurrence of pleural effusion on the side where the procedure was performed.

PNEUMOTHORAX

Air is not normally present between the visceral and parietal pleural surfaces. However, air can be introduced into the pleural space by a break in the surface of either pleural membrane, thus creating a *pneumothorax.* Because pressure within the pleural space is subatmospheric, air readily enters the space if there is any communication with air at atmospheric pressure.

Etiology and Pathogenesis

When a pneumothorax is created by the entry of air through the chest wall and the parietal pleura, the most common causes are (1) trauma (such as a knife or gunshot wound) and (2) introduction of air (either intentionally or unintentionally) via a needle or catheter inserted through the chest wall and into the pleural space. Alternatively, air may enter the pleura through a break in the visceral pleura, allowing communication between the airways or alveoli and the pleural space. Examples of the latter circumstance include rupture of a subpleural air pocket (such as a bleb, cyst, or bulla) into the pleural space or necrosis of the lung adjacent to the pleura by a destructive pneumonia or neoplasm.

A pneumothorax can result from a break in the parietal pleura (e.g., from trauma, needle or catheter insertion) or in the visceral pleura (e.g., from rupture of a subpleural air pocket, necrosis of lung adjacent to the pleura).

In some cases a reason for the pneumothorax is apparent, such as an underlying abnormality in the lung, a form of lung disease known to be associated with subpleural air pockets (emphysema or interstitial lung disease with honeycombing and subpleural cysts), or destruction of lung tissue adjacent to the pleural surface (necrotizing pneumonia or neoplasm). Pneumothorax in these clinical settings is said to be secondary to the known lung disease. In patients with acquired immunodeficiency syndrome, pneumothorax can develop as a complication of pulmonary infection with *Pneumocystis carinii,* presumably due to necrosis or cyst formation adjacent to the visceral pleura.

In contrast, other patients do not have a defined abnormality of the lung adjacent to the pleura and therefore are said to have a *primary spontaneous pneumothorax.* Even in this latter circumstance, there are frequently small subpleural pockets of air (blebs), especially at the lung apex, that have gone unrecognized clinically and on routine radiographic examination. If the bleb eventually ruptures, air is released from the lung parenchyma into the pleural space, creating a pneumothorax.

Patients who receive positive pressure to their tracheobronchial tree and alveoli—for example, with mechanical ventilation—are also subject to development of a pneumothorax. In this case, as a result of positive pressure, a preexisting subpleural bleb may rupture, or air may rupture through an alveolar wall into the interstitial space, track through the lung parenchyma to the subpleural surface, and then rupture into the pleural space. Alternatively, and perhaps more commonly, the air following alveolar rupture tracks retrograde to the mediastinum alongside blood vessels and airways, and produces a pneumomediastinum (see Chapter 16). A pneumothorax can then result when air ruptures through the mediastinal pleura into the pleural space.

Pathophysiology

The pathophysiologic consequences of a pneumothorax are variable, ranging from none to the development of acute cardiovascular collapse. The size of the pneumothorax—the amount of air within the pleural space—is an important determinant of the clinical effects. Because the lung is enclosed within a relatively rigid chest wall, accumulation of a substantial amount of pleural air is accompanied by collapse of the underlying lung parenchyma. In extreme cases, air in the pleural space occupies almost the entire hemithorax, and the lung is totally collapsed and functionless until the air is resorbed or removed.

A tension pneumothorax may be associated with total collapse of the underlying lung, mediastinal shift, and cardiovascular collapse.

Air in the pleural space is generally under atmospheric or subatmospheric pressure. In some cases the air may be under positive pressure, creating a *tension pneumothorax*. This tension within the pleural space is believed to occur as a result of a "check-valve" mechanism, by which air is free to enter the pleural space during inspiration, but the site of entry is closed during expiration. Therefore, only one-way movement of air into the pleural space is permitted, the intrapleural pressure increases, and the underlying lung collapses further. When pleural pressure is sufficiently high, the mediastinum and trachea may be shifted away from the side of the pneumothorax. In extreme cases, cardiovascular collapse may result, with a marked fall in cardiac output and blood pressure. It is commonly stated that these hemodynamic changes are due to inhibition of venous return into the superior and inferior venae cavae as a consequence of the positive intrathoracic pressure. However, an alternative explanation is that marked disturbances in gas-exchange are responsible for the hemodynamic changes. Whatever the mechanism, emergent treatment is necessary to release the air under tension and reverse the cardiovascular collapse. A particularly important risk factor for the development of a tension pneumothorax is positive pressure ventilation with a mechanical ventilator. When a pneumothorax occurs in this situation, the ventilator may continue to introduce air under high pressure through the site of rupture in the visceral pleura.

For most cases of pneumothorax, once the site of entry into the pleural space is closed, the air is spontaneously resorbed. The reason is that the partial pressure of air in a pneumothorax is higher than the partial pressure of gas in surrounding venous or capillary blood. For example, air within the pleural space might have a pressure a few torr below atmospheric, or approximately 755 to 758 torr. In contrast, gas pressures in mixed venous blood are approximately as follows: $P_{O_2} = 40$ torr, $P_{CO_2} = 46$ torr, $P_{N_2} = 573$ torr, and $P_{H_2O} = 47$ torr. The total gas pressure in mixed venous blood therefore is 706 torr, which is approximately 50 torr below that of air in the pleural space. Consequently, there is a gradient for diffusion of gas from the pleural space into mixed venous blood. With continued diffusion of gas in this direction, the size of the pneumothorax is slowly reduced, the gas pressures within the pleural space are maintained, and the gradient favoring absorption of gas continues until all the air is resorbed.

If pure O_2 is administered to the patient with a pneumothorax, the process of resorption can be hastened. In arterial blood, most of the nitrogen is replaced by O_2. As a result, the P_{N_2} in the capillary blood surrounding the pneumothorax becomes quite low, and the gradient for resorption of nitrogen from the pleural space has been increased considerably. At the same time, although the arterial P_{O_2} is high after inhalation of pure O_2, the P_{O_2} falls substantially in capillary and venous blood because of O_2 consumption by the tissues. Therefore, a large partial pressure gradient from pleural gas to pleural capillary blood is present for O_2 as well. The net result is that O_2 administration favors more rapid resorption of nitrogen (the main component of gas in the pneumothorax) without compromising the gradient promoting resorption of O_2.

Obviously, when a pneumothorax is causing significant clinical problems, the physician need not wait for spontaneous resorption of the air but can actively remove the air with a needle, catheter, or tube inserted into the pleural space.

Clinical Features

In many cases the clinical setting is appropriate for the development of a pneumothorax; for example, the patient may have predisposing underlying lung disease or may be receiving positive pressure ventilation with a mechanical ventilator. Interestingly, in the group of patients in whom a primary spontaneous pneumothorax develops, there is a striking predominance of males. In addition, the patients are often smokers, young adults, and frequently are tall and thin.

Clinical features of pneumothorax are the following:
Symptoms: chest pain, dyspnea
Physical signs: asymmetric (decreased) breath sounds, hyperresonance, tracheal deviation (tension), ↓ blood pressure (tension)

The most common complaint at the time of pneumothorax is the acute onset of chest pain or dyspnea, or both. However, some patients may be totally free of symptoms, particularly if the pneumothorax is small. On physical examination the findings depend to a large extent on the size of the pneumothorax. Because of decreased transmission of sound, breath sounds and tactile fremitus are diminished or absent. With a significant amount of air in the pleural space, there may be increased resonance to percussion over the affected lung.

When the pneumothorax is under tension, the patient is often in acute distress, and a decrease in blood pressure or even frank cardiovascular collapse may be present. Palpation of the trachea frequently demonstrates deviation away from the side of the pneumothorax.

Diagnostic Approach

The diagnosis of pneumothorax is made or confirmed by chest radiograph. The characteristic finding is a curved line representing the edge of the lung (the visceral pleura) separated from the chest wall. Between the edge of the lung and the chest wall, the pleural space is lucent, and none of the normal vascular markings of the lung are seen in this region (Figs. 15-5 and 15-6). When the pneumothorax is small, separation of the visceral and parietal pleura appears only at the apex of the lung, where the pleural air generally accumulates first. If the pneumothorax is substantial, the lung loses a significant amount of volume and therefore has a greater density than usual.

When both fluid and air are present in the pleural space *(hydropneumothorax)*, the fluid no longer appears as a meniscus tracking up along the lateral chest wall. Rather, the fluid falls to the most dependent part of the pleural space and appears as a liquid density with a perfectly horizontal upper

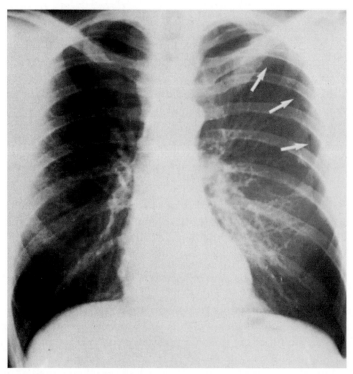

Figure 15-5 ■— Chest radiograph of patient with spontaneous pneumothorax on left. Arrows point to visceral pleural surface of lung. Beyond visceral pleura is air within pleural space; no lung markings can be seen in this region.

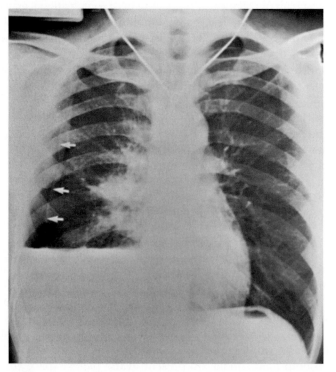

Figure 15-6 ■— Chest radiograph shows right hydropneumothorax. Horizontal line in lower right hemithorax is interface between air and liquid in pleural space. Arrows point to visceral pleura above level of effusion. There is air in pleural space between visceral pleura and chest wall.

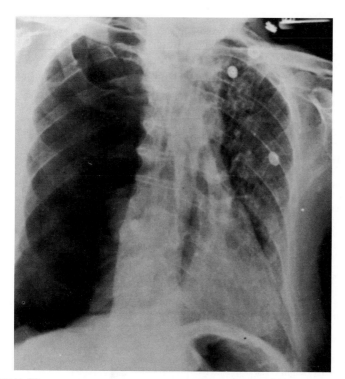

Figure 15-7 ■— Chest radiograph shows right-sided tension pneumothorax. There are no lung markings seen in right hemithorax, and the mediastinum is shifted left.

border (see Fig. 15-6). Finally, when gas in the pleural space is under tension, there is often evidence for structures (e.g., trachea and mediastinum) being "pushed" away from the side of the pneumothorax (Fig. 15-7).

Treatment

The treatment of a pneumothorax is determined by its size as well as by the ensuing clinical consequences. With a small pneumothorax causing few symptoms, it is best to wait for spontaneous resolution of the pneumothorax. As mentioned earlier, this process can be hastened by administration of 100 percent O_2, which alters the partial pressures of gases in capillary blood, favoring the resorption of pleural air. When the pneumothorax is large or the patient has significant clinical sequelae, the air is best removed, usually by a needle, a catheter, or a large-bore tube inserted into the pleural space. Occasionally, patients have recurrent spontaneous pneumothoraces, requiring obliteration of the pleural space by any one of a number of methods.

If a patient has hemodynamic compromise because of a tension pneumothorax, a needle, catheter, or tube must immediately be inserted to relieve the pressure. When this is performed, the sound of air under pressure escaping from the pleural space can readily be heard. The most important results of decompression are improvements in gas-exchange, venous return to the thorax, cardiac output, and arterial blood pressure.

References

General Reviews

Antony VB (ed): Diseases of the pleura. Clin Chest Med 19:229-417, 1998.
Colt HG: Thoracoscopy. Window to the pleural space. Chest 116:1409-1415, 1999.

Light RW: Pleural Diseases, 4th ed. Philadelphia, Lippincott Williams & Wilkins, 2001.

Loddenkemper R and Antony VB: Pleural diseases. Eur Respir Mon 7 (Monograph 22):1-326, 2002.

Pistolesi M, Miniati M, and Giuntini C: Pleural liquid and solute exchange. Am Rev Respir Dis 140:825-847, 1989.

Sahn SA: The pleura. Am Rev Respir Dis 138:184-234, 1988.

Wiener-Kronish JP and Broaddus VC: Interrelationship of pleural and pulmonary interstitial liquid. Annu Rev Physiol 55:209-226, 1993.

Zocchi L: Physiology and pathophysiology of pleural fluid turnover. Eur Respir J 20:1545-1558, 2002.

Pleural Effusion

American Thoracic Society: Management of malignant pleural effusions. Am J Respir Crit Care Med 162:1987-2001, 2000.

Bartter T, Santarelli R, Akers SM, and Pratter MR: The evaluation of pleural effusion. Chest 106:1209-1214, 1994.

Colice GL: Medical and surgical treatment of parapneumonic effusions. An evidence-based guideline. Chest 18:1158-1171, 2000.

Collins TR and Sahn SA: Thoracocentesis: clinical value, complications, technical problems, and patient experience. Chest 91:817-822, 1987.

Joseph J and Sahn SA: Connective tissue diseases and the pleura. Chest 104:262-270, 1993.

Light RW: Pleural effusion. N Engl J Med 346:1971-1977, 2002.

Light RW, MacGregor MI, Luchsinger PC, and Ball WC Jr: Pleural effusions: the diagnostic separation of transudates and exudates. Ann Intern Med 77:507-513, 1972.

Sokolowski JW Jr et al: Guidelines for thoracentesis and needle biopsy of the pleura. Am Rev Respir Dis 140:257-258, 1989.

Pneumothorax

Baumann MH et al: Management of spontaneous pneumothorax. An American College of Chest Physicians Delphi consensus statement. Chest 119:590-602, 2001.

Sahn SA and Heffner JE: Spontaneous pneumothorax. N Engl J Med 342:868-874, 2000.

Sepkowitz KA et al: Pneumothorax in AIDS. Ann Intern Med 114:455-459, 1991.

Weissberg D and Refaely Y: Pneumothorax. Experience with 1,199 patients. Chest 117:1279-1285, 2000.

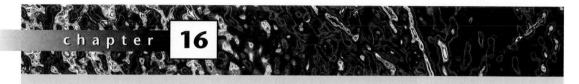

chapter 16

Mediastinal Disease

ANATOMIC FEATURES
MEDIASTINAL MASSES
  Etiology
  Clinical Features
  Diagnostic Approach
  Treatment

PNEUMOMEDIASTINUM
  Etiology and Pathogenesis
  Pathophysiology
  Clinical Features
  Diagnostic Approach
  Treatment

The mediastinum is the region of the thoracic cavity located between the two lungs. Included within the mediastinum are numerous structures, ranging from the heart and the great vessels (aorta, superior and inferior venae cavae) to lymph nodes and nerves. The physician dealing with diseases of the lung is confronted with mediastinal disease in two major ways—either because of a chest radiograph showing an abnormal mediastinum or because of symptoms similar to those originating from primary pulmonary disease. This chapter describes some of the anatomic features of the mediastinum and discusses two of its most common clinical problems: mediastinal masses and pneumomediastinum.

ANATOMIC FEATURES

The mediastinum is bounded superiorly by bony structures of the thoracic inlet and inferiorly by the diaphragm. Laterally, the mediastinal pleura on each side serves as a membrane separating the medial aspect of the lung (with its visceral pleura) from the structures contained within the mediastinum. The mediastinum is most frequently divided into three anatomic compartments: anterior, middle, and posterior (Table 16-1). This division is particularly useful for characterizing mediastinal masses, because specific etiologic factors often have a predilection for a particular compartment. In particular, normal structures located within or coursing through each of the compartments may serve as the origin of a mediastinal mass. Consequently, knowledge of the structures contained in each of the three compartments is quite important for the clinician evaluating a patient with a mediastinal mass.

It is easiest to visualize the borders of the three mediastinal compartments on a lateral chest radiograph, as shown in Figure 16-1. Several descriptions exist for the limits defining each compartment. According to the scheme used here, the anterior mediastinum extends from the sternum to the anterior border of the pericardium. Included within this region are the thymus, lymph nodes, and loose connective tissue.

The borders of the middle mediastinum are the anterior and posterior pericardium. This region includes the heart, pericardium, great vessels, trachea,

Table 16-1

Mediastinal Compartments: Anatomy and Pathology

Compartment	Borders	Normal Structures	Masses
Anterior	Anterior—sternum Posterior—pericardium, ascending aorta, brachiocephalic vessels	Lymph nodes Connective tissue Thymus (remnant in adults)	Thymoma Germ cell neoplasm Lymphoma Thyroid enlargement (intrathoracic goiter) Other tumors
Middle	Anterior—anterior pericardium, ascending aorta, brachiocephalic vessels Posterior—posterior pericardium	Pericardium Heart Vessels—ascending aorta, venae cavae, main pulmonary arteries Trachea Lymph nodes Nerves—phrenic, upper vagus	Carcinoma Lymphoma Pericardial cyst Bronchogenic cyst Benign lymph node enlargement (granulomatous disease)
Posterior	Anterior—posterior pericardium Posterior—posterior chest wall	Vessels—descending aorta Esophagus Vertebral column Nerves—sympathetic chain, lower vagus Lymph nodes Connective tissue	Neurogenic tumors Diaphragmatic hernias

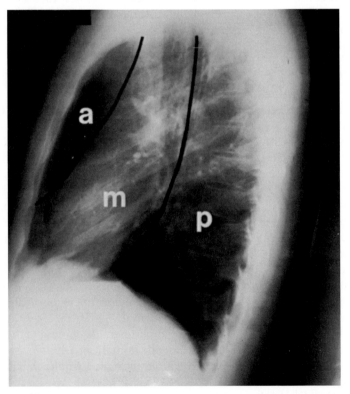

Figure 16-1 ■— Lateral chest radiograph shows borders of three mediastinal compartments. a = anterior; m = middle; p = posterior.

lymph nodes, and phrenic nerves. The upper portion of the vagus nerve also courses through the middle mediastinum.

Finally, the posterior mediastinum extends from the posterior pericardium to the posterior chest wall. This compartment normally includes the vertebral column, neural structures (including the chain of sympathetic nerves and the lower portion of the vagus nerves), the esophagus, and the descending aorta. In addition, some lymph nodes and loose connective tissue may be found.

MEDIASTINAL MASSES

Etiology

Because of the predilection for certain types of masses to occur in specific mediastinal compartments, it is easiest to consider separately masses occurring in each of the three anatomic regions. There is, however, a fair amount of overlap; that is, many types of mediastinal masses are not exclusively limited to the compartment in which they most frequently occur. A summary of the types of mediastinal masses, arranged by anatomic compartment, can be found in Table 16-1.

Anterior Mediastinal Masses

The major types of anterior mediastinal mass are thymoma, germ cell tumor, lymphoma, thyroid gland enlargement, and miscellaneous other tumors.

Thymomas, or tumors of the thymus gland, are the most common type of neoplasm originating in the anterior compartment. They may be benign or malignant in behavior, depending more on whether they are well encapsulated rather than on any particular histologic features. Thymomas are notable for their association with a variety of systemic syndromes. The best known and most common of these is myasthenia gravis, which is found in 10 to 50 percent of patients with thymic tumors. Myasthenia is characterized clinically by muscle weakness and pathophysiologically by a decreased number of acetylcholine receptors at neuromuscular junctions. The latter is frequently due to antibodies against the acetylcholine receptor. Other systemic syndromes associated with thymoma have included pure red blood cell aplasia, hypogammaglobulinemia, and several diseases that appear to have an autoimmune origin, such as systemic lupus erythematosus.

Germ cell tumors are believed to originate from primitive germ cells that probably underwent abnormal migration during an early developmental period. Several types of germ cell tumors have been described. The most common of these is the teratoma, a tumor composed of ectodermal, mesodermal, and endodermal derivatives. The types of tissue seen are clearly foreign to the area from which the tumor arose and may include such elements as skin, hair, cartilage, and bone. Like thymomas, these tumors may be benign or malignant, approximately 80 percent being described as benign. Other less common germ cell tumors include seminomas and choriocarcinomas.

Lymphoma may involve the mediastinum either as part of a disseminated process, in which the mediastinum is only one locus of the disease, or as a primary mediastinal mass without other clinically apparent tissue involvement. Hodgkin's disease, particularly the nodular sclerosis subtype, is well described as manifesting solely as a mediastinal mass, although other forms of

Myasthenia gravis occurs frequently in patients with thymoma.

Lymphoma and carcinoma commonly affect anterior or middle compartments; mediastinal disease may be isolated or part of more widespread involvement.

non-Hodgkin's lymphoma may also have a similar presentation. Like carcinoma, lymphoma involving the mediastinum is most common in the anterior or the middle mediastinal compartments.

Thyroid tissue may be the origin of a mediastinal mass, usually as a result of extension from thyroid tissue in the neck. Because these masses are generally not functional, the patients do not have clinical or laboratory evidence of hyperthyroidism. Only rarely do these masses of thyroid origin prove to be malignant.

Other tumors, including carcinomas, may produce a mediastinal mass. In many cases the mediastinal involvement is secondary to a primary neoplasm found elsewhere, particularly in the lung. In occasional cases, no other tumor is apparent, and the patients are believed to have a primary carcinoma originating in the mediastinum. Carcinomatous involvement of the mediastinum is not limited to the anterior mediastinum, but is also common in the middle mediastinal compartment.

A variety of less common neoplasms may occur in the anterior mediastinum, including parathyroid tumors and tumors of fatty or connective tissue origin. Given the infrequency of these tumors, they are not discussed in this book.

Middle Mediastinal Masses

In the middle mediastinum, carcinomas and lymphomas may be found, as mentioned in the discussion of anterior mediastinal masses. In addition, the middle mediastinum is frequently the location of benign cysts originating from structures found within this region. For example, fluid-filled pericardial and bronchogenic cysts originate from the pericardium and the tracheobronchial tree, respectively. However, these cysts are generally self-contained and usually do not directly communicate with either the pericardium or the airways. Benign enlargement of lymph nodes in the middle mediastinum, often associated with enlarged hilar nodes, is commonly found in granulomatous diseases, particularly sarcoidosis and tuberculosis.

Posterior Mediastinal Masses

The posterior mediastinum is characteristically the location of tumors of neurogenic origin. These tumors may arise from a variety of nerve elements found in the peripheral nerves, the sympathetic nervous system chain, or the paraganglionic tissue. Examples include neurilemomas (arising from Schwann's sheath), ganglioneuromas and neuroblastomas (respectively, benign and malignant lesions arising from the sympathetic nervous system), and pheochromocytomas. Diaphragmatic hernias, either congenital or acquired, are frequently posterior, with the herniated intra-abdominal organ appearing as a mediastinal mass.

Clinical Features

Almost half the patients with a mediastinal mass have no symptoms, and the mass is first detected on an incidentally performed chest radiograph. In the other patients, symptoms are frequently chest pain, cough, and dyspnea. Occasionally, there may be evidence of esophageal or superior vena caval compression, leading to difficulty swallowing (dysphagia) or to facial and upper extremity edema due to impairment of venous return (superior vena cava syndrome). Thymic tumors may manifest with one of the associated systemic syndromes, such as muscle weakness (from myasthenia gravis) or anemia (from pure red cell aplasia). Finally, a variety of systemic symptoms may be related to the presence of a lymphoma or other malignancy or to hormone production by hormonally active mediastinal tumors.

Diagnostic Approach

The initial diagnostic test in almost all cases is the chest radiograph, which generally shows the mass and allows determination of its location within the mediastinum (Fig. 16-2). Further characterization of the mass can be made by a variety of other techniques, but computed tomography (CT) has emerged so far as the most valuable of these. The CT scan is particularly useful for defining the cross-sectional appearance of the lesion, its density, and its relationship to other structures within the mediastinum. The newest of the major imaging procedures, magnetic resonance imaging (MRI), has been used in some centers for evaluation of mediastinal masses, but its overall usefulness compared with CT is not yet clear. Because blood vessels appear as hollow rather than solid structures, MRI can distinguish vessels from other mediastinal structures without the use of radiographic contrast. Unlike the traditional presentation of CT images as cross-sectional views, MRI also can display images in coronal and sagittal planes, as well as cross-sectional views.

CT is useful in the evaluation of mediastinal masses.

The definitive diagnosis of the type of mediastinal mass generally depends on the examination of tissue by histopathologic techniques. Tissue is frequently obtained either by mediastinoscopy, in which a rigid scope is inserted into the mediastinum via an incision at the suprasternal notch, or by exploration of the mediastinum by a surgical approach that is anterior and adjacent to the sternum (parasternal mediastinotomy). The technique of video-assisted thoracic surgery has also been used to obtain tissue from the

Techniques for biopsy of a mediastinal mass are the following:

1. Mediastinoscopy
2. Parasternal mediastinotomy
3. Percutaneous needle aspiration or biopsy

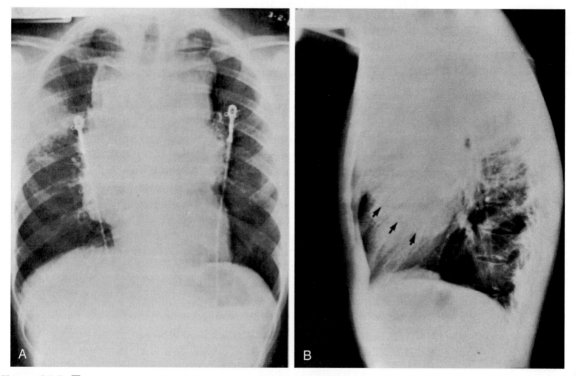

Figure 16-2 ▅▬ Chest radiograph of patient with large mediastinal mass. Mass, proved at surgery to be a germ cell tumor (seminoma), involves anterior and middle mediastinal compartments. Posteroanterior (*A*) and lateral (*B*) views. Arrows outline inferior border of mass on lateral view.

mediastinum. In some patients, aspiration or biopsy of the mass by a needle inserted percutaneously may provide sufficient tissue to make a diagnosis. In many cases the patient undergoes a more extensive procedure allowing biopsy and removal of the mass at the same time.

Treatment

Treatment of the various mediastinal masses depends to a large extent on the nature of the lesion. In many cases, complete removal of the mass by surgery is the preferred procedure. Because benign lesions may enlarge and compress vital mediastinal structures, excision of the mass is frequently indicated. In addition, there may be complicating hemorrhage or infection of a benign lesion and eventually even malignant transformation of an initially benign tumor.

In the case of malignant tumors, treatment depends on the type of tumor and the presence or absence of invasion of other mediastinal structures. Because surgical removal of the malignant lesion is often neither indicated nor possible, chemotherapy and radiotherapy are frequently the primary forms of treatment.

PNEUMOMEDIASTINUM

Normally, free air is not present within the mediastinum. When air enters the mediastinum for any number of reasons, a *pneumomediastinum* is said to be present.

Etiology and Pathogenesis

Sources of air entry in a pneumomediastinum are the following:
1. External (penetrating trauma)
2. Tracheal or esophageal tear
3. Alveolar rupture and tracking of air proximally

There are three major sources of air entry to the mediastinum: (1) through the skin and chest wall, as commonly seen in the setting of penetrating trauma, (2) from a tear or defect in the esophagus or the trachea, allowing air to enter the mediastinum directly, and (3) from the alveoli. In the last circumstance, an increase in intra-alveolar pressure may induce air entry into interstitial tissues of the alveolar wall. This interstitial air may then dissect alongside the wall of blood vessels coursing through the interstitium. Once air tracks back proximally, it may eventually enter the mediastinum at the site of origin of the vessels in the mediastinum.

Probably the most commonly occurring pathogenesis of a pneumomediastinum is the one just described. In some cases the reason for the increase in intra-alveolar pressure is obvious, for example, severe coughing, vomiting, or straining. In patients receiving assisted ventilation with a mechanical ventilator, the positive pressure produced by the ventilator may initiate alveolar rupture and a pneumomediastinum. A pneumomediastinum also may develop in asthmatic persons, presumably because of the development of high intra-alveolar pressure behind an obstructed bronchus. In other circumstances the immediate cause of the pneumomediastinum is not apparent, and the patient truly has a "spontaneous" pneumomediastinum.

Pathophysiology

With the accumulation of air in the mediastinum, an increase in pressure would be expected to cause a decrease in venous return to the great veins, with resulting cardiovascular compromise. However, when pressure builds up

Mediastinal Disease, page 223

within the mediastinum, air usually dissects further along fascial planes into the neck, allowing release of the pressure and preventing disastrous cardiovascular complications. In addition, an increase in mediastinal pressure sometimes results in rupture of the mediastinal pleura and escape of air into the pleural space.

Once air has entered the soft tissues of the neck, the patient is said to have *subcutaneous emphysema*. If there is continued entry of air from the mediastinum into the neck, the air dissects further over soft tissues of the chest and abdominal walls to produce more extensive subcutaneous emphysema.

Because of the escape route available for mediastinal air and the opportunity for decompression, major cardiovascular complications are quite uncommon. The development of subcutaneous emphysema, though unsightly, is also usually without major clinical sequelae.

Mediastinal air often results in subcutaneous emphysema.

Clinical Features

At the onset, patients with a pneumomediastinum often experience relatively sudden substernal chest pain. There may also be dyspnea and, rarely, cardiovascular compromise and hypotension. In some cases the pneumomediastinum causes no symptoms, and the problem is detected on chest radiograph—for example, on a film obtained during the course of an asthmatic attack.

Physical examination may reveal a crunching or clicking sound synchronous with the heartbeat on cardiac auscultation. If the patient has subcutaneous emphysema associated with the pneumomediastinum, popping and crackling sounds (crepitations) may be heard and felt when pressure is applied to the affected skin and subcutaneous tissue.

Diagnostic Approach

The chest radiograph is the most important study in documenting a pneumomediastinum. Gas may be seen within the mediastinal tissues and is usually

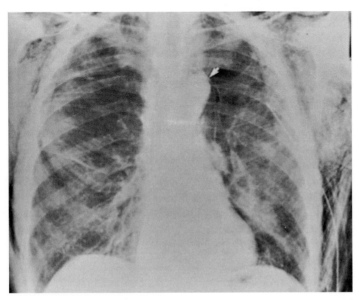

Figure 16-3 ▬ Chest radiograph shows pneumomediastinum and air in subcutaneous tissues (subcutaneous emphysema). Note numerous radiolucent stripes outlining mediastinal structures; these stripes represent air within mediastinum. Arrow points to air around aortic arch.

visible as one or more radiolucent stripes alongside and parallel to the heart border or the aorta (Fig. 16-3).

Treatment

Generally, no treatment is necessary for a pneumomediastinum, even when accompanied by subcutaneous emphysema. The air is usually resorbed spontaneously over time. When a pneumomediastinum is a consequence of tracheobronchial or esophageal rupture, surgery may be necessary for repair of the underlying tear. In the rare circumstance when pressure builds up within the mediastinum, an incision or tube may be necessary to allow escape of air from the mediastinum and release of the pressure.

References

Dulmet EM, Macchiarini P, Suc B, and Verley JM: Germ cell tumors of the mediastinum. Cancer 72:1894-1901, 1993.

Hoffman OA, Gillespie DJ, Aughenbaugh GL, and Brown LR: Primary mediastinal neoplasms (other than thymoma). Mayo Clin Proc 68:880-891, 1993.

Laurent F et al: Mediastinal masses: diagnostic approach. Eur Radiol 8:1148-1159, 1998.

Lin JC, Hazelrigg SR, and Landreneau RJ: Video-assisted thoracic surgery for disease within the mediastinum. Surg Clin North Am 80:1511-1533, 2000.

Maunder RJ, Pierson DJ, and Hudson LD: Subcutaneous and mediastinal emphysema: pathophysiology, diagnosis, and management. Arch Intern Med 144:1447-1453, 1984.

Morgenthaler TI et al: Thymoma. Mayo Clin Proc 68:1110-1123, 1993.

Ribet ME and Cardot GR: Neurogenic tumors of the thorax. Ann Thorac Surg 58:1091-1095, 1994.

Ribet ME, Copin MC, and Gosselin B: Bronchogenic cysts of the mediastinum. J Thorac Cardiovasc Surg 109:1003-1010, 1995.

Silverman NA (ed): Mediastinal tumors. Sem Thorac Cardiovasc Surg 12:260-306, 2000.

Strollo DC, Rosado de Christenson ML, and Jett JR: Primary mediastinal tumors. Part 1. Tumors of the anterior mediastinum. Chest 112:511-522, 1997.

Strollo DC, Rosado de Christenson ML, and Jett JR: Primary mediastinal tumors. Part 2. Tumors of the middle and posterior mediastinum. Chest 112:1344-1357, 1997.

chapter 17

Anatomic and Physiologic Aspects of Neural, Muscular, and Chest Wall Interactions with the Lungs

RESPIRATORY CONTROL
  Organization of Respiratory Control
  Ventilatory Response to Hypercapnia and Hypoxia

Ventilatory Response to Other Stimuli
RESPIRATORY MUSCLES

The movement of gas into and out of the lungs requires the action of a pump that is capable of creating negative intrathoracic pressure, expanding the lungs, and initiating airflow with each inspiration. This pump-like action is provided by the respiratory muscles, including the diaphragm, working in conjunction with the chest wall. However, the muscles themselves do not have any rhythmic activity in the way that cardiac muscle does, and they must be driven by rhythmic impulses provided by a "controller."

This chapter centers on a discussion of anatomic and physiologic features of the controlling system and the respiratory muscles in order to provide background for the discussion in the subsequent two chapters. In those chapters, disorders affecting respiratory control, respiratory musculature, and the chest wall are considered. Whereas much of the physiology and many of the clinical problems discussed here and in the next two chapters do not directly involve the lungs, they are so closely intertwined with respiratory function and dysfunction that they are appropriately considered in a textbook of pulmonary disease.

RESPIRATORY CONTROL

Although the process of breathing is a normal rhythmic activity that occurs without conscious effort, it involves an intricate controlling mechanism at the level of the central nervous system. The central nervous system transmits signals to the respiratory muscles, initiating inspiration approximately 12 to 20 times per minute. Remarkably, this controlling system is normally able to respond to varied needs of the individual, appropriately increasing ventilation during exercise and maintaining arterial blood gases within a narrow range.

This section begins with a description of the structural organization of neural control of ventilation and proceeds to a consideration of how various stimuli may interact with and adjust the output of the respiratory controller. Finally, there is a brief discussion of the ways in which the output of the controller can be quantified and how these techniques have proved useful in the evaluation of patients with a variety of clinical disorders.

Organization of Respiratory Control

The basic organization of the respiratory control system is diagrammed in Figure 17-1. Crucial to this system is the central nervous system "generator," from which signals originate that travel down the spinal cord to the various respiratory muscles. The inspiratory muscles, the most important of which is the diaphragm, respond to the signals by contracting and initiating inspiration. This process is described in more detail when the muscles are considered later in this chapter.

As a result of inspiratory muscular contraction, the diaphragm descends, the chest wall expands, and air flows from the mouth through the tracheo-bronchial tree to the alveolar spaces. Gas-exchange in the distal parenchyma allows movement of O_2 into the blood and a corresponding release of CO_2.

Although this sequence of events sounds relatively straightforward, it is complicated by an intricate feedback system that adjusts the output of the generator to achieve the desired effect. If there is an inadequate response of the respiratory muscles to the generator's signal, as judged by a variety of respiratory "reflexes," then the generator increases its output to compensate for the lack of expected effect. If the arterial blood gases deviate from the desired level, then chemosensors for O_2 and CO_2 alter their input to the respiratory generator, ultimately affecting its output. In addition, input from other regions of the central nervous system, particularly the cerebral cortex and the pons, can adjust the net output of the generator.

The Respiratory Generator

A central respiratory genera-tor within the medulla con-trols activity of the respiratory muscles.

Considering the importance of the respiratory generator in this scheme of respiratory control, its anatomy and its mode of action are described here. Much of the work clarifying the location of the respiratory generator involved animal experiments with transections at various levels of the central nervous system

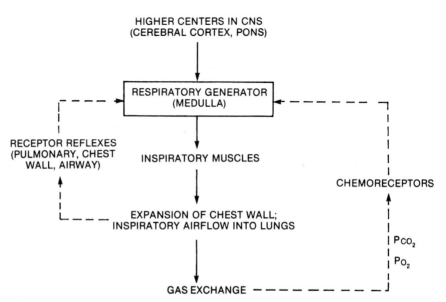

Figure 17-1 ━ Schematic diagram shows organization of respiratory control system. Dashed lines show feedback loops affecting respiratory generator.

and assessment of the effects on ventilation. Because transection between the brain and the brain stem does not significantly alter ventilation, the generator apparently resides somewhere at the level of the brain stem or lower and does not require interaction with higher cortical centers. When transections are made at various points within the brain stem, the breathing pattern is substantially altered but ventilation is not eliminated. It is only when a transection is made between the medulla and the spinal cord that ventilation ceases, indicating that the respiratory generator resides within the medulla.

Although the respiratory center (or the generator) has been referred to as a single region, it appears that more than one network of neurons within the medulla is involved in initiating and coordinating respiratory activity. According to a popular model, one group of neurons is responsible for initiating inspiration and regulating its speed as a result of the intensity of neuronal activity; another group of neurons controls the "switching off" of inspiration and hence determines the onset of expiration.

Therefore, there are two aspects of ventilatory control: the degree of inspiratory drive or central inspiratory activity (which regulates the inspiratory flow rate), and the timing mechanism (which controls the termination of inspiration). These two determining factors act in concert to set the respiratory rate and tidal volume and thus the minute ventilation and the specific pattern of breathing.

Input from Other Regions of the Central Nervous System

Even though the medullary respiratory center does not require additional input to drive ventilation, it does receive other information that contributes to a regular pattern of breathing and to more precise ventilatory control. For example, input from the pons appears to be necessary for a normal, coordinated breathing pattern. When the influence of the pons is lost, irregularities in the breathing pattern ensue.

In addition to pathways involved in the "automatic" or involuntary control of ventilation, the cerebral cortex exerts a conscious or voluntary control over ventilation. The cortical overriding of automatic control can be seen with either voluntary breath holding or hyperventilation. Its usefulness is readily apparent in people's need for voluntary control of breathing during such activities as speaking, eating, and swimming. Interestingly, the automatic control of ventilation may be disturbed while conscious control remains intact. In these cases, during wakefulness the cerebral cortex exerts sufficient voluntary control over ventilation to maintain normal arterial blood gas values. During periods when the patient is dependent on automatic ventilatory control—for example, during sleep—marked hypoventilation or apnea may occur. This rare condition is called *Ondine's curse* after a mythologic tale in which the suitor of Neptune's daughter was cursed to lose automatic control over all bodily functions.

Chemoreceptors

As shown in Figure 17-1, maintenance of arterial blood gases is the final goal of ventilatory control, and an important feedback loop exists to adjust respiratory center output if blood gases are not maintained at the desired level. Elevation of P_{CO_2} (hypercapnia) and depression of P_{O_2} (hypoxemia) are both capable of stimulating ventilation. In each case, one or more chemoreceptors "sense" alterations in P_{CO_2} or P_{O_2} and accordingly vary their input to the medullary respiratory center.

Changes in P_{CO_2} are sensed primarily at a central chemoreceptor in the medulla.

The primary sensor for CO_2 is located near the ventrolateral surface of the medulla and is called the *central chemoreceptor*. Even though it is located in the medulla, the central chemoreceptor is clearly separate from the medullary respiratory center and should not be confused with it. The central chemoreceptor does not appear to respond directly to blood P_{CO_2} but rather to the pH of the extracellular fluid (ECF) surrounding the chemoreceptor. The pH level, in turn, is determined by the level of hydrogen (H^+) and bicarbonate (HCO_3^-) ions as well as the P_{CO_2}. The blood-brain barrier, whose permeability properties govern the composition of cerebrospinal fluid (CSF) and brain ECF, prevents the free movement of either H^+ or HCO_3^- from blood to brain ECF, whereas CO_2 passes freely. The feedback loop for changes in P_{CO_2} can be summarized as follows:

Increased arterial blood P_{CO_2} → increased brain ECF P_{CO_2} → decreased brain ECF pH → decreased pH at central chemoreceptor → stimulation of central chemoreceptor → stimulation of medullary respiratory center → increased ventilation → decreased arterial blood P_{CO_2}.

The major sensors for P_{O_2} are the peripheral (carotid and aortic body) chemoreceptors.

The primary sensors for O_2 are not located in the central nervous system, but rather in two *peripheral chemoreceptors* called the *carotid body* and *aortic body chemoreceptors*. The carotid chemoreceptors, which are quantitatively much more important than aortic chemoreceptors, are located just beyond the bifurcation of each common carotid artery into internal and external branches. The aortic chemoreceptor is found between the pulmonary artery and the arch of the aorta. These chemoreceptors are sensitive to changes in P_{O_2}, with hypoxia stimulating chemoreceptor discharge. The peripheral chemoreceptors also have a minor role in sensing P_{CO_2}, but they are much less important for this purpose than are the central chemoreceptors. Peripheral chemoreceptor discharge is transmitted back to the central nervous system by cranial nerves: the glossopharyngeal in the case of the carotid bodies and the vagus nerve for the aortic bodies. The information is ultimately transmitted to the medullary respiratory center, so that its output is augmented as a result of hypoxemia.

Input from Other Receptors

In addition to chemoreceptor effects, input that originates from receptors in the lung (including the airways) and is carried via the vagus nerve to the central nervous system must be considered. Stretch receptors, located within the smooth muscle of airway walls, respond to changes in lung inflation; as the lung is inflated, receptor discharge increases. In animals, this stretch receptor reflex (the Hering-Breuer reflex) is responsible for apnea that occurs as a result of lung inflation. In contrast, conscious human adults do not readily demonstrate the Hering-Breuer reflex, and the role of the stretch receptors in ventilatory control is not entirely clear. Presumably, stretch receptors contribute to the "switching off" of inspiration, i.e., initiation of expiration, after a critical level of inspiratory inflation has been reached.

Irritant receptors, located superficially along the lining of airways, may also initiate tachypnea, usually in response to some noxious stimulus, such as a chemical or irritating dust. Juxtacapillary, or J, receptors are found within the pulmonary interstitium, adjacent to capillaries. One of their effects is to cause tachypnea, and they may be responsible for the respiratory stimulation caused by inflammatory processes or accumulation of fluid within the pulmonary interstitium.

Finally, receptors in the chest wall, particularly in the intercostal muscles, appear to play a role in the fine tuning of ventilation. The muscle spindles are part of a reflex arc that adjusts the output of respiratory muscles if the desired degree of muscular work has not been achieved.

Ventilatory Response to Hypercapnia and Hypoxia

Two of the stimuli for ventilation that have been best studied are well-defined chemical ones, hypercapnia and hypoxia. Hypercapnia is sensed primarily (but not exclusively) by the central chemoreceptor, and the stimulus appears to be the pH level of brain extracellular fluid. In contrast, hypoxia stimulates ventilation by acting on peripheral chemoreceptors, carotid much more than aortic.

When arterial PO_2 is held constant, ventilation increases in adults by approximately 3 L/min for each mm Hg rise in arterial PCO_2. This relatively linear response, the magnitude of which varies considerably among individuals, is shown in Figure 17-2. It can also be appreciated from Figure 17-2 that the response to increments in PCO_2 also depends on PO_2; at a lower PO_2, the response to hypercapnia is heightened.

With chronic hypercapnia, the ventilatory response to further increases in PCO_2 is diminished. The reason that CO_2 responsiveness is blunted is relatively straightforward. When CO_2 retention persists for days, the kidneys excrete less bicarbonate, and levels of bicarbonate rise in both plasma and brain ECF. The elevated bicarbonate can then buffer more successfully any acute changes in PCO_2, so that the brain ECF pH value changes less for any given increment in PCO_2.

Ventilatory responsiveness to CO_2 is blunted in patients with chronic hypercapnia.

With hypoxemia there is not the same linear relationship between alterations in partial pressure and ventilation. Rather, the ventilatory response is relatively small until PO_2 falls to approximately 60 torr, below which the rise in ventilation is much more dramatic (Fig. 17-3). The curvilinear relationship between PO_2 and ventilation can be made linear if ventilation is plotted against O_2 saturation instead of partial pressure (Fig. 17-4). However, despite the linear relationship between ventilation and O_2 saturation, it is the partial pressure of O_2, not the content or saturation, that is sensed by the chemoreceptor.

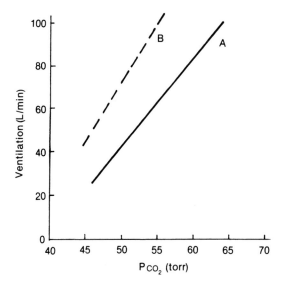

Figure 17-2 ■— Ventilatory response to progressive elevation of PCO_2 in normal individual. Solid line (A) shows response when simultaneous PO_2 is high (hyperoxic conditions); dashed line (B) shows heightened response when simultaneous PO_2 is low (hypoxic conditions).

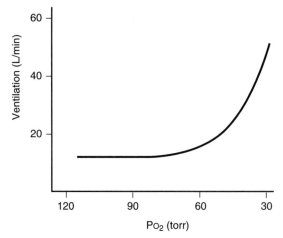

Figure 17-3 ▆— Ventilatory response to progressively decreasing P_{O_2} in normal individual (with P_{CO_2} kept constant). Ventilation does not rise significantly until P_{O_2} falls to approximately 60 torr.

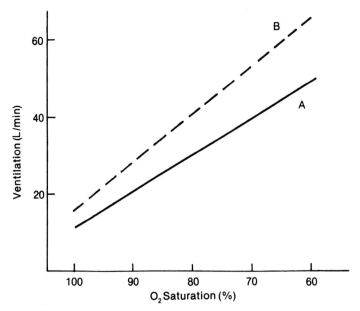

Figure 17-4 ▆— Ventilatory response to hypoxia, plotted using O_2 saturation rather than P_{O_2}. The relationship between ventilation and O_2 saturation during progressive hypoxia is linear. Solid line (A) shows response when measured at normal P_{CO_2}; dotted line (B) shows augmented response at elevated P_{CO_2}.

The P_{CO_2} also has an effect on a patient's response to hypoxia. The sensitivity to hypoxia is increased as P_{CO_2} is raised, or it is decreased as P_{CO_2} is lowered (see Fig. 17-4). This feature is important to consider in testing for responsiveness to hypoxia. As the patient hyperventilates in response to a low P_{O_2}, P_{CO_2} drops, and ventilation is stimulated less than it would be if P_{CO_2} were unchanged. Therefore, P_{CO_2} is best kept constant so that the condition for testing is actually "isocapnic" hypoxia.

When the clinician suspects a disorder of ventilatory control, quantitation of the ventilatory response to hypercapnia or hypoxia may be performed.

However, there is a wide range of responses to these stimuli even in seemingly normal individuals. This fact must be taken into account when ventilatory response data are interpreted.

Ventilatory Response to Other Stimuli

One of the most important times for a rapid and appropriate increase in ventilation is in response to a change in metabolic requirements. For example, with the metabolic needs of exercise, a normal individual can increase ventilation from a resting value of 5 L/min to 60 L/min or more, without any demonstrable change in arterial blood gas values. According to one popular theory, the initial rapid increase in ventilation at the onset of exercise is due to a neural stimulus, although the origin is not clear. After the initial rapid augmentation in ventilation, there is a later and slower rise that is probably due to a blood-borne chemical stimulus. However, there are many unanswered questions about the remarkably appropriate way that ventilation is capable of responding to the demands of exercise.

Another important ventilatory response is that to alterations in acid-base status. With excess metabolic acid production, i.e., metabolic acidosis, ventilation increases as the pH is lowered, and the elimination of additional CO_2 aids in returning the pH toward normal. The peripheral chemoreceptors appear to be primarily responsible for sensing acute metabolic acidosis and for stimulating the increase in ventilation. However, it is not entirely settled how much the central chemoreceptors modify or contribute to this response.

RESPIRATORY MUSCLES

The purpose of signals emanating from the respiratory generator is to initiate inspiratory muscle activity. Although the primary inspiratory muscle is the diaphragm, other muscle groups contribute to optimal movement of the chest wall in a variety of conditions and needs. Notable among these other inspiratory muscle groups are the scalene and the parasternal intercostal muscles, which display inspiratory activity even during normal quiet breathing. The so-called accessory muscles of inspiration—for example, sternocleidomastoid and trapezius muscles—are not normally used during quiet inspiration but can be recruited when necessary, either when diaphragm function is impaired or when ventilation is significantly increased. Another set of intercostal muscles, the external intercostal muscles, are also inspiratory muscles, but their overall importance during inspiration is less clear. Finally, there are additional muscles that coordinate upper airway activity during inspiration. Proper functioning of these muscles maintains patency of the upper airway, whereas dysfunction may be important in the pathogenesis of certain clinical disorders associated with upper airway obstruction.

During inspiration, contraction of the diaphragm and shortening of its muscle fibers occur. To understand the effect of this contraction, consider the configuration of the diaphragm within the chest. At its lateral aspect, the diaphragm is adjacent to the inner part of the lower rib cage; this portion of the chest wall and the diaphragm is known as the *zone of apposition* (Fig. 17-5). In this region, the muscle fibers of the diaphragm are oriented vertically. When the diaphragm contracts, shortening of these vertically oriented fibers diminishes the zone of apposition and causes the more medial dome of the diaphragm to descend and the lower rib cage to be lifted and rotated

The diaphragm is the major muscle of inspiration; the less important inspiratory and accessory muscles may increase their role in disease states.

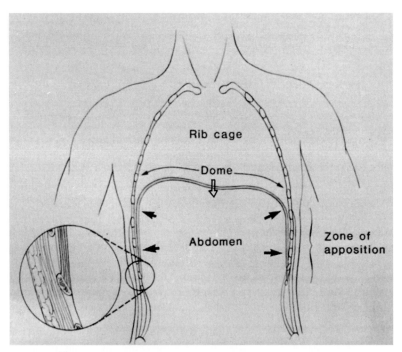

Figure 17-5 ■— Functional anatomy and action of diaphragm during breathing. At zone of apposition, fibers of diaphragm are oriented vertically alongside inner aspect of lower rib cage. During inspiration, descent of diaphragm *(open arrow)* causes increase in abdominal pressure that is transmitted through apposed diaphragm to expand lower rib cage *(solid arrows)*. (Adapted from De Troyer A and Estenne M: Clin Chest Med 9:175-193, 1988.)

outward. At the same time, by pushing abdominal contents downward, diaphragmatic contraction increases not only intra-abdominal pressure but also the lateral pressure on the lower rib cage transmitted through the apposed diaphragm. The effect of diaphragmatic contraction is thus to lift the lower ribs and expand the lower chest wall at the same time the abdominal wall also moves outward.

As the reader can now appreciate, the act of inspiration is more complex than it initially seemed. While the diaphragm acts on the abdomen and the lower chest wall, the scalene muscles and the parasternal intercostals (perhaps along with the external intercostals) act to expand the upper chest wall. The net effect is that abdominal contents are pushed downward, intra-abdominal pressure is increased, the chest wall expands, intrathoracic pressure is lowered, and air flows into the lungs. With normal resting breathing, the most apparent inspiratory motion is the outward movement of the abdomen, resulting from diaphragmatic descent and increased abdominal pressure. In the face of high workloads, increased ventilation, or certain disease states, the accessory muscles are additionally recruited to assist the primary inspiratory muscles.

An important determinant of the efficacy of diaphragmatic contraction is the initial shape and length of the diaphragm. For any muscle, the strength of contraction is decreased when its initial length is less, and the diaphragm is no exception. Therefore, at high lung volumes, the diaphragm is lower and foreshortened before its active contraction, so that the strength of contraction is diminished. At the same time, the lower, flatter diaphragm means that the zone of apposition is decreased, and there is less downward movement of the

The effectiveness of diaphragmatic contraction is decreased at high resting lung volumes, when the diaphragm is flatter and shorter.

diaphragm and outward movement of the lower chest wall associated with inspiration. At the extreme, the diaphragm is oriented horizontally, there is no zone of apposition, and contraction results in an indrawing of the lower rib cage but no useful inspiratory function. The importance of these factors will become apparent in the discussion of diaphragmatic function in obstructive lung disease, in which resting lung volume may be abnormally high.

In contrast to inspiration, expiration is a relatively passive process whereby the lung and chest wall return to the resting position. However, when breathing is deep and forceful or when there is increased airways resistance during expiration, the action of expiratory muscles may be important in aiding expiratory airflow. In particular, abdominal muscles (transverse abdominis, internal and external obliques) and internal intercostals are important in this role.

In summary, the normal operation of the respiratory apparatus depends on a signal generated by the respiratory center and eventually translated into an efficient pattern of respiratory muscle contraction. Although feedback and control systems ensure the optimal functioning of this system, this finely coordinated mechanism may fail in numerous ways. The goal in Chapters 18 and 19 is to examine clinically important dysfunction occurring at various levels of this complex system.

References

Respiratory Control

Berger AJ, Mitchell RA, and Severinghaus JW: Regulation of respiration. N Engl J Med 297:92-97; 138-143; 194-201, 1977.

Bianchi AL, Denavit-Saubié M, and Champagnat J: Central control of breathing in mammals: neuronal circuitry, membrane properties, and neurotransmitters. Physiol Rev 75:1-45, 1995.

Bonham AC: Neurotransmitters in the CNS control of breathing. Respir Physiol 101:219-230, 1995.

Calverley PMA: Control of breathing. *In* Hughes JMB and Pride NB (eds): Lung Function Tests: Physiological Principles and Clinical Applications. London, WB Saunders Co., 2000, pp 107-120.

Caruana-Montaldo B, Gleeson K, and Zwillich CW: The control of breathing in clinical practice. Chest 117:205-225, 2000.

Duffin J and Hung S: Respiratory rhythm generation. Can Anaesth Soc J 32:124-137, 1985.

Hedemark LL and Kronenberg RS: Chemical regulation of respiration. Chest 82:488-494, 1982.

Leff AR and Schumacker PT: Respiratory Physiology: Basics and Applications. Philadelphia, WB Saunders Co., 1993.

Lopata M and Lourenço RV: Evaluation of respiratory control. Clin Chest Med 1:33-45, 1980.

Mitchell RA: Neural regulation of respiration. Clin Chest Med 1:3-12, 1980.

Mitchell RA and Berger AJ: Neural regulation of respiration. Am Rev Respir Dis 111:206-224, 1975.

von Euler C: Neural organization and rhythm generation. *In* Crystal RG, West JB, Weibel ER, and Barnes PJ (eds): The Lung: Scientific Foundations, 2nd ed. Philadelphia, Lippincott-Raven, 1997, pp 1711-1724.

West JB: Respiratory Physiology—The Essentials, 6th ed. Philadelphia, Lippincott Williams & Wilkins, 2000.

Respiratory Muscles

American Thoracic Society and European Respiratory Society: ATS/ERS statement on respiratory muscle testing. Am J Respir Crit Care Med 166:518-624, 2002.

Derenne J-P, Macklem PT, and Roussos C: The respiratory muscles: mechanics, control, and pathophysiology. Am Rev Respir Dis 118:119-133; 373-390; 581-601, 1978.

De Troyer A: The mechanism of inspiratory expansion of the rib cage. J Lab Clin Med 114:97-104, 1989.

De Troyer A and Estenne M: Functional anatomy of the respiratory muscles. Clin Chest Med 9:175-193, 1988.

Epstein SK: An overview of respiratory muscle function. Clin Chest Med 15:619-639, 1994.

Guenter CA and Whitelaw WA: The role of diaphragm function in disease. Arch Intern Med 139:806-808, 1979.

Macklem PT: Respiratory muscles: the vital pump. Chest 78:753-758, 1980.

Moxham J: Respiratory muscle testing. Monaldi Arch Chest Dis 51:483-488, 1996.

Polkey MI and Moxham J: Terminology and testing of respiratory muscle dysfunction. Monaldi Arch Chest Dis 54:514-519, 1999.

Rochester DF: The respiratory muscles. *In* Tierney DF (ed): Current Pulmonology, vol. 16. St. Louis, Mosby-Year Book, 1995, pp 87-119.

Roussos C and Macklem PT: The respiratory muscles. N Engl J Med 307:786-797, 1982.

Supinski GS: The respiratory muscles. *In* Simmons DH (ed): Current Pulmonology, vol. 10. Chicago, Year Book Medical Publishers, 1989, pp 25-72.

chapter **18**

Disorders of Ventilatory Control

PRIMARY NEUROLOGIC DISEASE Presentation with Hyperventilation Presentation with Hypoventilation Abnormal Patterns of Breathing **CHEYNE-STOKES BREATHING**	**CONTROL ABNORMALITIES** **SECONDARY TO LUNG DISEASE** **SLEEP APNEA SYNDROME** Types Clinical Features Pathophysiology Treatment

The finely tuned system of ventilatory control described in the last chapter is altered in a variety of clinical circumstances. In some cases a primary disorder of the nervous system may affect the neurologic network involved in ventilatory control and may therefore either diminish or increase the "drive" to breathe. In other instances the controlling system undergoes a process of adaptation in response to primary lung disease, and any alteration in function is therefore a secondary phenomenon.

In this chapter, primary and secondary disturbances in ventilatory control are considered. Of the secondary disorders, the one most commonly seen is that associated with chronic obstructive pulmonary disease; therefore, the discussion of secondary disorders of ventilatory control will stress this particular disorder. Also covered is a common disturbance in the pattern of breathing, termed *Cheyne-Stokes breathing,* with a brief discussion of its pathogenesis. The final topic is ventilatory disorders associated with sleep, because alteration of ventilatory control may be an important component of the pathogenesis of sleep-related respiratory dysfunction.

PRIMARY NEUROLOGIC DISEASE

Several diseases of the nervous system alter ventilation, apparently by affecting regions involved in ventilatory control. However, the results are variable, depending on the particular type of disorder and the region involved. In some cases hyperventilation is prominent, whereas in others hypoventilation is significant. In a third category the most apparent change is in the pattern of breathing.

Presentation with Hyperventilation

With certain acute disorders of the central nervous system, hyperventilation (i.e., decreased PCO_2 and respiratory alkalosis) is relatively common. Acute infections (meningitis, encephalitis), strokes, and trauma affecting the central nervous system are notable examples. The exact mechanism of hyperventilation in these situations is not known with certainty.

Many acute disorders of the central nervous system are associated with hyperventilation.

Presentation with Hypoventilation

A presentation with hypoventilation presumably results from a primary insult to the nervous system that affects centers involved with control of breathing. In such circumstances, patients have an elevated PCO_2, but because the clinical problems are generally not acute, the pH level has returned toward normal as a result of renal compensation with retention of bicarbonate. When no specific etiologic factor or prior event can be found to explain the hypoventilation, the patient is said to have *idiopathic hypoventilation* or *primary alveolar hypoventilation*. Other patients have had a significant insult to the nervous system at some time in the past, such as encephalitis, and chronic hypoventilation is presumably a sequela of the past event.

Patients with these syndromes of hypoventilation are characterized by depressed ventilatory responses to the chemical stimuli of hypercapnia and hypoxia. Measurement of arterial blood gases generally reveals an elevation in arterial PCO_2 accompanied by a decrease in PO_2, the latter being primarily due to hypoventilation. As in other disorders associated with these blood gas abnormalities, cor pulmonale may result and may represent the presenting problem in these syndromes. The term *Ondine's curse,* mentioned in Chapter 17, has been applied to some of these patients with alveolar hypoventilation—specifically when automatic control of ventilation is impaired but voluntary control remains intact.

Treatment of alveolar hypoventilation has generally centered around two modalities, drugs (most commonly the hormone progesterone) and electrical stimulation of the phrenic nerve. Progesterone is well known to be a respiratory stimulant and in some cases may improve respiratory drive and decrease CO_2 retention. As another approach, the diaphragm may be induced to contract by repetitive electrical stimulation of the phrenic nerve, which can be achieved by intermittent current applied to an implanted electrode. An alternative to these two modes of therapy involves assisted ventilation, especially at night, with any of several assist devices. These provide either positive pressure to the airway or negative pressure around the chest, thus augmenting minute ventilation without altering the patient's own respiratory drive.

Treatment of alveolar hypoventilation due to depressed central respiratory drive consists of the following:
1. Pharmacologic (e.g., progesterone)
2. Electrical stimulation of phrenic nerve
3. Assisted ventilation

Abnormal Patterns of Breathing

In addition to disturbances in overall alveolar ventilation, patients with neurologic disease may demonstrate abnormal patterns of breathing. The term *ataxic breathing* is applied to a grossly irregular breathing pattern observed with some types of lesions in the medulla. In contrast, certain lesions in the pons result in a breathing pattern characterized by a prolonged inspiratory pause; this pattern is called *apneustic breathing*.

Another type of abnormal breathing pattern is termed *Cheyne-Stokes breathing*. Unlike the other patterns just mentioned, Cheyne-Stokes breathing is quite common and warrants a special section to describe it and discuss what is known about its pathogenesis.

CHEYNE-STOKES BREATHING

Cheyne-Stokes breathing is a cyclic pattern in which periods of gradually increasing ventilation alternate with periods of gradually decreasing ventilation (even to the point of apnea). This type of ventilation is schematized in Figure 18-1. It has been known for many years that two main types of

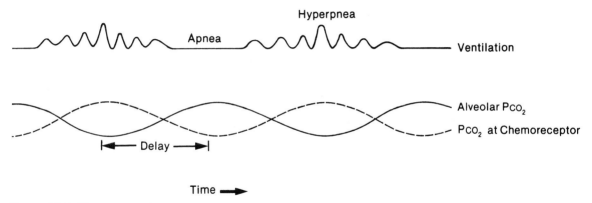

Figure 18-1 ━ Cheyne-Stokes breathing, showing cyclic pattern of ventilation. In patients with prolonged circulation time, delay between signal to chemoreceptor (PCO_2 at chemoreceptor) and ventilatory output (reflected by alveolar PCO_2) is shown.

disorders are associated with this type of breathing: congestive heart failure and some forms of central nervous system disease. Cheyne-Stokes breathing can also be seen under certain physiologic situations even in the absence of underlying disease. Examples include the onset of sleep and exposure to high altitude.

> Common causes of Cheyne-Stokes ventilation are congestive heart failure and some forms of central nervous system disease.

Central to the pathogenesis of Cheyne-Stokes ventilation is a problem with the feedback system of ventilatory control. Normally, the controlling system is able to adjust its output to compensate for arterial blood gas values that differ from the ideal or desired state. For example, with an elevated arterial PCO_2, the central chemoreceptor signals the medullary respiratory center to increase its output in order to augment ventilation and restore PCO_2 to normal. Similarly, the peripheral chemoreceptor responds to hypoxemia by increasing its output, signaling the medullary respiratory center to augment ventilation and restore PO_2 to normal.

At times, however, this feedback system may fail, especially if there is a delayed response to the signal or if the system responds more than necessary and overshoots the mark. Such defects in the feedback process appear to be at work in Cheyne-Stokes breathing. This section touches on a few aspects of theories proposed to explain Cheyne-Stokes ventilation, but for further discussion the interested reader is referred to the references at the end of this chapter.

A prolongation in circulation time, which is one of the mechanisms postulated to play a role in congestive heart failure, results in an abnormal delay between events in the lung and the sensing of PCO_2 changes by the central chemoreceptor. Hence, medullary respiratory output is out of phase with gas-exchange at the lungs, and oscillations in ventilation occur as the central chemoreceptor and the medullary respiratory center make belated attempts to maintain a stable PCO_2 (see Fig. 18-1).

An alternative explanation for Cheyne-Stokes breathing occurring with congestive heart failure is an accentuated ventilatory response to hypercapnia. This type of heightened responsiveness of the feedback system produces "instability" of respiratory control and a cyclical overshooting and undershooting of ventilation. Such increased responsiveness of the ventilatory control system may also play a role in patients with central nervous system disease who exhibit periods of Cheyne-Stokes respiration.

A similar type of instability of ventilatory control occurs when hypoxia is driving the feedback system, as is seen upon exposure to high altitude. The ventilatory response to hypoxia is alinear, so that, for the same drop in P_{O_2}, the increment in ventilation is larger at a lower absolute P_{O_2} (see Fig. 17-3). This means that at a relatively high initial P_{O_2}, the system is less likely to respond to small changes in P_{O_2}, but is then apt to overshoot as the P_{O_2} falls further. This instability of the respiratory control system results in a widely oscillating output from the respiratory center and thus a cyclic pattern of ventilation.

CONTROL ABNORMALITIES SECONDARY TO LUNG DISEASE

Ventilatory control mechanisms often respond to various forms of primary lung disease by altering respiratory center output. Either stimulation of peripheral chemoreceptors by hypoxemia or stimulation of receptors by diseases affecting the airways or the pulmonary interstitium can induce the respiratory center to increase its output, resulting in a respiratory alkalosis. Patients with asthma, for example, commonly demonstrate increased respiratory drive and hyperventilation during acute attacks as a consequence of stimulation of airway receptors. Similarly, patients with acute pulmonary embolism, pneumonia, or chronic interstitial lung disease often hyperventilate, presumably as a result of stimulation of one or more types of intrathoracic receptors, with or without the additional ventilatory stimulus contributed by hypoxemia.

In contrast, patients with chronic obstructive lung disease have variable levels of P_{CO_2}. As mentioned in Chapter 6, some patients with COPD (type A pathophysiology) do not generally demonstrate CO_2 retention, whereas the condition of others (type B) is often characterized by hypercapnia. In the latter group, the ventilatory control mechanism appears to be reset to operate at a higher setpoint for P_{CO_2}. When responsiveness to increased levels of P_{CO_2} is measured in hypercapnic patients, it is apparent that their ventilatory response is diminished. However, these patients with chronic, compensated respiratory acidosis have higher levels of plasma (as well as cerebrospinal fluid) bicarbonate because of bicarbonate retention by the kidneys. Therefore, for any increment in P_{CO_2}, the effect on pH at the medullary chemoreceptor is attenuated by the increased buffering capacity available. A "chicken and egg" question then becomes important: Is the CO_2 retention secondary to an underlying ventilatory control abnormality in these patients, or is the diminution in ventilatory sensitivity merely secondary to chronic CO_2 retention? Although this question remains unanswered, there is some evidence to suggest that familial factors may be important and that CO_2 retention is more likely to develop in patients with lower respiratory sensitivity (on a genetic basis).

Whatever the answer to this question, there is a clinically important corollary to this depression in CO_2 sensitivity, irrespective of the cause of CO_2 retention. When O_2 is administered to the chronically hypoxemic and hypercapnic patient, the P_{CO_2} may rise even further. At the extreme, if very high levels of inspired O_2 are administered, even life-threatening CO_2 retention may occasionally be seen. This phenomenon has frequently been ascribed to loss of sensitivity to CO_2 as a ventilatory stimulus, resulting from chronic CO_2 retention. Such patients therefore are thought to be primarily dependent on hypoxic drive as a ventilatory stimulus; when this stimulus is removed after

Administration of O_2 to the chronically hypoxemic and hypercapnic patient may elevate P_{CO_2}.

administration of high levels of inspired O_2, hypoventilation, and sometimes apnea, occurs.

However, this phenomenon is actually more complicated, because the degree of further CO_2 retention does not necessarily correlate with the depression in minute ventilation. It is thought that other factors, including alterations in the pattern of breathing, in the CO_2-hemoglobin dissociation curve (from the Haldane effect), and in ventilation-perfusion relationships as a result of O_2 administration, may be more important than depressed ventilation in contributing to this well-recognized clinical phenomenon. For example, when impaired ventilation to a particular region of the lung leads to alveolar hypoxia in that region, localized vasoconstriction occurs as a compensatory response to diminish the perfusion and minimize the amount of ventilation-perfusion mismatch. However, administration of supplemental O_2 may alleviate alveolar hypoxia in these poorly ventilated regions, thus aborting the compensatory localized vasoconstriction. Ventilation-perfusion mismatch becomes more marked in the absence of hypoxic vasoconstriction, leading to less efficient elimination of CO_2 and to increased levels of P_{CO_2}.

Fortunately, significant elevations in P_{CO_2} upon administration of supplemental O_2 to the chronically hypercapnic patient can generally be prevented by avoiding excessive concentrations of supplemental O_2 beyond those needed to raise oxygen saturation to approximately 90 percent. The clinician should therefore not withhold supplemental O_2 from hypoxemic patients who have chronic hypercapnia, since significant hypoxemia poses more of a risk than does a further increase in P_{CO_2}. Nevertheless, such patients are usually given relatively limited amounts of supplemental O_2 (often called "low-flow O_2" because of the low flow rate of O_2 given via nasal prongs) in order to minimize the degree of further hypercapnia.

SLEEP APNEA SYNDROME

Sleep apnea syndrome is a comparatively recently recognized disorder of respiration during sleep. Although a number of factors contribute to its pathogenesis, sleep-related changes in ventilatory control, specifically control of upper airway muscles, constitute an important component.

In this syndrome, patients have repetitive periods of apnea—i.e., cessation of breathing—occurring during sleep. A period of more than 10 seconds without airflow is generally considered to constitute an apneic episode, and patients with this syndrome often have hundreds of such episodes during the course of a night's sleep. The term *hypopnea* is used to describe a reduction in airflow of 50 percent or more, but without the complete cessation of airflow implied by the term apnea. Since episodes of apnea and hypopnea commonly coexist, the broader term *sleep apnea-hypopnea syndrome* is sometimes used. Sleep apnea syndrome is surprisingly common, with estimates suggesting a prevalence of 2 to 4 percent in middle-aged adults. Men are affected more commonly than women, and those women who are affected are typically postmenopausal.

Types

Sleep apnea syndrome is commonly divided into several types—obstructive, central, and mixed—depending on the nature of the episodes. In obstructive apnea the drive to breathe is still present during the apneic episode, but

Categories of sleep apnea syndrome are the following:

1. Obstructive
2. Central
3. Mixed

transient obstruction of the upper airway prevents inspiratory airflow. Inspiratory muscles are active during obstructive apnea; however, their attempts at initiating airflow are to no avail. In central apnea, there is no drive to breathe during the apneic period—i.e., there is no signal from the respiratory center to initiate inspiration. Hence, no respiratory muscle activity can be observed when airflow ceases. Frequently, patients may have episodes of apnea that have features of both central and obstructive apnea, and are therefore called mixed apnea. Typically, such episodes start without ventilatory effort (central apnea), but upper airway obstruction is present when ventilatory effort resumes (obstructive apnea). Because clinically significant episodes of obstructive apnea are more frequent than those of central apnea, the focus here is on the clinical features, pathophysiology, and treatment of obstructive apnea.

Clinical Features

Patients with sleep apnea syndrome may seek medical consultation because of (1) symptoms or signs that they or their partner have noticed during a night's sleep, (2) daytime symptoms, or (3) complications that arise from the repetitive apneic episodes. During sleep, patients with episodes of obstructive apnea are often noted to have a markedly deranged sleep pattern. Loud snoring is particularly prominent, and patients may have obvious snorting and agitation as a result of trying to breathe against the obstructed airway. They may also have violent movements during periods of obstruction; not uncommonly, the sleep partner complains of being hit or injured as a result of these violent movements. On waking, patients often complain of a severe headache, presumably related to the derangements in gas-exchange that occur during the apneic episodes.

Clinical features of sleep apnea syndrome are the following:
1. Disordered respiration during sleep
2. Daytime hypersomnolence
3. Cardiovascular complications

With such a disordered pattern of sleep, these patients are effectively sleep-deprived, and it is not surprising that they may be overly somnolent during the normal waking hours. The degree of somnolence can be debilitating and even dangerous; patients commonly fall asleep while driving, eating, or working or during a variety of other usual daytime activities. Patients are also often considered to have a personality disorder, partially because of their extreme hypersomnolence and partially because of psychologic changes that have presumably resulted from their disease.

Secondary cardiovascular complications of obstructive sleep apnea are believed to be mediated in part by increased sympathetic nervous system activity. During the episodes of apnea, patients may have a variety of cardiac arrhythmias or conduction disturbances, although they are rarely life-threatening. As a result of episodes of prolonged hypoxemia at night, pulmonary hypertension can result, and unexplained cor pulmonale may be the presenting clinical problem. Systemic hypertension also appears to be associated with and perhaps a consequence of obstructive sleep apnea.

Pathophysiology

During the last two decades, a great deal has been learned about the pathogenesis and the risk factors leading to obstructive sleep apnea syndrome. Normally, inspiration is characterized not only by contraction of the diaphragm, resulting in negative airway pressure, but also by increased activity of a number of upper airway muscles acting to keep the pharynx patent.

The genioglossus muscle is particularly important in this regard, because it prevents the tongue from falling against the posterior pharyngeal wall and occluding the pharynx.

In patients with obstructive sleep apnea, structural and functional factors often work together to allow the upper airway to close during inspiration. In most patients, an excess of soft tissue in the upper airway, often as a consequence of obesity, compromises the size of the pharyngeal opening. During sleep, particularly rapid-eye-movement sleep, a loss of activity of the upper airway muscles allows inspiratory collapse of the soft tissues and obstruction of the upper airway. Airflow eventually resumes following each episode of obstruction as the patient arouses (although these "micro-arousals" are often not evident to the patient), when activity of the upper airway muscles is restored, and when the airway temporarily becomes patent. However, as the patient then falls asleep again, inspiratory muscle activity is again lost, and the cycle repeats itself. Because of the importance of structural factors contributing to a small upper airway, patients who are obese (with short, fat necks) or who have a small jaw (micrognathia), a large tongue, or large tonsils are at particular risk for obstructive sleep apnea.

During an episode of central apnea, monitoring of chest wall motion reveals no movement, corresponding to cessation of airflow and a fall in O_2 saturation (Fig. 18-2A). With obstructive apnea, chest wall and abdominal movement can be detected during a fruitless attempt to move air through the obstructed airway. Airflow measured simultaneously is found to be absent (tidal volume = 0), and the O_2 saturation drops, often to profoundly low levels (see Fig. 18-2B). When O_2 saturation drops significantly during sleep, disturbances in cardiac rhythm occur, and elevation of pulmonary artery pressure may be seen as a consequence of hypoxia-induced pulmonary vasoconstriction.

Treatment

In patients with central apnea, treatment generally revolves around the use of respiratory stimulants or an electrical, implanted phrenic nerve pacemaker to stimulate the diaphragm. In obstructive apnea, a variety of forms of therapy have been used. With patients who are markedly obese, an attempt at significant weight loss is often made. Although weight loss can sometimes dramatically improve the number and severity of the apneic episodes, long-term weight reduction is difficult for most patients to maintain, making other forms of therapy necessary. In all patients, respiratory depressants, including alcohol and sedative-hypnotic drugs, should be avoided, because they may worsen obstructive sleep apnea.

The first-line therapy used in most patients with obstructive sleep apnea syndrome is nasal continuous positive airway pressure, commonly called *nasal CPAP.* A mask connected to an air compressor is placed over the nose of the patient at bedtime. The compressor maintains positive pressure in the upper airway throughout the respiratory cycle, thus providing a pneumatic splint to keep the airway open.

Nasal continuous positive airway pressure (CPAP) is often applied at night to patients with obstructive sleep apnea to prevent upper airway closure.

An alternative but less common form of therapy involves nocturnal use of an oral appliance to maintain the tongue and/or the jaw in a relatively anterior position. This mechanical form of therapy facilitates airway patency by keeping the tongue away from the posterior pharyngeal wall.

Because nasal CPAP and oral appliances are so often effective, other forms of previously utilized therapy are now used less frequently.

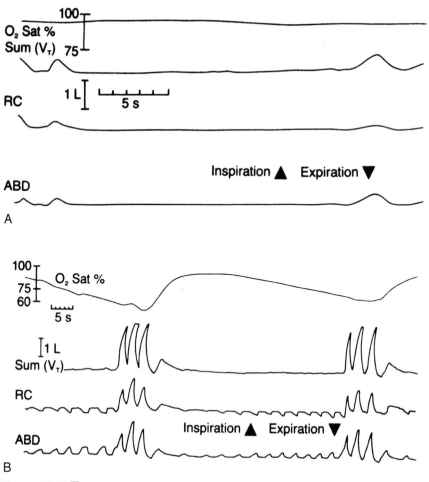

Figure 18-2 ■— Examples of recordings in sleep apnea syndrome. O_2 Sat = O_2 saturation, RC = rib cage, ABD = abdominal movement, and V_T = tidal volume (monitored as sum of rib cage and abdominal movements). *A*, Central sleep apnea. Absence of abdominal, rib cage, and sum movements are associated with small fall in arterial oxygen saturation. *B*, Obstructive sleep apnea. Apneas at beginning and midportion of recording are marked by absence of sum movements (V_T) despite respiratory efforts. When diaphragm contracts and upper airway is obstructed during attempted inspiration, abdomen moves out (upward on tracing) while rib cage moves inward (downward). Each apnea shown is associated with marked fall in O_2 saturation and is terminated by three deep breaths. (From Tobin MJ, Cohn MA, and Sackner MA: Arch Intern Med 143:1221–1228, 1983. Copyright 1983, American Medical Association.)

Nevertheless, surgical modes of therapy may be beneficial in selected patients. For example, some patients are treated by means of a surgical procedure called *uvulopalatopharyngoplasty,* which involves removal of redundant soft tissue in the upper airway. Patients with particularly severe obstructive apnea whose disease is refractory to other forms of therapy can be treated with a tracheostomy, which involves placement of a tube in the trachea to allow air to bypass the site of upper airway obstruction. Despite the apparent drastic nature of tracheostomy as a form of treatment, the therapeutic response is often quite gratifying. Patients may have a dramatic reversal of their symptoms and a striking improvement in their lifestyle, which was previously limited by intractable daytime sleepiness.

References

Primary Neurologic Disease

Farmer WC, Glenn WWL, and Gee JBL: Alveolar hypoventilation syndrome: studies of ventilatory control in patients selected for diaphragm pacing. Am J Med 64:39-49, 1978.

Garay SM, Turino GM, and Goldring RM: Sustained reversal of chronic hypercapnia in patients with alveolar hypoventilation syndromes: long-term maintenance with noninvasive nocturnal mechanical ventilation. Am J Med 70:269-274, 1981.

Krachman S and Criner GJ: Hypoventilation syndromes. Clin Chest Med 19:139-155, 1998.

Mellins RB, Balfour HH, Turino GM, and Winters RW: Failure of automatic control of ventilation (Ondine's curse). Medicine 49:487-504, 1970.

Reichel J: Primary alveolar hypoventilation. Clin Chest Med 1:119-124, 1980.

Cheyne-Stokes Breathing

Cherniack NS and Longobardo GS: Abnormalities in respiratory rhythm. *In* Fishman AP, Cherniack NS, Widdicombe JG, and Geiger SR (eds): Handbook of Physiology. Section 3: The Respiratory System, vol. II. Control of Breathing, part 2. Bethesda, MD, American Physiological Society, 1986, pp 729-749.

Cherniack NS and Longobardo GS: Cheyne-Stokes breathing: an instability in physiologic control. N Engl J Med 288:952-957, 1973.

Naughton MT: Pathophysiology and treatment of Cheyne-Stokes respiration. Thorax 53:514-518, 1998.

Control Abnormalities Secondary to Lung Disease

Aubier M et al: Effects of the administration of O_2 on ventilation and blood gases in patients with chronic obstructive pulmonary disease during acute respiratory failure. Am Rev Respir Dis 122:747-754, 1980.

Caruana-Montaldo B, Gleeson K, and Zwillich CW: The control of breathing in clinical practice. Chest 117:205-225, 2000.

Dunn WF, Nelson SB, and Hubmayr RD: Oxygen-induced hypercarbia in obstructive pulmonary disease. Am Rev Respir Dis 144:526-530, 1991.

Milic-Emili J and Aubier M: Some recent advances in the study of the control of breathing in patients with chronic obstructive lung disease. Anesth Analg 59:865-873, 1980.

Mountain R, Zwillich C, and Weil J: Hypoventilation in obstructive lung disease: the role of familial factors. N Engl J Med. 298:521-525, 1978.

Park SS: Respiratory control in chronic obstructive pulmonary diseases. Clin Chest Med 1:73-84, 1980.

Weinberger SE, Schwartzstein RM, and Weiss JW: Hypercapnia. N Engl J Med 321:1223-1231, 1989.

Sleep Apnea Syndrome

American Academy of Sleep Medicine Task Force: Sleep-related breathing disorders in adults: recommendations for syndrome definition and measurement techniques in clinical research. Sleep 22:667-689, 1999.

Badr MS: Pathogenesis of obstructive sleep apnea. Prog Cardiovasc Dis 41:323-330, 1999.

Cartwright R: Obstructive sleep apnea: a sleep disorder with major effects on health. Dis Mon 47:109-147, 2001.

Flemons WW: Obstructive sleep apnea. N Engl J Med 347:498-504, 2002.

Kuna ST and Sant'Ambrogio G: Pathophysiology of upper airway closure during sleep. JAMA 266:1384-1389, 1991.

Netzer N, Eliasson AH, Netzer C, and Kristo DA: Overnight pulse oximetry for sleep-disordered breathing in adults: a review. Chest 120:625-633, 2001.

Roux F, D'Ambrosio C, and Mohsenin V: Sleep-related breathing disorders and cardiovascular disease. Am J Med 108:396-402, 2000.

Simonds AK: New developments in the treatment of obstructive sleep apnea. Thorax 55 (Suppl 1):S45-S50, 2000.

Skomro RP and Kryger MH: Clinical presentations of obstructive sleep apnea syndrome. Prog Cardiovasc Dis 41:331-340, 1999.

Strollo PJ Jr and Rogers RM: Obstructive sleep apnea. N Engl J Med 334:99-104, 1996.

Strollo PJ Jr and Sanders MH (eds): Sleep disorders. Clin Chest Med 19:1-222, 1998.

Teran-Santos J, Jimenez-Gomez A, and Cordero-Guevera J: The association between sleep apnea and the risk of traffic accidents. N Engl J Med 340:847-851, 1999.

Disorders of the Respiratory Pump

The chest wall, diaphragm, and related neuromuscular apparatus moving the chest wall act in concert to translate signals from the ventilatory controller into expansion of the thorax. Together, these structures constitute the respiratory pump, an important system that may fail as a result of diseases affecting any of its parts. Because disorders of the respiratory pump include a variety of problems, this discussion is limited to those disorders that are most common and most important clinically: (1) neuromuscular disease affecting the muscles of respiration (Guillain-Barré syndrome, myasthenia gravis, poliomyelitis, amyotrophic lateral sclerosis), (2) diaphragmatic fatigue, (3) diaphragmatic paralysis, and (4) diseases affecting the chest wall (kyphoscoliosis, obesity).

NEUROMUSCULAR DISEASE AFFECTING THE MUSCLES OF RESPIRATION

A number of neuromuscular diseases have the potential for affecting the muscles of respiration. In some cases the underlying process is acute and generally reversible—for example, Guillain-Barré syndrome—and the muscles of respiration are transiently affected for a variable amount of time. In other cases the neuromuscular damage is permanent, and any consequences that affect the muscles of respiration are chronic and irreversible. In this section, brief definitions of some specific neurologic disorders with respiratory sequelae are followed by a discussion of the pathophysiology and clinical consequences of these diseases as they relate to the respiratory system.

Specific Diseases

The major neuromuscular diseases that can affect the muscles of respiration are listed in Table 19-1; several are discussed here.

Guillain-Barré syndrome is a disorder that is characterized by demyelination of peripheral nerves. It is thought to be triggered by exposure to an antigen (typically an infectious agent), and the resulting immune response gets

Table	19-1		
	Disorders of the Respiratory Pump		
Neuromuscular Diseases			**Chest Wall Diseases**
Guillain-Barré syndrome			Kyphoscoliosis
Myasthenia gravis			Obesity
Poliomyelitis			Ankylosing spondylitis
Post-polio syndrome			
Amyotrophic lateral sclerosis			
Quadriplegia			
Polymyositis			
Muscular dystrophy			

misdirected to similar antigenic determinants (epitopes) on neural tissue. Frequently, patients have a history of a recent viral or bacterial illness, followed by development of an ascending paralysis and variable sensory symptoms. Classically, weakness or paralysis starts symmetrically in the lower extremities and progresses or ascends proximally to the upper extremities and trunk. In severe cases, respiratory muscle weakness or paralysis accompanies the more usual limb and trunk symptoms. Generally, the natural history of this disease leads to recovery, and permanent sequelae are frequently absent. When respiratory muscles are affected, respiratory failure often supervenes but is usually reversible over the course of weeks to months.

In *myasthenia gravis,* patients experience weakness and fatigue of voluntary muscles, most frequently those innervated by cranial nerves, but peripheral (limb) and, potentially, respiratory muscles are also affected. The primary abnormality is found at the neuromuscular junction, where transmission of impulses from nerve to muscle is impaired by a decreased number of receptors on the muscle for the neurotransmitter acetylcholine and by the presence of antibodies against these receptors. Although myasthenia gravis is a chronic illness, the manifestations can often be controlled by appropriate therapy, and individual episodes of respiratory failure are potentially reversible.

Poliomyelitis is a viral disease in which the polio virus attacks motor nerve cells of the spinal cord and brain stem. Both the diaphragm and intercostal muscles can be affected, with resulting weakness or paralysis and respiratory failure. Surviving patients generally recover respiratory muscle function, although occasional patients have chronic respiratory insufficiency from prior disease. As the result of mass vaccination of the population, new cases are quite rare.

In *post-polio syndrome,* patients develop new or progressive symptoms of weakness occurring decades after the initial episode of poliomyelitis. Involvement occurs in muscles originally affected by the disease, and respiratory muscle involvement is therefore more likely in those patients who had respiratory failure with their initial disease.

Amyotrophic lateral sclerosis is a degenerative disease of the nervous system that involves both upper and lower motor neurons. Commonly, muscles innervated by either cranial nerves or spinal nerves are affected. Clinically, progressive muscle weakness and wasting develop, eventually leading to profound weakness of respiratory muscles and death. Although the time course of the disease is variable from patient to patient, the natural history is one of irreversibility and progressive deterioration. As a result, patients and families must confront the difficult decision of how aggressively to provide some form of ventilatory support when the patient is in respiratory failure, considering the lack of available treatment to arrest the progressive neurologic deterioration.

Pathophysiology and Clinical Consequences

Weakness of respiratory muscles is the hallmark of respiratory involvement in the neuromuscular diseases. Depending on the specific disease, chest wall (intercostal) muscles, diaphragm, and expiratory muscles of the abdominal wall are each affected to a variable extent.

Because of the impairment of inspiratory muscle strength, patients may be unable to maintain sufficient minute ventilation for adequate CO_2 elimination. In addition, patients often alter their pattern of breathing, taking more shallow and more frequent breaths. Although this pattern of breathing may be easier and more comfortable, it is also less efficient, because a greater proportion of each breath is wasted on ventilating the anatomic dead space. Therefore, even if total minute ventilation is maintained, alveolar ventilation (and thus CO_2 elimination) is impaired by the altered pattern of breathing.

The respiratory difficulty that develops in patients with neuromuscular disease is also complicated by weakness of expiratory muscles and by an ineffective cough. Recurrent respiratory tract infections, accumulation of secretions, and areas of collapse or atelectasis thus contribute to the clinical problems seen in these patients.

Symptoms include dyspnea and anxiety; patients may also have a feeling of suffocation. Often, the presence of generalized muscle weakness severely limits patients' activity and lessens the degree of dyspnea that would be present if they were capable of more exertion.

Features of neuromuscular disease are the following:
1. Altered pattern of breathing (↑ rate, ↓ tidal volume)
2. Ineffective cough
3. Restrictive pattern on pulmonary function tests
4. Decreased maximal inspiratory/expiratory pressures
5. ↑ P_{CO_2}, often with ↓ P_{O_2}

With severe neuromuscular disease, pulmonary function tests show a restrictive pattern of impairment. Although muscle weakness is the primary cause for the restriction, the compliance of the lung and the chest wall may be secondarily affected, further contributing to the restrictive pattern. The decrease in pulmonary compliance is presumably due to microatelectasis, i.e., alveolar collapse, resulting from the shallow tidal volumes. At the same time, stiffening of various components of the chest wall—for example, tendons, ligaments, and joints—is thought to be responsible for decreased distensibility of the chest wall. Functional residual capacity (FRC) is normal or decreased, depending on how much respiratory system compliance is altered. Total lung capacity is decreased primarily as a result of inspiratory muscle weakness, but changes in respiratory system compliance may contribute as well. Residual volume (RV) is frequently increased as a result of expiratory muscle weakness (Fig. 19-1). The degree of muscle weakness can be quantitated by measuring the maximal inspiratory and expiratory pressures the patient is able to generate with a maximal inspiratory and expiratory effort against a closed mouthpiece. Both maximal inspiratory pressure (MIP) and maximal expiratory pressure (MEP) may be significantly depressed.

In the setting of severe muscle weakness, arterial blood gases are most notable for the presence of alveolar hypoventilation, i.e., hypercapnia. Hypoxemia also occurs as a result of alveolar hypoventilation and the associated depression in alveolar P_{O_2}. When hypoventilation is the sole cause of hypoxemia, the alveolar-arterial oxygen difference is normal. However, complications of atelectasis, respiratory tract infections, and inadequately cleared

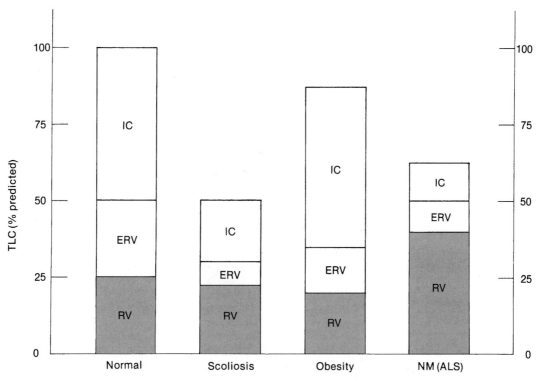

Figure 19-1 ▪— Examples of lung volumes (total lung capacity and its subdivisions) in patients with chest wall and neuromuscular (NM) disease compared with those of normal subject. Clear area represents vital capacity and its subdivisions: IC = inspiratory capacity, ERV = expiratory reserve volume. Shaded area is RV = residual volume. ALS = amyotrophic lateral sclerosis. (Adapted from Bergofsky EH: Am Rev Respir Dis 119:643–669, 1979.)

secretions may add a component of ventilation-perfusion mismatch that further depresses Po_2 and increases $AaDo_2$.

DIAPHRAGMATIC DISEASE

Although diaphragmatic involvement is a significant component of many of the neuromuscular diseases described above that affect the muscles of respiration, there are additional etiologic and clinical considerations that justify a separate discussion of diaphragmatic disease. We will first consider diaphragmatic fatigue, a potential consequence of disorders affecting other parts of the respiratory system that significantly increase the workload placed on the diaphragm. We will then discuss diaphragmatic paralysis, with separate considerations of unilateral and bilateral paralysis, since the causes and the clinical manifestations are often quite different.

Diaphragmatic Fatigue

Excluding cardiac muscle, the diaphragm is the single muscle used most consistently and repetitively throughout the course of a lifetime. It is well suited for sustained activity and for aerobic metabolism, and under normal circumstances the diaphragm does not become fatigued.

However, if the diaphragm is required to perform an excessive amount of work or if its energy supplies are limited, fatigue may develop and may contribute to respiratory dysfunction in certain clinical settings. For example, if a normal individual repetitively uses the diaphragm to generate 40 percent or more of its maximal force, fatigue develops and prevents this degree of effort from being sustained indefinitely. For patients with diseases that increase the work of breathing, particularly obstructive lung disease and diseases of the chest wall (described in the next section), the diaphragm works at a level much closer to the point of fatigue. When a superimposed acute illness further increases the work of breathing, or when an intercurrent problem (e.g., depressed cardiac output, anemia, or hypoxemia) decreases the energy supply available to the diaphragm, then diaphragmatic fatigue may contribute to the development of hypoventilation and respiratory failure.

Inefficient diaphragmatic contraction is an additional factor that may contribute to diaphragmatic fatigue, especially in the patient with obstructive lung disease. When the diaphragm is flattened and its fibers are shortened as a result of hyperinflated lungs, the force or pressure developed during contraction is less for any given level of diaphragmatic excitation (see Chapter 17). Therefore, a higher degree of stimulation is necessary to generate comparable pressure by the diaphragm, and increased energy consumption results.

Diaphragmatic fatigue is often difficult to detect because the force generated by the diaphragm cannot be measured conveniently. Ideally, diaphragmatic fatigue is documented by measuring the pressure across the diaphragm (i.e., the difference between abdominal and pleural pressure, called the *transdiaphragmatic pressure*) during diaphragmatic stimulation or contraction. As an alternative to measurement of transdiaphragmatic pressure, the strength of the inspiratory muscles in general can be assessed by measuring the pressure that a patient can generate with a maximal inspiratory effort against a closed mouthpiece, i.e., the MIP. A useful finding on physical examination is the pattern of motion of the abdomen during breathing when the patient is supine. If diaphragmatic contraction is especially weak or absent, pleural pressure falls mainly as a result of contraction of other inspiratory muscles. The negative pleural pressure is transmitted across the relatively flaccid diaphragm to the abdomen, which then moves paradoxically inward during inspiration.

Along with investigation of the role of diaphragmatic fatigue in respiratory failure, there have also been attempts to improve or reverse fatigue. Use of assisted ventilation with a mechanical ventilator to rest the diaphragm is one potential method for reversing fatigue. Alternatively, use of theophylline has been shown experimentally to increase the strength of diaphragmatic contraction. However, whether this type of pharmacologic therapy produces a clinically beneficial effect has yet to be proved.

Factors contributing to diaphragmatic fatigue are the following:
1. Increased work of breathing
2. Decreased energy supply to diaphragm
3. Inefficient diaphragmatic contraction

Diaphragmatic weakness can be demonstrated in the supine position by inward motion of the abdomen during inspiration.

Unilateral Diaphragmatic Paralysis

Paralysis of a single diaphragm (also called a hemidiaphragm) typically results from disease affecting the ipsilateral phrenic nerve. A particularly common cause of unilateral diaphragmatic paralysis is invasion of the phrenic nerve by malignancy. The underlying tumor is frequently lung cancer which has invaded or metastasized to the mediastinum, and either the primary tumor itself or mediastinal lymph nodes affected by tumor invade the phrenic nerve somewhere along its course through the mediastinum.

Paralysis of the left diaphragm is also seen relatively commonly following cardiac surgery. In these cases, a cold solution is instilled in the pericardium during the procedure to stop cardiac contraction (cold cardioplegia) and allow surgery on a nonbeating heart, while circulation is maintained by cardiopulmonary bypass. However, the cold solution causes temporary paralysis of the left phrenic nerve, leading to diaphragmatic paralysis of variable duration. Finally, in some patients with unilateral diaphragmatic paralysis, no underlying reason for the paralysis can be identified, and the problem is considered idiopathic. It has been postulated that a viral infection affecting the phrenic nerve may be responsible in such cases.

The possibility of unilateral diaphragmatic paralysis is usually first suggested by a characteristic appearance on the chest radiograph (Fig. 19-2). The affected diaphragm is elevated above its usual position, in the absence of any associated lobar atelectasis or other reason for volume loss on the affected side. Since chest radiographs are taken during a full inspiration (to total lung capacity), the normal diaphragm descends during inspiration, while the paralyzed diaphragm cannot. Patients may or may not be symptomatic with dyspnea as a result of the paralyzed hemidiaphragm, often depending upon the presence or absence of additional underlying lung disease.

Because there are other causes of an elevated diaphragm besides diaphragmatic paralysis (e.g., processes below the diaphragm, such as a subphrenic abscess), it is generally useful to confirm objectively that diaphragmatic paralysis is the cause of diaphragmatic elevation. This can be done relatively easily by real-time observation of diaphragmatic movement during a "sniff test." With this technique, the radiologist observes diaphragmatic motion under fluoroscopy while the patient sniffs. During the act of sniffing, which is a rapid inspiratory activity, the normal diaphragm contracts and therefore descends, while the paralyzed diaphragm moves passively (and paradoxically) upward as a result of the rapid development of negative intrathoracic pressure during the sniff.

Bilateral Diaphragmatic Paralysis

Paralysis of both diaphragms has much more serious clinical implications than unilateral paralysis, as the patient must depend upon the accessory muscles of inspiration to maintain minute ventilation. The causes of bilateral diaphragmatic paralysis are those neuromuscular diseases listed in Table 19-1,

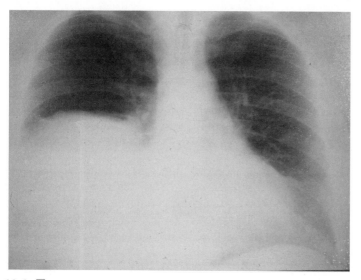

Figure 19-2 ■━ Chest radiograph demonstrating elevation of the right hemidiaphragm due to unilateral (right) phrenic nerve paralysis.

with bilateral diaphragmatic paralysis being the most severe consequence of respiratory involvement by these disorders.

A characteristic clinical manifestation of bilateral diaphragmatic paralysis is dyspnea that is significantly exacerbated by assuming the recumbent position, i.e., severe orthopnea. When the patient is supine, the abdominal contents push on the flaccid diaphragm, as the beneficial effects of gravity on abdominal contents and on lowering the position of the diaphragm are lost. On physical examination, patients typically demonstrate paradoxical inward motion of the abdomen during inspiration while they are supine, as also described in the earlier discussion on diaphragmatic fatigue. The deleterious effect of assuming the recumbent position is also seen with pulmonary function testing, as the vital capacity measured in the supine position is significantly lower than that measured in the upright position.

DISEASES AFFECTING THE CHEST WALL

With certain diseases of the chest wall, difficulty in expanding the chest may impede normal inspiration (see Table 19-1). The focus in this section is on two specific disorders that pose the greatest clinical problems: kyphoscoliosis and obesity.

Kyphoscoliosis

Kyphoscoliosis is an abnormal curvature of the spine in both the lateral and anteroposterior directions (Fig. 19-3). As a result of this deformity, the rib cage becomes stiffer and more difficult to expand; i.e., chest wall compliance is decreased. In patients with significant kyphoscoliosis, respiratory difficulties

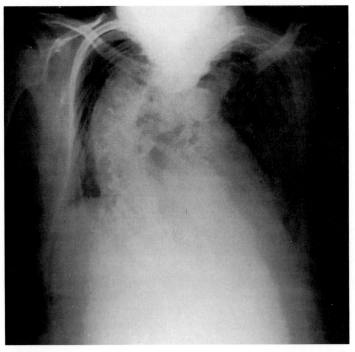

Figure 19-3 ┣━ Chest radiograph of patient with severe kyphoscoliosis. Note marked spinal curvature and chest wall distortion.

are common. In particularly severe cases, chronic respiratory failure is the consequence. Although some cases of kyphoscoliosis are actually secondary to neuromuscular disease such as poliomyelitis, the majority of severe cases associated with respiratory impairment are idiopathic.

Several pathophysiologic features contribute to respiratory dysfunction in patients with kyphoscoliosis. A crucial underlying problem is the increased work of breathing resulting from the poorly compliant chest wall. To maintain even a normal minute ventilation, the work expenditure of the respiratory muscles is greatly increased. In addition, however, patients decrease their tidal volume and increase respiratory frequency because of difficulty expanding the abnormally stiff chest wall. Consequently, the proportion of wasted ventilation rises, and alveolar ventilation falls unless total ventilation undergoes a compensatory increase. Hence, the increased work of breathing acts together with the altered pattern of breathing to decrease alveolar ventilation and to increase P_{CO_2}.

In addition, the marked distortion of the chest wall causes underventilation of some regions of the lung, microatelectasis, ventilation-perfusion mismatch, and hypoxemia. Therefore, there are frequently two causes for hypoxemia in kyphoscoliosis: hypoventilation and ventilation-perfusion mismatch.

A common complication of severe kyphoscoliosis is pulmonary hypertension and cor pulmonale. Hypoxemia and, to a lesser extent, hypercapnia are important for the development of pulmonary hypertension. However, increased resistance of the pulmonary vessels also results from compression and possibly from impaired development in regions in which the chest wall is especially distorted. Long-standing pulmonary hypertension itself also causes structural changes in the vessels, with thickening of the walls of pulmonary arteries. This thickening is not acutely reversible, even with correction of the hypoxemia.

Exertional dyspnea is probably the most common symptom experienced by patients with severe kyphoscoliosis and respiratory impairment. Unlike patients with neuromuscular disease, those with a chest wall deformity such as kyphoscoliosis have normal muscle strength and therefore are otherwise capable of normal levels of exertion. Patients with kyphoscoliosis also are not subject to the same difficulty in generating an effective cough as are patients with neuromuscular disease. Expiratory muscle function is preserved, an effective cough is maintained, and problems with secretions and recurrent respiratory tract infections are not prominent clinical features.

Pulmonary function tests in patients with kyphoscoliosis are notable for a restrictive pattern of impairment, with a decrease in the total lung capacity. Vital capacity is also significantly decreased, whereas RV tends to be relatively preserved. Functional residual capacity, determined by the outward recoil of the chest wall balanced by the inward recoil of the lung, is decreased, because the poorly compliant chest wall has a diminished propensity to recoil outward (see Fig. 19-1).

As mentioned earlier, severe cases of kyphoscoliosis are generally characterized by hypercapnia and hypoxemia. The latter is usually due to both hypoventilation and ventilation-perfusion mismatch. Chronic respiratory insufficiency and cor pulmonale are the end results of severe kyphoscoliosis, and the level of respiratory difficulty appears to correlate with the severity of the chest wall deformity.

Surgical therapy aimed at improving or correcting the spinal deformity may be useful in children or adolescents, but it is rarely effective in adults.

Features of severe kyphoscoliosis are the following:

1. Increased work of breathing
2. Altered pattern of breathing ($\uparrow$ rate, $\downarrow$ tidal volume)
3. Exertional dyspnea
4. Ventilation-perfusion mismatch
5. $\uparrow$ P_{CO_2}, often with $\downarrow$ P_{O_2}
6. Pulmonary hypertension, cor pulmonale
7. Restrictive pattern on pulmonary function tests

Supportive therapy that may be beneficial includes a variety of measures that provide ventilatory assistance to the patient. Treatments with an intermittent positive-pressure breathing machine augment tidal volume by delivering positive pressure to the patient during inspiration. The increase in tidal volume improves microatelectasis and lung compliance, affording the patient several hours with decreased work of breathing after each treatment. At night, ventilatory assistance with either inspiratory positive pressure delivered at the mouth or negative pressure around the chest wall allows the respiratory muscles to rest. Nocturnal ventilatory support may provide sufficient rest for the inspiratory muscles to diminish daytime respiratory muscle fatigue. Further discussion of these types of ventilatory support is presented in Chapter 29.

Obesity

Obesity has many consequences for health, and respiratory symptoms are one aspect. Obesity can produce a wide spectrum in severity of respiratory impairment, ranging from no symptoms to marked limitation in function. Surprisingly, the degree of obesity does not appear to correlate with the presence or severity of respiratory dysfunction. Some patients who are massively obese have no difficulty in comparison with much less obese patients who may be severely limited. An explanation of these discrepancies is based on the several factors that contribute to respiratory dysfunction; obesity is only one of these factors.

The problem of respiratory impairment in obesity was popularly known for years as the *pickwickian syndrome,* or *obesity-hypoventilation syndrome.* The name pickwickian was applied because of the description of the fat boy, Joe, in Dickens' *Pickwick Papers,* who had many of the characteristics described in this syndrome. Specifically, Joe had features of massive obesity, somnolence, and peripheral edema, the latter presumably related to cor pulmonale and right ventricular failure. With the accumulation of knowledge about the pathogenesis of respiratory impairment in obesity, the term pickwickian syndrome has become less meaningful.

Obesity appears to exert two effects on the respiratory system. As a result of excess soft tissue, the chest wall becomes stiffer or less compliant, and thus more work is necessary for expansion of the thorax. In addition, the massive accumulation of soft tissue in the abdominal wall exerts pressure on abdominal contents, forcing the diaphragm up to a higher resting position.

In a fashion similar to that of kyphoscoliosis, the stiff chest wall results in lower tidal volumes and increased wasted or dead space ventilation. Therefore, in order to maintain adequate alveolar ventilation, overall minute ventilation must increase in the face of increased work of breathing. Some patients are able to compensate appropriately by increasing their overall minute ventilation, and Pco_2 remains normal. Others do not compensate fully, and hypercapnia is the necessary consequence.

Exactly what distinguishes these two types of patients is not really known. Perhaps patients in the latter group, for whom the term obesity-hypoventilation syndrome can be applied, started out with a central nervous system respiratory controller that was relatively hyporesponsive. Output of the controller might not have responded sufficiently to keep pace with increased ventilatory requirements, and CO_2 retention would then result. Once hypercapnia actually develops, it is much more difficult to assess the innate responsiveness of the patient's ventilatory controller, because chronic

hypercapnia—i.e., chronic respiratory acidosis with a compensatory metabolic alkalosis—blunts the responsiveness of the central chemoreceptor.

An additional distinguishing feature between normocapnic and hypercapnic obese patients may relate to inspiratory muscle strength. Whereas
inspiratory muscle strength is normal in obese patients with a normal P_{CO_2},
it is reduced by approximately 30 percent in patients with the obesity-
hypoventilation syndrome, perhaps as a result of respiratory muscle fatigue.

The high resting position of the diaphragm in obesity, occurring as a
result of pressure from the obese abdomen, is associated with decreased
expansion of the lung and closure of small airways and alveoli at the bases.
The dependent regions are thus hypoventilated relative to their perfusion, and
this ventilation-perfusion mismatch results in arterial hypoxemia.

An additional factor that contributes to the overall clinical picture in
many massively obese patients is upper airway obstruction during sleep, i.e.,
the obstructive form of sleep apnea syndrome. Presumably, soft tissue deposition in the neck and tissues surrounding the upper airway predisposes the
person to episodes of complete upper airway obstruction during sleep. In a
large percentage of cases, somnolence that occurs in patients who supposedly
have the obesity-hypoventilation syndrome is related to the presence of
obstructive sleep apnea.

Although obesity, depressed respiratory drive, respiratory muscle weakness, and sleep apnea syndrome contribute to respiratory dysfunction, exactly
how they interact in individual patients is often difficult to assess. Because
sleep apnea syndrome and depressed respiratory drive also occur in patients
who are not obese, it is reasonable to view some of the contributing pathophysiologic factors in terms of a Venn diagram (Fig. 19-4). Probably the most
marked symptoms and respiratory dysfunction are seen in patients who are
represented at the intersection of the three circles.

The symptoms that may occur in the obese patient can be associated
with the increased work of breathing (e.g., dyspnea) or with the sleep apnea
syndrome (e.g., daytime somnolence and disordered sleep with profound
snoring). Patients may also have clinical manifestations related to the complications of pulmonary hypertension, cor pulmonale, and right ventricular
failure. These complications are largely related to arterial hypoxemia both
during the day and at night, particularly if the patient has sleep apnea
syndrome.

Features of obesity are the
following:

1. Decreased chest wall
   compliance
2. High diaphragm (low
   FRC)
3. Altered pattern of
   breathing (↑ rate, ↓ tidal
   volume)
4. Ventilation-perfusion
   mismatch
5. Variable ↑ P_{CO_2}, ↓ P_{O_2}
6. Obstructive apnea
   (common)

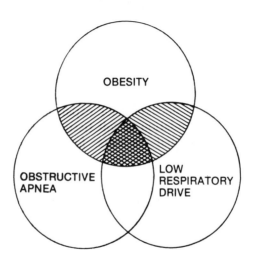

Figure 19-4 ■— Venn diagram shows
hypothetical indication of the way obesity
interacts with obstructive apnea and
low respiratory drive. Overlap on left indicates obese, normocapnic patients with
obstructive apnea. Overlap on right indicates hypercapnic obese patients without
obstructive apnea. Overlap at center indicates obese, hypercapnic patients with
obstructive apnea.

Pulmonary function tests frequently demonstrate a restrictive pattern of dysfunction, with a decrease in the total lung capacity. As mentioned earlier, the diaphragm is pushed up in the massively obese patient, reducing FRC, which in these patients is much closer to RV; thus, spirometric examination shows the expiratory reserve volume to be greatly reduced. This pattern of functional impairment is shown in Figure 19-1.

In most obese patients, arterial blood gases show a decrease in the P_{O_2} and an increase in the AaD_{O_2} as a consequence of high diaphragms, airway and alveolar closure, and ventilation-perfusion mismatch. If P_{CO_2} is not elevated, these patients are sometimes said to have "simple obesity." When the P_{CO_2} is elevated, the term *obesity-hypoventilation syndrome* is often used, and in these cases superimposed hypoventilation is an additional factor contributing to hypoxemia. Obviously, if the patient has sleep apnea syndrome, arterial blood gas values become even more deranged at night during episodes of apnea.

In the treatment of obese patients with respiratory dysfunction, weight loss is theoretically crucial. If weight loss is successful, many of the clinical problems may resolve. Unfortunately, attempts at significant and sustained weight loss are often futile, and other modes of therapy must be instituted. In patients who hypoventilate, respiratory stimulants, especially progesterone, have been used with some success. If the patient has obstructive sleep apnea syndrome, therapy aimed at eliminating the episodes of nocturnal upper airway obstruction (see Chapter 18) is crucial.

References

Neuromuscular Disease Affecting the Muscles of Respiration

Benditt JO: Management of pulmonary complications in neuromuscular disease. Phys Med Rehabil Clin N Am 9:167-185, 1998.

Derenne J-P, Macklem PT, and Roussos C: The respiratory muscles: mechanics, control, and pathophysiology. Am Rev Respir Dis 118:581-601, 1978.

Kaplan LM and Hollander D: Respiratory dysfunction in amyotrophic lateral sclerosis. Clin Chest Med 15:675-681, 1994.

Luce JM and Culver BH: Respiratory muscle function in health and disease. Chest 81:82-90, 1982.

Mansel JK and Norman JR: Respiratory complications and management of spinal cord injuries. Chest 97:1446-1452, 1990.

Roussos C and Macklem PT: The respiratory muscles. N Engl J Med 307:786-797, 1982.

Smith PEM et al: Practical problems in the respiratory care of patients with muscular dystrophy. N Engl J Med 316:1197-1205, 1987.

Sunderrajan EV and Davenport J: The Guillain-Barré syndrome: pulmonary-neurologic correlations. Medicine 64:333-341, 1985.

Teener JW and Raps EC: Evaluation and treatment of respiratory failure in neuromuscular disease. Rheum Dis Clin North Am 23:277-292, 1997.

Tobin MJ: Respiratory muscles in disease. Clin Chest Med 9:263-286, 1988.

Zulueta JJ and Fanburg BL: Respiratory dysfunction in myasthenia gravis. Clin Chest Med 15:683-691, 1994.

Diaphragmatic Disease

Aldrich TK: Respiratory muscle fatigue. Clin Chest Med 9:225-236, 1988.

Aubier M et al: Aminophylline improves diaphragmatic contractility. N Engl J Med 305:249-252, 1981.

Belman MJ and Sieck GC: The ventilatory muscles: fatigue, endurance and training. Chest 82:761-766, 1982.

Celli B: The diaphragm and respiratory muscles. Chest Surg Clin N Am 8:207-224, 1998.

Cohen CA et al: Clinical manifestations of inspiratory muscle fatigue. Am J Med 73:308-316, 1982.

Mador MJ: Respiratory muscle fatigue and breathing patterns. Chest 100:1430-1435, 1991.

Pacia EB and Aldrich TK: Assessment of diaphragm function. Chest Surg Clin N Am 8:225-236, 1998.

Roussos C and Macklem PT: The respiratory muscles. N Engl J Med 307:786-797, 1982.

Tripp HF and Bolton JW: Phrenic nerve injury following cardiac surgery: a review. J Card Surg 13:218-223, 1998.

Diseases Affecting the Chest Wall

Berger KI et al: Obesity hypoventilation syndrome as a spectrum of respiratory disturbances during sleep. Chest 120:1231-1238, 2001.

Bergofsky EH: Respiratory failure in disorders of the thoracic cage. Am Rev Respir Dis 119:643-669, 1979.

Kafer ER: Respiratory and cardiovascular functions in scoliosis. Bull Eur Physiopathol Respir 13:299-321, 1977.

Koenig SM: Pulmonary complications of obesity. Am J Med Sci 321:249-279, 2001.

Libby DM, Briscoe WA, Boyce B, and Smith JP: Acute respiratory failure in scoliosis or kyphosis. Am J Med 73:532-538, 1982.

Luce JM: Respiratory complications of obesity. Chest 78:626-631, 1980.

Mohsenin V and Gee JBL: Effect of obesity on the respiratory system and pathophysiology of sleep apnea. *In* Tierney DF (ed): Current Pulmonology, vol. 14. St. Louis, Mosby-Year Book, 1993, pp 179-197.

Sutton FD et al: Progesterone for outpatient treatment of pickwickian syndrome. Ann Intern Med 83:476-479, 1975.

chapter 20

Lung Cancer: Etiologic and Pathologic Aspects

ETIOLOGY AND PATHOGENESIS
  Smoking
  Occupational Factors
  Genetic Factors
  Parenchymal Scarring
  Miscellaneous Factors
  Concepts in the Pathogenesis of
    Lung Cancer

PATHOLOGY
  Squamous Cell Carcinoma
  Small Cell Carcinoma
  Adenocarcinoma
  Large Cell Carcinoma

Carcinoma of the lung, a public health problem of immense proportions, has been a source of great frustration to individual physicians and to the medical profession in general. Several decades ago, its primary cause—cigarette smoking—was identified without a shadow of a doubt. Fortunately, the prevalence of smoking in developed countries has been gradually falling after having peaked in the mid-1970s. Unfortunately, any optimism is tempered by the following concerns: (1) approximately 25 percent of all American adults still smoke, (2) though smoking prevalence declined substantially in the years before 1990, it has remained unchanged since then, and (3) tobacco use is continuing to increase in Third World countries as the tobacco industry focuses its marketing efforts on developing nations.

A few statistics put the magnitude of the problem of lung cancer into perspective. In the United States, there are nearly 170,000 new cases of lung cancer diagnosed annually, and more than 150,000 individuals each year die as a result of this disease. For many years, carcinoma of the lung has been the leading cause of cancer deaths among men, and it more recently surpassed breast cancer as the leading cause among women. Lung cancer is responsible for 25 to 30 percent of all deaths due to cancer and approximately 5 percent of all deaths from any cause. It is a sobering thought to realize that during the last 5 years more Americans were killed by lung cancer than were killed in all the wars in the nation's history.

The number of cases and the number of deaths related to lung cancer have increased dramatically over the last several decades. For no other form of cancer has the increase approached that of lung cancer. For men, the death rate appears to have reached a peak in 1990 and fortunately has been decreasing since then. In women the death rate increased 5-fold in the 30 years from 1960 to 1990, but appears to have reached a plateau in the late 1990s. Despite the magnitude of the problem, our ability to treat carcinoma of the lung has improved only minimally. Five-year survival has increased from approximately 7 to 14 percent during the last several decades, making the prognosis of this disease still dismal in the vast majority of cases.

This discussion of carcinoma of the lung is presented in two parts. In this chapter, a consideration of what is known about the etiology and pathogenesis of lung cancer is followed by a description of the pathologic aspects and classification of the different types of tumors. Chapter 21 continues with a discussion of the clinical aspects of the disease, including diagnostic and therapeutic considerations. Finally, Chapter 21 concludes with a brief discussion of two additional types of neoplastic disease affecting the respiratory system, bronchial carcinoid tumor (bronchial adenoma) and mesothelioma, along with a consideration of the common problem of the patient with a solitary pulmonary nodule.

ETIOLOGY AND PATHOGENESIS

For no other common cancer affecting humans have the causative factors been worked out so well as for lung cancer. Cigarette smoking is clearly responsible for the vast majority of cases (more than 85 percent, according to some estimates), and additional risk factors associated with occupational exposure have also been identified. After a discussion of these two major risk factors, genetic factors are considered as a potential contributor to the risk of lung cancer. Next is a brief description of the importance of previous scarring within the pulmonary parenchyma, which has been implicated in the development of "scar carcinomas," and several miscellaneous proposed risk factors are also mentioned. Finally, the role of oncogenes and tumor suppressor genes in the pathogenesis of lung cancer is discussed.

Smoking

Cigarette smoking is the single most important risk factor for development of carcinoma of the lung. As might be expected, the duration of the smoking history, the number of cigarettes smoked each day, the depth of inhalation, and the amount of each cigarette smoked all correlate with the risk for development of lung cancer. As a rough but easy way to quantitate prior cigarette exposure, the number of years of smoking can be multiplied by the number of packs smoked per day, giving the number of "pack years."

Although the evidence incriminating smoking with lung cancer is incontrovertible, the responsible component of cigarette smoke has not been identified with certainty. Cigarette smoke consists of a gaseous phase and a particulate phase, and potential carcinogens have been found in both phases, ranging from nitrosamines to benzo[a]pyrene and other polycyclic hydrocarbons. Filters appear to decrease but certainly not eliminate the potential carcinogenic effects of cigarettes. There is also a substantially lower risk for lung cancer associated with cigar or pipe smoking, presumably related to the fact that cigar and pipe smoke is generally not inhaled.

The actual development of lung cancer as a result of smoking takes many years of exposure. However, histologic abnormalities before the development of a frank carcinoma have been well documented in the bronchial epithelium of smokers. These changes, including loss of bronchial cilia, hyperplasia of bronchial epithelial cells, and nuclear abnormalities, may be the histologic forerunners of a true carcinoma. If a person stops smoking, many of these precancerous changes are reversible. Epidemiologic studies have suggested that the risk for development of lung cancer decreases progressively after cessation of smoking but probably never returns to the level in nonsmokers, even

Histologic abnormalities in the bronchial epithelium induced by smoking precede the development of carcinoma.

after more than 10 to 15 years have elapsed. In many cases, the initial cellular changes leading to or predisposing to malignant transformation have already developed by the time the patient stops smoking, and it is merely a matter of time before the carcinoma develops or becomes clinically apparent.

Data indicate that the risk of lung cancer is also increased for nonsmoking spouses because of their exposure to sidestream smoke. Although the risk due to "passive smoking" is relatively small compared with the risk of active smoking, involuntary exposure to cigarette smoke is likely responsible for some cases of lung cancer seen in nonsmokers.

Occupational Factors

A number of potential environmental risk factors have been identified, most of which occur with occupational exposure. Perhaps the most widely studied of the environmental or occupationally related carcinogens is asbestos, a fibrous silicate formerly in wide use due to its properties of fire resistance and thermal insulation. Shipbuilders, construction workers, and those who work with insulation and brake linings are among those who may be exposed to asbestos.

The risk of lung cancer is markedly increased by the combined risk factors of asbestos exposure and smoking.

Carcinoma of the lung is the most likely malignancy to result from asbestos exposure, although other tumors, especially mesothelioma (see Chapter 21), are also strongly associated with prior asbestos exposure. The risk for development of lung cancer is particularly high in a smoker exposed to asbestos, in which case these two risk factors probably have a multiplicative effect. Specifically, asbestos alone appears to confer a 2- to 5-fold increase in risk for lung cancer, whereas smoking alone is associated with an approximately 10-fold increased risk. Together, the two risk factors make the person who smokes and has an asbestos exposure 20 to 50 times more likely to have carcinoma of the lung than a nonsmoking, nonexposed counterpart. Like other forms of asbestos-related disease, there is a long time lapse before the development of the complication. In the case of lung cancer, more than 2 decades generally elapse after exposure before the tumor becomes apparent.

Several other types of occupational exposure have also been implicated. Examples include exposure to arsenic (in workers making pesticides, glass, pigments, and paints), ionizing radiation (especially in uranium miners), haloethers (bis-chloromethyl ether and chloromethyl methyl ether in chemical industry workers), and polycyclic aromatic hydrocarbons (in petroleum, coal tar, and foundry workers). As is the case with asbestos, there is generally a long latent period of at least 2 decades from the time of exposure until presentation of the tumor.

Genetic Factors

Why lung cancer develops in some heavy smokers and not in others is a question that has great importance but no answer. The assumption is that genetic factors must place some individuals at higher risk for lung cancer after exposure to carcinogens. The finding of an increased risk of lung cancer among first-degree relatives of lung cancer patients, even after confounding factors have been taken into account, supports this hypothesis. Candidate genetic factors have primarily included specific enzymes of the cytochrome P-450 system. These enzymes may have a role in metabolizing products of cigarette smoke to potent carcinogens, so that genetically determined increased activity or expression of the enzymes is associated with a greater risk of developing lung cancer following exposure to cigarette smoke.

One such example is the enzyme aryl hydrocarbon hydroxylase, which can convert hydrocarbons to carcinogenic metabolites. This enzyme is induced by smoking, and it has been suggested that genetically determined inducibility of this enzyme by smoking may correlate with the risk for lung cancer. Another enzyme of the cytochrome P-450 system is one that can be identified by its ability to metabolize the antihypertensive drug debrisoquine. Some data suggest an association between extensive metabolism of debrisoquine and the development of lung cancer. Presumably, the action of this enzyme on a potentially carcinogenic substrate from cigarette smoke affects an individual's risk for developing lung cancer. However, for both of these cytochrome P-450 enzymes, the available data are inconsistent, and a role for these enzymes has therefore not been universally accepted.

Other as yet unidentified genetic factors potentially affect the susceptibility to environmental carcinogens. If such factors are eventually recognized and the individuals at risk are identified, it might be possible to prevent susceptible individuals from being exposed to the known environmental carcinogens.

Parenchymal Scarring

Scar tissue within the lung can be a locus for the subsequent occurrence of lung cancer, called a *scar carcinoma*. The scarring may be either localized (e.g., resulting from an old focus of tuberculosis or another infection) or diffuse (e.g., from pulmonary fibrosis, whether idiopathic or associated with a specific cause). Most frequently, scar carcinomas of the lung are adenocarcinomas and often a specific subtype called *bronchioloalveolar carcinoma*. These cell types are discussed in the next section of this chapter.

Although it is easy to consider carcinomas occurring within or adjacent to scar tissue to be scar carcinomas, it also appears that adenocarcinomas of the lung may develop fibrotic areas within the tumor. Therefore, in some cases it may be impossible to know whether the scar preceded or followed development of the carcinoma.

Miscellaneous Factors

There has been a great deal of interest and publicity in the lay press regarding the risk of lung cancer from exposure to radon, a gas that is a decay product of radium-226. Exposure to this known carcinogen may occur indoors in homes built on soil that has a high radium content and is releasing radon into the surrounding environment. Although the finding of unacceptably high levels of radon in some home environments has sparked concern about the risk of lung cancer and interest in widespread testing of houses, uncertainty remains about the overall risk posed by exposure to radon. At the extreme, it has been suggested that radon is the second most important factor contributing to lung cancer and is potentially responsible for 20,000 lung cancer deaths per year in the United States. However, this magnitude of risk has not been universally accepted.

Finally, there is some evidence suggesting that at least one dietary factor may affect the risk of lung cancer. Low intake and serum levels of beta-carotene, the provitamin form of vitamin A, have been associated in some studies with an increased risk of lung cancer. However, the data relating to this issue are controversial, and if there is truly an increased risk associated with low dietary intake of beta-carotene, it is a relatively minor one compared with the risk posed by cigarette smoking. In fact, the issue has been further complicated by data suggesting a slight increase in the incidence of lung cancer in individuals given supplemental beta-carotene.

Concepts in the Pathogenesis of Lung Cancer

There has been a great deal of interest in identifying the cell(s) of origin, i.e., the histogenesis, of the various types of lung cancer and in elucidating the genetic changes involved in the malignant transformation of these cells. For many years, it was assumed that the different histopathologic types of lung cancer (which are described in the next section) were each associated with a different cell of origin. It was thought that previously well-differentiated normal cells underwent a process of dedifferentiation and unrestricted growth when exposed to a carcinogenic stimulus. However, based in part on the common finding of cellular heterogeneity, i.e., more than one cell type within a single tumor, it is currently believed that all types of lung cancer arise from an undifferentiated precursor or stem cell. In the course of this cell's undergoing malignant transformation, it then differentiates along one or more particular pathways that determine its ultimate histologic appearance, i.e., its cell type(s).

Alterations in genes that code for proteins controlling or regulating cell growth have been found in a high proportion of patients with lung cancer. It is believed that these molecular changes may play a central role in the pathogenesis of lung cancer. Two types of oncogenes have been identified—proto-oncogenes (which code for growth-promoting factors) and tumor suppressor genes (which code for factors having a negative regulatory effect on cell proliferation). A mutation in one of the paired alleles of a proto-oncogene can result in production of a protein with a growth-promoting effect, so that a "dominant" behavior or effect would be observed. In contrast, both alleles of a tumor suppressor gene need to be altered before the absence of the gene product would be clinically manifest as increased cell growth or malignant transformation; this requirement produces a "recessive" pattern of clinical expression.

Specific common alterations in proto-oncogenes that have been identified in lung cancer include mutations in the *ras* and *myc* families of dominant oncogenes. A variety of mutations in recessive tumor suppressor genes have also been identified, including the retinoblastoma (*rb*) and *p53* genes. In addition, deletion of genetic material from chromosome 3p (the short arm of chromosome 3) has been recognized in lung cancer, and it is thought that deletion may involve loss of one or more tumor suppressor genes. Particularly interesting experimental data link a carcinogenic metabolite of benzo[a]pyrene, which is found in cigarette smoke, to those mutations of the *p53* gene which are most commonly seen in lung cancer.

PATHOLOGY

The term *bronchogenic carcinoma* is often used interchangeably with the term lung cancer, implying that lung cancers arise from bronchi or bronchial structures. Many if not most lung cancers do originate within airways, but other tumors arise in the periphery of the lung and may not necessarily originate in an airway. In this section the focus is on the currently accepted classification of lung cancer and a summary of what is known about the behavior patterns of the various types of tumors.

> Alterations in proto-oncogenes and tumor suppressor genes have been found in many patients with lung cancer.

Almost all lung cancers fall within one of four histologic categories: (1) squamous cell carcinoma, (2) small cell carcinoma, (3) adenocarcinoma, and (4) large cell carcinoma. Within each category are several subcategories that, for our purposes, are less important. However, two of these subcategories are discussed—bronchioloalveolar carcinoma (a type of adenocarcinoma) and oat cell carcinoma (a type of small cell carcinoma)—because these are frequent diagnoses and often-used terms in the clinical setting.

One of the most important distinctions to make is between small cell carcinoma and all the other cell types, which are grouped together as *non-small cell carcinoma.* The importance of this distinction relates to the propensity for clinical and subclinical metastasis in small cell carcinoma, which affects the approaches to staging and treatment of this tumor compared with those of all the other cell types.

Each of the four major categories of lung cancer is associated with cigarette smoking. However, the statistical association between smoking and the individual cell types is greatest for squamous and small cell carcinomas, which are seen almost exclusively in smokers. Even though smoking also increases the risk for adenocarcinoma and large cell carcinoma, these cell types also occur in nonsmokers.

Squamous Cell Carcinoma

Approximately one-third of all bronchogenic carcinomas are of the squamous cell type. These tumors originate within the epithelial layer of the bronchial wall, in which a series of progressive histologic abnormalities result from chronic or repetitive cigarette smoke–induced injury.

Initially, there is metaplasia of the normal bronchial columnar epithelial cells, which are replaced by squamous epithelial cells. Over time these squamous cells become more and more atypical in appearance, until there is development of a well-localized carcinoma, i.e., carcinoma in situ. Eventually, the carcinoma extends beyond the bronchial mucosa and becomes frankly invasive. At this stage the tumor generally comes to clinical attention by producing either symptoms or radiographic changes. In some cases, detection of the carcinoma is made at the earlier in situ stage, usually by recognition of the malignant cells in a specimen of sputum obtained for cytologic examination.

Specific histologic features of squamous cell carcinoma allow the pathologist to make this diagnosis. These tumors are characterized by the presence of keratin, "squamous pearls," and intercellular bridges (Fig. 20-1).

Squamous cell carcinomas tend to be located in relatively large or proximal airways, most commonly at the subsegmental, segmental, or lobar level. With growth of the tumor into the bronchial lumen, the airway may become obstructed; the lung distal to the obstruction frequently collapses (becomes atelectatic), and a postobstructive pneumonia may develop. Sometimes a cavity develops within the tumor mass; this finding of cavitation is much more common with squamous cell than with other types of bronchogenic carcinoma.

Spread of squamous cell carcinoma beyond the airway usually involves (1) direct extension to the pulmonary parenchyma or to other neighboring structures or (2) invasion of lymphatic vessels, with spread to local lymph nodes in the hilum or mediastinum. These tumors have a general tendency to remain within the thorax and to cause problems by intrathoracic complications rather than by distant metastasis. The overall prognosis in terms of the

Major histologic categories of lung cancer are the following:

1. Squamous cell carcinoma
2. Small cell carcinoma
3. Adenocarcinoma
4. Large cell carcinoma

Features of squamous cell carcinomas are the following:

1. Generally arise in proximal airways
2. May cause airway obstruction, leading to distal atelectasis or pneumonia
3. May cavitate
4. Intrathoracic spread rather than distant metastases

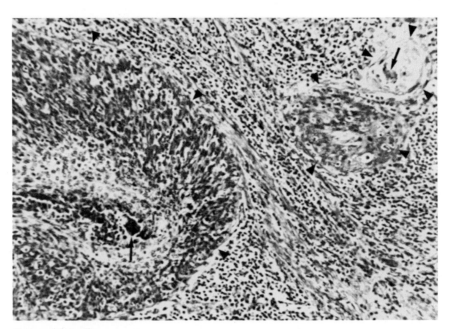

Figure 20-1 ▪— Low-power photomicrograph of squamous cell carcinoma. Note three foci of tumor, each highlighted by arrowheads. Intervening regions show connective tissue and inflammatory cells. Arrows point to two areas of keratin formation by the tumor. (Courtesy of Dr. Earl Kasdon.)

potential for 5-year survival is better for patients with squamous cell carcinoma than for patients with any of the other cell types.

Small Cell Carcinoma

Small cell carcinoma, comprising approximately 20 percent of all lung cancers, was previously considered to have several subtypes, of which *oat cell carcinoma* was the most important. The most recent (1999) classification of lung cancer simplifies the classification and no longer includes oat cell carcinoma as a separate subtype. Like squamous cell carcinoma, small cell carcinomas generally originate within the bronchial wall, most commonly at a proximal level. There is dispute about the cell of origin of small cell carcinoma. An older theory proposed that these tumors arise from a neurosecretory type of epithelial cell termed the *Kulchitsky cell* or *K cell.* These cells have the capacity for polypeptide production and are considered a type of APUD cell (i.e., capable of *a*mine *p*recursor *u*ptake and *d*ecarboxylation). As mentioned earlier, a more recent theory suggests that small cell carcinomas, like other lung cancers, have their origin from a pluripotent stem cell. The eventual cell type then depends on the pattern and degree of differentiation from this precursor cell. Molecular and chromosomal studies have shown that almost all small cell carcinomas demonstrate deletions on the short arm of chromosome 3 (3p).

In small cell carcinoma, the malignant cells appear as small, darkly stained cells with sparse cytoplasm (Fig. 20-2). The local growth of the tumor often follows a submucosal pattern, but the tumor quickly invades lymphatics and submucosal blood vessels. Hilar and mediastinal nodes are involved early in the course of the disease and are frequently the most prominent aspect of the radiographic presentation.

Because of the rapid dissemination of small cell carcinoma, metastatic spread to distant sites is also a common early complication. Distant disease,

Features of small cell carcinomas are the following:

1. Generally arise in proximal airways
2. Commonly produce polypeptide hormones
3. Hilar and mediastinal node involvement
4. Early, distant metastatic disease

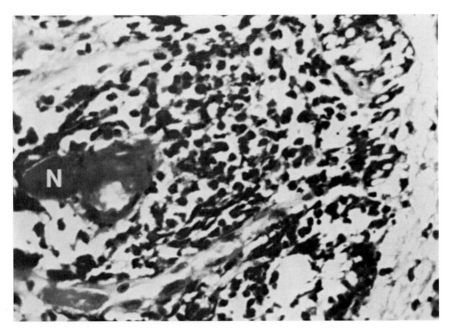

Figure 20-2 ▬— High-power photomicrograph of small cell carcinoma. Malignant cells have irregular, darkly stained nuclei and sparse cytoplasm. Note small area of necrosis (N) within tumor. (Courtesy of Dr. Earl Kasdon.)

which may be clinically occult at the time of presentation, often affects the brain, liver, bone (and bone marrow), and adrenal glands. It is this propensity for early metastatic involvement that gives small cell carcinoma the worst prognosis among the four major categories of bronchogenic carcinoma.

Adenocarcinoma

Adenocarcinoma appears to have reached or surpassed squamous cell carcinoma as the most frequent cell type, accounting for more than one-third of all lung tumors. Because the majority of adenocarcinomas occur in the periphery of the lung, it is much harder to relate their origin to the bronchial wall. At present, it is believed that these tumors probably arise at the level of bronchioles or the alveolar walls. Adenocarcinomas sometimes appear at a site of parenchymal scarring that is either localized or part of a diffuse fibrotic process.

The characteristic appearance defining adenocarcinoma is the tendency to form glands and in many cases to produce mucus (Fig. 20-3). In the bronchioloalveolar subcategory of adenocarcinoma, the malignant cells seem to grow and spread along the preexisting alveolar walls, almost as though they were using the alveolar wall as a scaffolding for their growth (Fig. 20-4).

The usual presenting pattern of adenocarcinoma is a peripheral lung nodule or mass. Occasionally, the tumors can arise within a relatively large bronchus and may therefore be observed clinically because of complications of localized bronchial obstruction, as seen with squamous cell carcinoma. The bronchioloalveolar subcategory can manifest in several ways: as a nodule or mass lesion, as a localized infiltrate simulating a pneumonia, or as widespread parenchymal disease.

Although adenocarcinoma may spread locally to adjacent regions of lung or to pleura, it also has a propensity for nodal involvement (hilar and

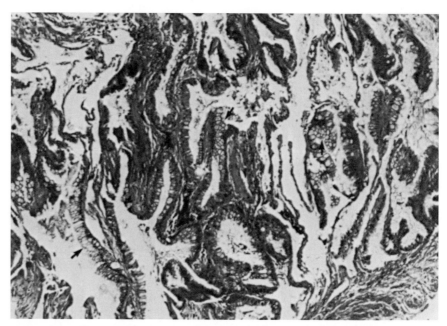

Figure 20-3 ■— Low-power photomicrograph of adenocarcinoma of lung. Malignant cells form gland-like structures and produce mucus (*arrows*). (Courtesy of Dr. Earl Kasdon.)

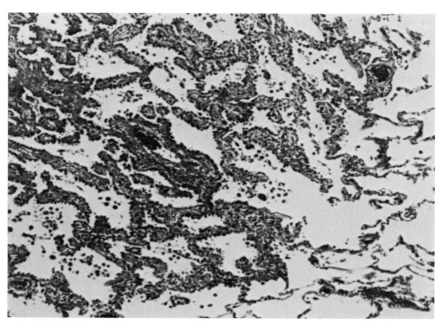

Figure 20-4 ■— Low-power photomicrograph of bronchioloalveolar carcinoma. Tumor cells appear to be growing along preexisting alveolar walls. Lower right corner of photograph shows normal alveolar walls, which can be contrasted with areas of tumor. (Courtesy of Dr. Earl Kasdon.)

Features of adenocarcinomas are the following:

1. Often manifest as a solitary, peripheral pulmonary nodule
2. May arise in an old parenchymal scar
3. Generally localized when manifest as a peripheral lung nodule
4. Spread to hilar and mediastinal nodes and to distant sites

mediastinal) and for distant metastatic spread. Like small cell carcinoma, it spreads to liver, bone, central nervous system, and adrenal glands. In comparison with small cell carcinoma, however, adenocarcinoma is more likely to be localized at the time of presentation, particularly when it manifests as a solitary peripheral lung nodule. The overall prognosis for adenocarcinoma is not surprising given this behavior; its natural history and survival rates are intermediate between those of squamous cell and small cell carcinomas.

Large Cell Carcinoma

Large cell carcinoma accounts for approximately 15 to 20 percent of all lung cancers. It is the most difficult carcinoma to define well, because the tumors are often defined by the characteristics they lack, i.e., the specific features that would otherwise classify them as one of the other three cell types.

The behavior of these tumors is relatively similar to that of adenocarcinoma. They often appear in the periphery of the lung as mass lesions, although they tend to be somewhat larger than adenocarcinomas. Their natural history is also similar to that of adenocarcinoma, both in terms of propensity for spread and overall prognosis.

For a summary of the distinguishing features of each cell type, Table 21-1 in Chapter 21 reiterates many of the points discussed so far.

References

Etiology and Pathogenesis

Alberg AJ and Samet JM: Epidemiology of lung cancer. Chest 123 (Suppl):21S-49S, 2003.

Davila DG and Williams DE: The etiology of lung cancer. Mayo Clin Proc 68:170-182, 1993.

Denissenko MF, Pao A, Tang M, and Pfeifer GP: Preferential formation of benzo[a]pyrene adducts at lung cancer mutational hotspots in p53. Science 274:430-432, 1996.

Giaccone G: Oncogenes and antioncogenes in lung cancer. Chest 109:130S-134S, 1996.

Goodman GE: Prevention of lung cancer. Thorax 57:994-999, 2002.

Hackshaw AK, Law MR, and Wall NJ: The accumulated evidence on lung cancer and environmental tobacco smoke. BMJ 315:980-988, 1997.

Lubin JH and Boice JD Jr: Lung cancer risk from residential radon: meta-analysis of eight epidemiologic studies. J Natl Cancer Inst 89:49-57, 1997.

Rom WN et al: Molecular and genetic aspects of lung cancer. Am J Respir Crit Care Med 161:1355-1367, 2000.

Smith RA and Glynn TJ: Epidemiology of lung cancer. Radiol Clin North Am 38:453-470, 2000.

Whitesell PL and Drage CW: Occupational lung cancer. Mayo Clin Proc 68:183-188, 1993.

Pathology

Brambilla E, et al: The new World Health Organization classification of lung tumors. Eur Respir J 18:1059-1068, 2001.

Franklin WA: Diagnosis of lung cancer: pathology of invasive and preinvasive neoplasia. Chest 117 (Suppl):80S-89S, 2000.

Müller K-M: Lung cancer: morphology. Eur Respir Mon 17:34-47, 2001.

Verbeken EK and Brambilla E: WHO classification of lung and pleural tumours. The WHO/IASLC 1999 revision. Eur Respir Rev 12 (review 84):172-176, 2002.

Lung Cancer: Clinical Aspects

In this chapter the goal is to extend the discussion of lung cancer into the clinical realm and to relate how the pathologic processes considered in Chapter 20 are encountered in a clinical setting. An outline of the major clinical features of lung cancer is followed by a discussion of the diagnostic approach and general principles of management. The chapter concludes with a brief discussion of bronchial carcinoid tumors, malignant mesothelioma, and the clinical problem of the solitary pulmonary nodule.

CLINICAL FEATURES

Because lung cancer presumably starts with a single malignant cell, there must be a long period of repetitive divisions and doubling of cell number before the tumor becomes clinically apparent. During this preclinical period, it has been estimated that approximately 30 divisions take place before the tumor reaches 1 cm in diameter. This process most likely requires a number of years, during which time the patient and the physician are unaware of the tumor.

In general, the possibility of lung cancer is raised because of findings on imaging studies (chest radiography or CT scan) or sputum cytology, or because of an assortment of symptoms that may ensue. The focus in this section is primarily on symptoms; imaging studies and sputum cytology are discussed in the section on diagnostic approach. The symptoms at the time of presentation may relate to the primary lung lesion, to metastatic disease (either in intrathoracic lymph nodes or at distant sites), or to what are commonly called "paraneoplastic syndromes."

Symptoms Relating to Primary Lung Lesion

Perhaps the most common symptoms associated with lung cancer are cough and hemoptysis. Because bronchogenic carcinoma generally develops in smokers, these patients often dismiss their symptoms (particularly cough) as routine complications of smoking and chronic bronchitis. With tumors originating in large airways, such as squamous or small cell carcinoma, patients may also have problems related to bronchial obstruction, e.g., pneumonia behind the obstruction or shortness of breath secondary to occlusion of a major bronchus. In contrast, with tumors that arise in the periphery of the lung, including many adenocarcinomas and large cell carcinomas, patients tend not to have symptoms related to bronchial involvement, and their lesions are often found on a routinely obtained chest radiograph.

When tumors involve the pleural surface, either by direct extension or by metastatic spread, patients may have chest pain, often pleuritic in nature, or dyspnea resulting from substantial accumulation of pleural fluid. Other adjacent structures, particularly the heart and esophagus, can be involved by direct invasion or extrinsic compression by the tumor; resulting complications include pericardial effusion, arrhythmias, and dysphagia.

Tumors originating in the most apical portion of the lung, which are called *superior sulcus* or *Pancoast tumors,* often produce a characteristic constellation of symptoms and physical findings caused by direct extension to adjacent structures. Involvement of the nerves comprising the brachial plexus can result in pain and weakness of the shoulder and arm. Involvement of the cervical sympathetic chain produces the typical features of Horner's syndrome—ptosis (drooping upper eyelid), miosis (constricted pupil), and anhidrosis (loss of sweat) over the forehead and face—all occurring on the same side as the lung mass. Invasion of neighboring bony structures, i.e., ribs and vertebrae, is a common additional complication.

Symptoms Relating to Nodal and Distant Metastasis

When the mediastinum has metastatic lymph nodes from a primary lung cancer, symptoms often arise from invasion or compression of important structures within the mediastinum, such as the phrenic nerve, the recurrent laryngeal nerve, and the superior vena cava. As a consequence, the following conditions, respectively, may develop: diaphragmatic paralysis (often with accompanying dyspnea), vocal cord paralysis (with hoarseness), or superior vena cava obstruction (with edema of the face and upper extremities resulting from obstruction to venous return).

Distant metastases, most commonly to the brain, bone or bone marrow, liver, and adrenal gland(s), are frequently asymptomatic. In other cases, symptoms depend on the particular organ system involved. As mentioned in Chapter 20, small cell carcinoma is the cell type most likely to generate distant metastases. Squamous cell carcinoma is least likely, and both adenocarcinoma and large cell carcinoma occupy an intermediate position.

Paraneoplastic Syndromes

Finally, many lung tumors are capable of producing clinical syndromes that are not readily attributable to the space-occupying nature of the tumor or to direct invasion of other structures or organs. These syndromes are sometimes called the "paraneoplastic" manifestations of malignancy and are frequently due to production of a hormone or a hormone-like substance by the tumor. When a detectable hormone is produced by the lung tumor (or, for that matter, by any type of tumor), the patient is said to have "ectopic" hormone production. Sometimes clinical symptoms result from high circulating levels of the hormone; in other cases, only sensitive techniques of measurement are capable of demonstrating production of the hormone.

Potential clinical problems with lung cancer are the following:
1. Symptoms from an endobronchial tumor: cough, hemoptysis
2. Problems of bronchial obstruction: postobstructive pneumonia, dyspnea
3. Pleural involvement: chest pain, pleural effusion, dyspnea
4. Involvement of adjacent structures: heart, esophagus
5. Complications of mediastinal involvement: phrenic or recurrent laryngeal nerve paralysis, superior vena cava obstruction
6. Distant metastases: brain, bone or bone marrow, liver, adrenals
7. Ectopic hormone production: ACTH, ADH, parathyroid hormone-related peptide
8. Other paraneoplastic syndromes: neurologic, clubbing, hypertrophic osteoarthropathy
9. Nonspecific systemic effects: anorexia, weight loss

Why some tumors are capable of hormone production is not clear. It has been hypothesized that genetic information coding for the particular hormone is present but not expressed in the normal, nonmalignant cell. In the course of becoming malignant, the cell undergoes a process of gene derepression, during which it regains the ability to express this normally silent genetic material coding for hormone production.

The cell type most frequently associated with ectopic production of humoral substances is small cell carcinoma, presumably because of its similarity or relationship to a type of neuroendocrine cell in the airway (the Kulchitsky cell) with secretory granules and the potential for peptide synthesis. Adrenocorticotropic hormone (ACTH) and antidiuretic hormone (ADH) are the best described hormones produced by small cell carcinoma, potentially giving rise to the ectopic ACTH syndrome or to the syndrome of inappropriate ADH (SIADH), respectively. In addition, squamous cell carcinoma is capable of causing hypercalcemia, due to production of a peptide with parathyroid hormone–like activity, called parathyroid hormone–related peptide. Production of other hormones, such as calcitonin and human chorionic gonadotropin, has also been well described with bronchogenic carcinoma.

Some of the other paraneoplastic syndromes cannot be attributed to a known hormone, and our understanding of their mechanisms varies. Examples range from a wide variety of neurologic syndromes (some of which appear to be due to autoimmune antibody production) to the soft tissue and bony manifestations of clubbing and hypertrophic osteoarthropathy (described in Chapter 3). The nonspecific systemic effects of malignancy, such as anorexia and weight loss, are also potential consequences of lung cancer, and it has been hypothesized that production of various mediators, such as tumor necrosis factor, may mediate these systemic effects.

DIAGNOSTIC APPROACH

A wide variety of diagnostic methods are utilized in evaluating cases of known or suspected lung cancer. Some of these techniques have also been proposed for screening of asymptomatic individuals with risk factors for lung cancer, in an attempt to detect early, preclinical lesions. However, a beneficial effect of screening on mortality has not yet been objectively demonstrated.

Many of the studies that assess the lung on a macroscopic level are used to demonstrate the presence, location, and possibility of spread of a bronchogenic carcinoma. Evaluation on a microscopic level is essential for defining the histologic type of lung cancer, which is an important factor in determining what modalities of therapy are most appropriate. Finally, functional assessment of the patient with lung cancer plays a role primarily in quantitating the severity of underlying lung disease, particularly chronic obstructive lung disease resulting from prior heavy smoking. Knowledge of a patient's functional limitation from lung disease is essential before the clinician can decide whether operative removal of a lung cancer is even feasible without precipitating disabling respiratory insufficiency.

Macroscopic Evaluation

The initial test for detection and macroscopic evaluation of bronchogenic carcinoma is generally the chest radiograph. The presence on chest radiograph of a nodule or mass within the lung always raises the question of lung cancer, especially when the patient has a history of heavy smoking. The location of the lesion may also give an indirect clue about its histology: peripheral lesions are more likely to be large cell carcinoma or adenocarcinoma, whereas central lesions are statistically more likely to be squamous or small cell carcinoma (Figs. 21-1 and 21-2). The chest radiograph is also most useful for determining whether there are additional suspicious lesions, such as a second primary tumor or metastatic spread from the original carcinoma. Involvement of hilar or mediastinal nodes or the pleura (with resulting pleural effusion) may be detected on the chest radiograph and will substantially affect the overall approach to therapy.

Computed tomography (CT) has become a relatively standard part of the diagnostic evaluation of patients with lung cancer. Besides helping to define the location, extent, and spread of tumor within the chest, this technique has been particularly useful for the detection of enlarged, potentially malignant, lymph nodes within the mediastinum, which are often not seen with conventional radiography. However, even though CT effectively identifies enlarged mediastinal nodes, it cannot determine whether such nodes are just hyperplastic or are enlarged because of tumor involvement. Consequently, histologic sampling of enlarged mediastinal nodes is often necessary to confirm tumor involvement of the nodes.

A relatively new technique that has gained increasing popularity in the evaluation of patients with known or suspected lung cancer is positron emission tomographic (PET) scanning, which is described in Chapter 3. Because of their high metabolic activity, malignant lesions typically exhibit uptake of the tracer [18]fluoro-deoxyglucose (FDG). Focal uptake in the region of a

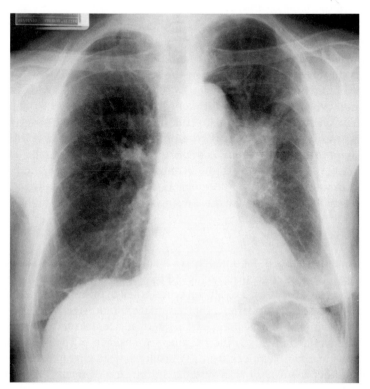

Figure 21-1 ■— Chest radiograph shows small cell carcinoma of lung manifesting as left hilar mass.

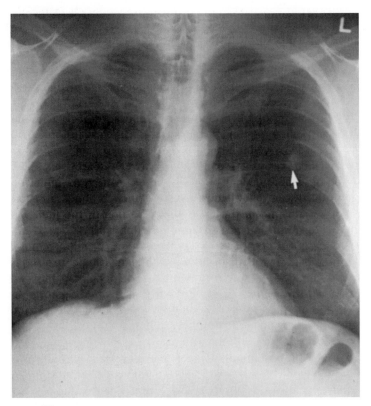

Figure 21-2 ■— Chest radiograph shows adenocarcinoma of lung manifesting as solitary pulmonary nodule (*arrow*).

parenchymal nodule or mass suggests (but does not prove) that the lesion is malignant, and uptake in the mediastinum or at distant sites often reflects spread of the tumor to those sites.

The best way to directly examine the airways of a patient with presumed or known bronchogenic carcinoma is by bronchoscopy, either with a rigid or, much more frequently, a flexible bronchoscope (see Chapter 3). The location and intrabronchial extent of many tumors can be directly observed, and samples can be obtained from the lesion, either for cytologic or histologic examination. These specimens can be obtained even when the lesion is beyond direct visualization with the bronchoscope. In addition, the bronchoscopist can assess whether an intrabronchial carcinoma is impinging significantly on the bronchial lumen and causing either partial or complete airway occlusion.

Staging of Lung Cancer

Basis for staging of non-small cell lung cancer includes the following:

1. Size, location, and local complications of the primary tumor
2. Hilar and mediastinal lymph node involvement
3. Distant metastasis

Once a tumor has been documented, evaluation of the extent and spread of the malignancy is often formally achieved by staging. In the case of non-small cell carcinoma of the lung (i.e., all cell types other than small cell carcinoma), staging is based on (1) the primary intrathoracic tumor—its size, location, and local complications such as direct extension to adjacent structures or obstruction of the airway lumen, (2) the presence or absence of tumor within hilar and mediastinal lymph nodes, and (3) distant spread of tumor beyond the thorax to other tissues or organ systems. In the case of small cell carcinoma, the disease is classified as either limited (localized within one hemithorax) or extensive (beyond the limits of one hemithorax).

The first component of staging, taking into account characteristics of the primary tumor itself, is generally accomplished with a combination of chest radiography and bronchoscopy, sometimes with additional information obtained from CT.

The second component, based on involvement of mediastinal lymph nodes by tumor, is often initially assessed by CT, sometimes complemented by PET scanning. Definitive evaluation has generally been based on direct examination (and biopsy) of the nodes by either of two techniques, mediastinoscopy or mediastinotomy. In the procedure called *suprasternal mediastinoscopy*, the mediastinum is visualized with a scope placed through an incision made just above the sternal notch. Biopsy specimens can be obtained by this technique if there is any suspicion that abnormal nodes are present. The other procedure, *parasternal mediastinotomy*, involves examining the mediastinum through a small incision made adjacent to the sternum, and samples of suspicious nodes can be taken. In selected cases, the technique of transbronchial needle aspiration is an option for needle sampling of cellular material from lymph nodes adjacent to major airways. This technique, which is performed as part of fiberoptic bronchoscopy, has been especially useful for sampling nodes in the subcarinal region.

The third component involves determining whether the tumor has disseminated to distant sites. Spread of a lung tumor to other organs is often documented with either radioisotope or CT scanning. For instance, metastatic disease in bone can be well demonstrated with radioisotope bone scanning. CT is particularly suitable for detection of metastases to the liver, brain, and adrenal glands.

Microscopic Evaluation

Evaluation of lung cancer on a microscopic level is crucial for establishing the specific cell type of the tumor. Some of the techniques used were mentioned briefly in Chapter 3. Specimens are obtained either for cytologic examination of abnormal cells shed from the tumor or for histologic examination of a biopsy specimen obtained directly from the lesion. Cytologic examination can be performed on sputum, on washings or brushings obtained through a bronchoscope, or on material aspirated from the tumor with a small-gauge needle. Biopsy material can be obtained by passing a biopsy forceps through a bronchoscope, by using a cutting needle passed through the chest wall directly into the tumor, or by directly sampling tissue at the time of a surgical procedure. The staining techniques for processing these materials are discussed in Chapter 3.

Functional Assessment

Functional assessment of the patient with lung cancer provides important information for guiding the clinician in the choice of treatment. As will be seen in the following section on principles of therapy, surgery is usually the procedure of choice if staging techniques have shown that the disease is limited and approachable surgically. However, when surgery is performed, usually a lobe and sometimes even an entire lung may need to be removed. Because these patients are generally smokers, they are at high risk for having significant underlying chronic obstructive pulmonary disease, and they may not tolerate removal of a substantial amount of lung tissue. Useful studies for the clinician in evaluating these patients include pulmonary function tests, measurement of arterial blood gases, and sometimes additional tests to determine exercise tolerance or the relative amount of function contributed by the

Assessment of pulmonary function helps determine whether surgical resection can be tolerated in the functionally compromised patient.

area of lung to be removed. Further specification of guidelines precluding surgery is beyond the scope of this discussion but may be found in the references listed at the end of the chapter.

Diagnostic Screening for Lung Cancer

Given that the likelihood of "curing" lung cancer through surgical resection is greatest when the lesion has not yet metastasized to lymph nodes or distant sites, it seems logical that screening high-risk individuals for early, small lesions that have not yet caused symptoms would improve overall survival. Nevertheless, controlled studies of sputum cytology and chest radiography in a high-risk population of smokers have not been able to demonstrate improved mortality from lung cancer with the use of these screening techniques. As a result, and despite some methodologic problems with these studies, routine screening of high-risk current or former smokers by sputum cytology or chest radiography is not currently recommended.

More recently, low-dose fast helical chest CT has been shown to be more sensitive than chest radiography for detecting small lung cancers. However, whether screening with chest CT will improve mortality from lung cancer remains unknown. In addition, such scans detect many benign lesions, potentially resulting in unnecessary diagnostic procedures with some associated morbidity. At present, this important public health issue of screening for lung cancer has generated great interest as well as controversy, and it remains a subject of active investigation.

PRINCIPLES OF THERAPY

Although many advances have been made during the last 2 decades in the treatment of a variety of malignancies, patients with lung cancer have seen only a minor improvement in their prognosis during the same time. The 5-year survival of all patients with lung cancer is approximately 14 percent, certainly a dismal overall outlook.

The three major forms of treatment available for lung cancer are surgery, radiation therapy, and chemotherapy. During the last 10 to 15 years, somewhat more radical approaches have been used, particularly combination modalities of therapy. General guidelines for the clinician suggest when and how to use these modalities, but it is still often not known with certainty what therapy or combination of therapies will prove the most beneficial for a given patient. There appear to be two primary factors determining how a particular tumor should be treated—its staging (i.e., size, location, and extent of spread) and its cell type.

According to current practice for the treatment of bronchogenic carcinoma, surgery is the treatment of choice for localized tumors. When the tumor has extended directly to the pleura (with malignant cells found in the pleural fluid) or to the mediastinum, it is usually considered unresectable, and alternative therapy is used. Similarly, when contralateral mediastinal nodes are involved, the tumor is generally considered unresectable. At present, there is great interest in trying to determine the best modes of therapy in patients for whom the benefit of surgery is debatable, e.g., patients with ipsilateral mediastinal node involvement or with chest wall involvement. Combining surgery with another modality, either chemotherapy or radiation therapy, has been a promising approach to this subcategory of patients. Finally, if metastases to distant tissues or organs have occurred, then surgery is not an appropriate form of therapy.

The cell type is an important consideration in deciding about management, because small cell carcinoma has a high likelihood of having already metastasized by the time it is detected. Because of the early spread of small cell carcinoma, surgery is not considered the treatment of choice, unless the particular small cell tumor is a solitary peripheral nodule without any evidence of mediastinal or distant spread. In the more usual presentation of small cell carcinoma as a central mass, unresectable disease is virtually ensured, and chemotherapy (with or without radiotherapy) is considered the primary mode of therapy.

When one of the non–small cell tumors is unresectable on the basis of any criteria, the clinician is faced with a choice of no treatment, radiotherapy, or chemotherapy. The final choice is often a highly individual one, depending not only on the particular patient but also on the physician's preferences. In some cases, radiation therapy treatments are instituted early, in an attempt to shrink the tumor and delay local complications. In other circumstances, therapy is withheld until a complication ensues, such as bleeding or airway obstruction. Radiation treatments are then given with the goal of palliation, or reducing the tumor size for temporary alleviation of the acute problem. Unfortunately, palliation is by definition not curative therapy, and further problems with the tumor are certain to develop.

Other palliative forms of therapy are now being used to establish patency of an airway that has been partially or completely occluded or compressed by tumor. The treatment is typically accomplished with either fiberoptic or rigid bronchoscopy, using such techniques as LASER, cryotherapy, or electrocautery to diminish the size of the endobronchial tumor and re-establish a lumen. Alternatively or as a combined approach used in addition to the above techniques, an endobronchial stent, i.e., a hollow and relatively rigid plastic or metal tube, can be positioned within the airway lumen to maintain its patency.

As mentioned earlier, the overall 5-year survival in patients with carcinoma of the lung is less than 15 percent. The patients who survive are those whose disease was localized at presentation and amenable to surgical therapy. In this latter group, 5-year survival approaches 50 percent.

Table 21-1 summarizes many of the specific features about lung cancer discussed in Chapters 20 and 21. Each of the major cell types is considered separately, with emphasis placed on clinical, radiographic, and therapeutic aspects of each category of tumor.

BRONCHIAL CARCINOID TUMORS

Bronchial carcinoid tumors have often been called *bronchial adenomas,* because they were thought to represent a benign or adenomatous form of neoplasm involving the bronchial tree. In fact, although many patients with these tumors have an excellent prognosis and are cured by surgical removal, it is more accurate to view these tumors as low-grade malignancies, and they are currently classified as such. They constitute approximately 5 percent of primary lung tumors.

Bronchial carcinoid tumors arise most commonly in relatively central airways of the tracheobronchial tree. Although the cell of origin is not known with certainty, it has been postulated that these tumors arise from the

Table 21-1

Lung Cancer: Comparative Features

Cell Type	Frequency* (%)	Location†	Radiographic Appearance‡	Spread	Treatment	Relative Prognosis§	Miscellaneous
Squamous cell	30–35	Proximal, endobronchial	1. Central mass 2. Obstructive atelectasis 3. Postobstructive pneumonia 4. Normal	Contiguous intrathoracic spread; nodal metastasis	Surgery, combined modality therapy, or palliative therapy	Best	Hypercalcemia (occasional)
Small cell (including oat cell)	20	Proximal, endobronchial (submucosal)	1. Central mass 2. Hilar, mediastinal adenopathy	Hilar, mediastinal nodes; distant metastasis	Chemotherapy (± radiation therapy)	Worst	Ectopic hormone production (ADH, ACTH) relatively common
Adenocarcinoma (including bronchioloalveolar cell)	35	Peripheral	Solitary peripheral nodule or mass	Contiguous intrathoracic spread; nodal and distant metastasis	Surgery, combined modality therapy, or palliative therapy	Intermediate	
Large cell	15–20	Variable	Variable; often large peripheral mass	Contiguous intrathoracic spread; nodal and distant metastasis	Surgery, combined modality therapy, or palliative therapy	Intermediate	

*Approximate percent of all lung cancers.
†Most common location; for all cell types, variable locations are seen.
‡Common presentations on chest radiograph.
§For all cell types, the overall prognosis is generally poor.

neurosecretory Kulchitsky cells (K cells). Alternatively, they may arise from undifferentiated stem cells within the airway wall. It has also been suggested that bronchial carcinoid tumors may represent a more benign variant of small cell carcinoma, which has similarly been considered by some pathologists to arise from the K cell. In some carcinoid tumors, the histology has atypical features more suggestive of frank malignancy; these tumors have a poorer overall prognosis than those without such features.

Two important epidemiologic features distinguish bronchial carcinoid tumors from the other pulmonary neoplasms discussed here. First, smoking does not appear to be a risk factor. Second, as a group, patients with bronchial carcinoid tumors are younger than those with other pulmonary malignancies; frequently, young adults are the ones affected.

Bronchial carcinoid tumors are often discovered on either an abnormal chest radiograph or during episodes of hemoptysis or pneumonia distal to an obstructing airway tumor. Ectopic hormone production may also be found, probably relating to the presumed neurosecretory origin of the neoplastic cells. The carcinoid syndrome, due to the effects of serotonin produced by the tumor, is quite uncommon, being found in less than 5 percent of all cases of bronchial carcinoid tumors.

> Common features of bronchial carcinoid tumors are the following:
> 1. Often found in young adults
> 2. Hemoptysis
> 3. Pneumonia distal to an obstructing endobronchial mass

The treatment of these tumors is surgical resection if at all possible. For many patients the prognosis is excellent, and recurrent or distant disease is not a problem after surgical removal. However, metastatic disease is commonly found in patients whose tumors have atypical histology; the prognosis is worse for these patients.

MALIGNANT MESOTHELIOMA

Unlike the other tumors discussed, *malignant mesothelioma* primarily involves the pleura rather than the airways or the pulmonary parenchyma. Like bronchial carcinoid tumors, it is not associated with smoking as a risk factor. Although malignant mesothelioma is relatively uncommon, it is important at least partially because a specific etiologic factor in many of the cases can be identified.

The primary risk factor for development of malignant mesothelioma is a prior history of exposure to asbestos, generally in the range of 30 to 40 years earlier. Individuals who have worked in the types of jobs that expose them to asbestos (see Chapter 20) are obviously the ones at highest risk, but a heavy exposure is not necessary for predisposing a person to malignant mesothelioma. In fact, mesothelioma has been noted to develop even in wives of asbestos workers, presumably because of inhalation of asbestos dust while cleaning their husbands' clothes.

The main symptoms of patients with malignant mesothelioma are chest pain and dyspnea; cough may also be present. The chest radiograph is usually most notable for the presence of pleural fluid, and there is often irregular or lobulated thickening of the pleura (Fig. 21-3). Diagnosis requires biopsy of the pleura and histologic demonstration of the malignancy. Because the tumor originates in the pleura and does not directly communicate with airways, malignant cells are not shed into the tracheobronchial tree and cannot be found on cytologic examination of sputum.

> Mesothelioma is suggested by pleural fluid, irregular or lobulated pleural thickening, and a distant history of asbestos exposure.

The prognosis for malignant mesothelioma is quite poor. The tumor eventually entraps the lung and spreads to mediastinal structures. Death results, generally from respiratory failure. No clearly effective form of therapy

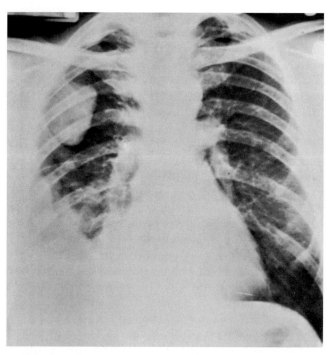

Figure 21-3 ■— Chest radiograph of patient with mesothelioma. Note several lobulated, pleural-based masses in right hemithorax accompanied by right pleural effusion.

is available, and fewer than 10 percent of patients survive 3 years. A radical surgical approach, extrapleural pneumonectomy, has sometimes been used in conjunction with chemotherapy and/or radiotherapy. This procedure involves removal of the entire ipsilateral lung along with both the visceral and parietal pleura. Alternatively, obliteration of the pleural space (pleurodesis) with a sclerosing agent can be done in an attempt to prevent re-accumulation of large amounts of pleural fluid. Because of the poor prognosis, mesothelioma has also become a target for a variety of new types of investigational therapy, including immunotherapy, use of biologic response modifiers (such as interferons and interleukin-2), and gene therapy.

THE SOLITARY PULMONARY NODULE

Although the solitary pulmonary nodule on chest radiograph (defined as a single, rounded lesion 3 cm or less in diameter) is a common presentation of lung cancer, there is actually a broad differential diagnosis for this radiographic abnormality. The physician is therefore faced with judging the likelihood that a nodule is malignant and choosing the appropriate pathway for diagnosis and management. Because lung cancer that manifests as a pulmonary nodule may be curable by surgical resection, it is undesirable to neglect management of such a lesion until it is no longer curable. On the other hand, to subject a patient to thoracotomy, a major surgical procedure, for removal of a benign lesion requiring no therapy is also undesirable.

The diagnostic possibilities for the solitary pulmonary nodule are presented in Table 21-2. Besides primary lung cancer, the major alternative diagnoses are benign pulmonary neoplasms, solitary metastases to the lung from a distant primary carcinoma, and infections (especially healed granulomatous

Table 21-2

Differential Diagnosis of the Solitary Pulmonary Nodule

Neoplasms
Malignant
  Primary lung cancer
  Solitary pulmonary metastasis
    from distant carcinoma
  Bronchial carcinoid (bronchial adenoma)
Benign neoplasms
  Hamartoma
  Miscellaneous (fibroma, lipoma, etc.)

Vascular Abnormality
Arteriovenous malformation

Infection
Infectious granuloma
    Tuberculosis ("tuberculoma")
    Histoplasmosis ("histoplasmoma")
  Bacterial abscess
  Miscellaneous (e.g., hydatid cyst, dog
    heartworm)

Miscellaneous
Rounded atelectasis
Hematoma
Pseudotumor (fluid loculated in a fissure)

lesions from tuberculosis or fungal disease). Estimating the likelihood of a malignant versus a benign lesion from its radiographic appearance is based on the following three major factors:

1. Growth. One of the most helpful pieces of information is an old chest radiograph. Comparison of old and new films shows whether a lesion is stable and gives an approximation of the rate of growth. Although it is difficult to say with certainty whether a lesion is benign or malignant based on the rate of growth, the absence of any increase in size for at least 2 years is an extremely good indication that a lesion is benign.

2. Calcification. The presence of calcification within a pulmonary nodule, best demonstrated on CT scan, potentially may favor the diagnosis of a benign lesion, especially a granuloma or hamartoma. If certain patterns of calcification are found—diffuse speckling, dense calcification, laminated (onion-skin) calcification, or "popcorn" calcification—then the lesion is almost assuredly benign. On the other hand, calcification at the periphery of a lesion or amorphous calcification within the lesion may actually be suggestive of malignancy. A peripheral area of calcification, for example, is entirely consistent with a scar carcinoma arising in the region of an old, calcified parenchymal scar (such as an old calcified granuloma).

3. Border appearance. An irregular or spiculated margin is suggestive of a malignant lesion, whereas a benign lesion commonly has a smooth and discrete border.

Additional clinical features may be more suggestive of a benign versus a malignant lesion but are somewhat less reliable. In individuals younger than 35 years of age, primary lung cancer is an unlikely although certainly not impossible diagnosis. The presence of a heavy smoking (and/or asbestos) history indicates a high risk for a malignant lesion; however, the absence of a smoking history does not rule out the diagnosis of lung cancer, particularly a peripheral adenocarcinoma. The size of a lesion may also be helpful, as those larger than 3 cm in diameter (usually called masses rather than nodules when they exceed 3 cm) are much more likely to be malignant than are nodules less than 2 cm in diameter. Finally, the presence of a previously diagnosed distant carcinoma obviously raises the possibility that a lung nodule represents a metastatic focus of tumor.

Criteria for assessing the likelihood that a solitary pulmonary nodule is malignant are the following:

1. Stability or change in size of the lesion
2. Presence or absence of calcification; pattern of calcification
3. Smooth versus irregular appearance of the border

The practical question of how to evaluate and manage these cases is often a difficult one, and the decision-making process must be individualized for each patient. A simple, noninvasive test such as sputum cytologic examination is most helpful if results are positive; however, the yield is low, even with peripheral nodules that are eventually proven to be carcinoma. Unless the lesion has been stable on chest radiograph for more than two years, chest CT scanning is done routinely to look at border characteristics, assess the presence and pattern of calcification, and identify other abnormalities, especially lymph nodes within the mediastinum. PET scanning (see Chapter 3), when available, is being performed increasingly when the diagnosis is uncertain after evaluating the clinical information and other imaging studies. Uptake of labeled fluoro-deoxyglucose suggests that the lesion has a high metabolic activity and is malignant, whereas lack of uptake suggests a metabolically inactive benign lesion.

More invasive procedures, such as percutaneous needle aspiration or biopsy and transbronchial biopsy (through a fiberoptic bronchoscope), are available and may be used in an attempt to make a histologic diagnosis. However, in many cases biopsy findings that are negative for malignancy do not obviate the need for surgery, because malignant cells may be missed by the limited sampling of a needle or biopsy forceps. Hence, a commonly used approach with a lesion suspicious for carcinoma is to proceed directly with resection, assuming no contraindications to surgery and no clinical evidence that the lesion has spread elsewhere or has metastasized from a distant primary malignancy. With the increasing availability of video-assisted thoracic surgery using a thoracoscope, this procedure is commonly used as a less invasive means of removing and therefore diagnosing small peripheral lung nodules. A more definitive resection, such as a lobectomy performed by thoracotomy, is then commonly performed if the nodule is found to be malignant.

When lung cancer manifests as a solitary peripheral nodule, the prognosis is much better than for the general group of patients with lung cancer. As a result of frequently curative surgical resection, more than 50 percent of patients with an initial solitary peripheral lung cancer survive 5 years, compared with the less than 15 percent, 5-year survival rate of all lung cancer patients.

References

Lung Cancer: General Reviews and Clinical Aspects

American College of Chest Physicians: Diagnosis and management of lung cancer: ACCP evidence-based guidelines. Chest 123 (suppl):1S-337S, 2003.
Matthay RM (ed): Lung cancer. Clin Chest Med 23:1-277, 2002.
Patel AM, Davila DG, and Peters SG: Paraneoplastic syndromes associated with lung cancer. Mayo Clin Proc 68:278-287, 1993.
Patel AM and Peters SG: Clinical manifestations of lung cancer. Mayo Clin Proc 68:273-277, 1993.
Spiro SG (ed): Lung cancer. Eur Respir Mon 17:1-329, 2001.

Lung Cancer: Diagnostic Approaches

American Thoracic Society/European Respiratory Society: Pretreatment evaluation of non–small cell lung cancer. Am J Respir Crit Care Med 156:320-332, 1997.
Boiselle PM, Ernst A, and Karp DD: Lung cancer detection in the 21st century: potential contributions and challenges of emerging technologies. AJR Am J Roentgenol 175:1215-1221, 2000.
Deslauriers J and Grégoire J: Clinical and surgical staging of non–small cell lung cancer. Chest 117 (Suppl):96S-103S, 2000.
Henschke CI, et al: Early Lung Cancer Action Project: overall design and findings from baseline screening. Lancet 354:99-105, 1999.
Hollings N and Shaw P: Diagnostic imaging of lung cancer. Eur Respir J 19:722-742, 2002.
Hyer JD and Silvestri G: Diagnosis and staging of lung cancer. Clin Chest Med 21:95-106, 2000.

Marshall MC and Olsen GN:The physiologic evaluation of the lung resection candidate. Clin Chest Med 14:305-320, 1993.

Mulshine JL and Smith RA: Screening and early diagnosis of lung cancer. Thorax 57:1071-1078, 2002.

Patz EF Jr: Imaging bronchogenic carcinoma. Chest 117 (Suppl):90S-95S, 2000.

Patz EF Jr, Goodman PC, and Bepler G: Screening for lung cancer. N Engl J Med 343:1627-1633, 2000.

Peterman RM et al: Preoperative staging of non-small-cell lung cancer with positron-emission tomography. N Engl J Med 343:254-261, 2000.

Petty TL:The early diagnosis of lung cancer. Dis Mon 47:204-264, 2001.

Van Klaveren RJ, et al: Lung cancer screening by low-dose spiral computed tomography. Eur Respir J 18:857-866, 2001.

Lung Cancer: Treatment

Adjei AA, Marks RS, and Bonner JA: Current guidelines for the management of small cell lung cancer. Mayo Clin Proc 74:809-816, 1999.

Bunn PA et al: New therapeutic strategies for lung cancer: biology and molecular biology come of age. Chest 117 (Suppl):163S-168S, 2000.

Bunn PA, Kelly K, and Bunn PA Jr: New combinations in the treatment of lung cancer: a time for optimism. Chest 117 (Suppl):138S-143S, 2000.

Deslauriers J and Grégoire J: Surgical therapy of early non–small cell lung cancer. Chest 117 (Suppl):104S-109S, 2000.

Johnson DH: Management of small cell lung cancer: current state of the art. Chest 116 (Suppl):525S-530S, 1999.

Spiro SG and Porter JC: Lung cancer—where are we today? Current advances in staging and non-surgical treatment. Am J Respir Crit Care Med 166:1166-1196, 2002.

Bronchial Carcinoids

Davila DG, Dunn WF, Tazelaar HD, and Pairolero PC: Bronchial carcinoid tumors. Mayo Clin Proc 68:795-803, 1993.

Fink G et al: Pulmonary carcinoid: presentation, diagnosis, and outcome in 142 cases in Israel and review of 640 cases from the literature. Chest 119:1647-1651, 2001.

Hasleton PS: Histopathology and prognostic factors in bronchial carcinoid tumors. Thorax 49:S56-S62, 1994.

Kulke MH and Mayer RJ: Carcinoid tumors. N Engl J Med 340:858-868, 1999.

Malignant Mesothelioma

Aisner J: Current approach to malignant mesothelioma of the pleura. Chest 107:332S-344S, 1995.

Boutin C, Schlesser M, Frenay C, and Astoul PH: Malignant pleural mesothelioma. Eur Respir J 12:972-981, 1998.

British Thoracic Society Standards of Care Committee: Statement on malignant mesothelioma in the United Kingdom. Thorax 56:250-265, 2001.

Sterman DH, Kaiser LR, and Albelda SM:Advances in the treatment of malignant pleural mesothelioma. Chest 116:504-520, 1999.

Upham JW, Garlepp MJ, Musk AW, and Robinson BWS: Malignant mesothelioma: new insights into tumour biology and immunology as a basis for new treatment approaches. Thorax 50:887-893, 1995.

Solitary Pulmonary Nodule

Cummings SR, Lillington GA, and Richard RJ: Managing solitary pulmonary nodules. Am Rev Respir Dis 134:453-460, 1986.

Midthun DE, Swensen SJ, and Jett JR:Approach to the solitary pulmonary nodule. Mayo Clin Proc 68:378-385, 1993.

Ost D and Fein A: Evaluation and management of the solitary pulmonary nodule. Am J Respir Crit Care Med 162:782-787, 2000.

Shaffer K: Role of radiology for imaging and biopsy of solitary pulmonary nodules. Chest 116 (Suppl):519S-522S, 1999.

Swensen SJ et al:The probability of malignancy in solitary pulmonary nodules. Arch Intern Med 157:849-855, 1997.

Yankelevitz DF and Henschke CI: Small solitary pulmonary nodules. Radiol Clin North Am 38:471-478, 2000.

Lung Defense Mechanisms

In the process of exchanging thousands of liters of air each day for O_2 uptake and CO_2 elimination, the lung is exposed to a wide variety of foreign substances transported with the inhaled air. Some of these are potentially injurious; others are relatively harmless. Inhaled air is not the only source of foreign material; secretions from the mouth and pharynx are also frequently aspirated into the tracheobronchial tree, even in normal individuals. This myriad of foreign substances is perhaps best classified into three major categories: small particulate material, noxious gases, and microorganisms. Because the oropharynx is rich with bacteria, aspirated secretions are particularly important as a source of unwanted bacteria entering the airways.

To protect itself against potentially toxic inhaled material, the respiratory system has evolved complex protective mechanisms that can be dissected into different components. Each component appears to have a distinct role, but there is a tremendous degree of interaction and "cooperation" among different components. That the distal lung parenchyma normally is sterile serves as testimony to the effectiveness of the defense system. However, the protective mechanisms can break down, either as a result of certain diseases or frequently as a consequence of treatment, especially medication administered to patients.

Before the discussion of infectious disorders of the respiratory system beginning with Chapter 23, it is appropriate to consider first how the lung protects itself against the infectious agents to which it is exposed. Although the focus is on protective mechanisms against infection, defenses against noninfectious substances, especially inhaled particulate material, are also addressed. The major categories of defense mechanisms to be discussed include: (1) physical or anatomic factors relating to deposition and clearance of inhaled material, (2) phagocytic and inflammatory cells that interact with the inhaled material, and (3) immune responses, which depend on prior exposure to, and recognition of, the foreign material. The chapter then proceeds with a discussion of several ways that the system breaks down, resulting in an inability to handle microorganisms and an increased risk for certain types of respiratory tract infection. We conclude by briefly considering how we can activate or augment specific immune responses through vaccination, thus enhancing our defenses against selected respiratory pathogens.

PHYSICAL OR ANATOMIC FACTORS

The pathway from the mouth or nose down to the lung parenchyma requires that inhaled air traverse a series of progressively branching airways. Hence, it is possible for inhaled particulate material to be deposited at various points in the airway, never reaching the most distal region of lung, the alveolar spaces. Particle size is an important determinant of deposition along the airway and thus affects the likelihood of a particle's reaching the distal parenchyma. When an inhaled particle is greater than 10 μm in diameter, it is likely to settle high in the upper airway—for example, in the nose. For particles 5 to 10 μm in diameter, settling tends to occur somewhat lower, in the trachea or the conducting airways but not down to the level of the small airways and alveoli. The particles most likely to reach the distal lung parenchyma range in size from 0.5 to 5 μm. Many bacteria fall within this size range, so that deposition along the airways is not very effective for excluding bacteria from the lower respiratory tract. However, large particles of dust and other inhaled material are effectively excluded from the distal lung parenchyma by virtue of their size.

When particles are deposited in the trachea or bronchi, two major processes, cough and mucociliary transport, are responsible for physical removal of these particles from the airways. Cough is an important protective mechanism, frequently triggered by stimulation of airway irritant receptors that are activated by inhaled or aspirated foreign material. The rapid acceleration and high flow rates of air achieved by a cough are often effective in clearing irritating foreign material from the airways.

The term *mucociliary transport* or *mucociliary clearance* refers to a process of waves of beating cilia moving a blanket of mucus (and any material trapped within the mucus) progressively upward along the tracheobronchial tree. From the trachea down to the respiratory bronchioles, the most superficial layer of epithelial cells lining the airway has cilia projecting into the airway lumen. These cilia have a structure identical to that of cilia found elsewhere in the body, consisting of longitudinal microtubules arranged in a characteristic way. Specifically, a cross-sectional view of cilia shows two central microtubules, surrounded by nine pairs of microtubules arranged around the periphery (Fig. 22-1). Small projecting sidearms from each doublet, called *dynein arms,* are believed to be crucial to the contractile function of the microtubules and hence to the beating of the cilia.

Strikingly, the movement of cilia on a particular cell and the movement between cells are quite coordinated, producing actual "waves" of ciliary motion. How such a pattern of ciliary motion is coordinated from cell to cell or even within the same cell is not known. What this wave-like motion accomplishes is movement of the overlying mucous layer in a cephalad direction (i.e., from distal to more proximal parts of the tracheobronchial tree), at a speed in the trachea estimated at 6 to 20 mm/min. If inhaled particles are

Factors affecting deposition and physical clearance of particles are the following:
1. Particle size
2. Cough
3. Mucociliary transport

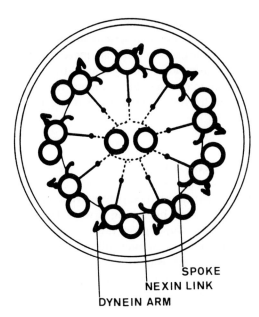

Figure 22-1 ■— Schematic diagram of cross section of cilium. Two central microtubules and nine pairs of peripheral microtubules are shown. Dynein arm projects from each peripheral doublet, and nexin links and radial spokes provide connections within microtubular structure. (From Eliasson R, Mossberg B, Camner P, and Afzelius BA: N Engl J Med 297:1-6, 1977. Copyright 1977 Massachusetts Medical Society. All rights reserved.)

SPOKE
NEXIN LINK
DYNEIN ARM

trapped in the mucous layer, they too are transported upward and eventually are either expectorated or swallowed.

There are actually two layers comprising the mucous blanket bathing the epithelial cells. Directly adjacent to the cells is the *sol layer,* within which the cilia are located. Superficial to the sol layer is the more viscous *gel layer,* which is produced by both submucosal mucous glands and goblet cells. In contrast, the origin of the periciliary sol layer is unknown. One can picture the viscous gel layer floating on top of the sol layer and being propelled upward as the cilia are able to beat more freely within the less viscous sol layer.

PHAGOCYTIC AND INFLAMMATORY CELLS

Dendritic Cells and Pulmonary Alveolar Macrophages

In the airways and at the level of the alveoli, particles and bacteria can be scavenged by mononuclear phagocytic cells, including *dendritic cells* and *pulmonary alveolar macrophages.* These cells constitute a major form of defense against material that has escaped deposition in the upper airway and has reached the intrathoracic airways or the alveolar structures.

Dendritic cells, which are closely related in lineage to monocytes and macrophages, are located in the airway epithelium as well as in alveolar walls and peribronchial connective tissue. These cells have long and irregular cytoplasmic extensions, and are believed to have an important role in processing and presenting antigenic material to lymphocytes, a critical step for the later immunologic defense provided by lymphocytes. *Langerhans' cells,* a type of dendritic cell with a particular ultrastructural appearance, are the cells whose abnormal proliferation appears to be responsible for eosinophilic granuloma of the lung (also called Langerhans' cell histiocytosis), as described in Chapter 11.

Pulmonary alveolar macrophages, which are large, mobile cells approximately 15 to 50 μm in diameter, are descendants of circulating monocytes derived from the bone marrow. Their cytoplasm contains a variety of granules of various shapes and sizes, many of which are packages of digestive enzymes that can dispose of ingested foreign material. Alveolar macrophages have a major role in killing microorganisms that have reached the lower respiratory tract, and they also release chemoattractant cytokines (chemokines) that recruit other inflammatory cells.

Phagocytosis

When an alveolar macrophage is exposed to inhaled particles or bacteria, attachment of the foreign material to the surface of the macrophage is the first step in the processing sequence. The particles or bacteria are then engulfed within the plasma membrane, which invaginates and pinches off within the cell to form a cytoplasmic phagosome containing the now isolated foreign material. In some circumstances, this sequence of attachment and phagocytosis is facilitated by opsonins, which coat the foreign material. Opsonins are proteins that bind to extracellular materials and make them more adherent to phagocytic cells and more amenable to engulfment or ingestion. Opsonins can be specific for the particular foreign substance, such as antibodies directed against antigenic material, or they may demonstrate nonspecific binding to a variety of substances. Particularly important specific opsonins are antibodies of the immunoglobulin (Ig) G class directed against antigenic foreign material, either bacteria or other antigenic particles. These opsonins greatly promote attachment to and ingestion by macrophages.

Once bacteria or other foreign material is isolated within phagosomes, a process of intracellular digestion occurs within the macrophage. Often the phagosomes combine with lysosomes, forming phagolysosomes, in which proteolytic enzymes supplied by the lysosome digest, detoxify, or destroy the phagosomal contents. In addition to lysosomal enzymes, there are a variety of oxidation products, such as hydrogen peroxide and other intermediate products of oxidative metabolism, that are toxic to bacteria and may play a role in the ability of the macrophage to kill ingested microorganisms.

The macrophage does not always kill or totally eliminate inhaled foreign material to which it is exposed. In some cases, such as with inhaled silica particles, the ingested material is toxic to the macrophage and may eventually kill the cell. In other cases, ingested material is inert but essentially indigestible and may persist indefinitely in the form of an indigestible residue. Organisms that are especially capable of persistent infection of macrophages without being killed include *Mycobacterium tuberculosis* and the human immunodeficiency virus.

Finally, there is mutual cooperation between macrophages and lymphocytes in the handling of foreign antigens. As noted in the earlier description of dendritic cells, intracellular processing of antigenic material by macrophages is often a prerequisite for further steps in the immune process provided by lymphocytes. On the other hand, soluble mediators (cytokines) produced by sensitized lymphocytes upon exposure to specific antigens are capable of activating macrophages and facilitating their ability to digest and kill microorganisms.

Polymorphonuclear Leukocytes

Another important cell involved in pulmonary defense is the polymorphonuclear leukocyte (PMN). This cell is a particularly important component of the defense mechanism for an established bacterial infection of the lower

---

Major phagocytic and inflammatory cells are the following:

1. Dendritic cells (airway and parenchymal)
2. Pulmonary alveolar macrophages
3. Polymorphonuclear leukocytes

respiratory tract. Normally, few PMNs reside in the small airways and alveoli. When bacteria have overwhelmed the initial defense mechanisms already discussed, they may replicate within alveolar spaces, causing a bacterial pneumonia. An examination of the histologic features of a bacterial pneumonia reveals that a prominent component of the inflammatory response is an outpouring of PMNs into the alveolar spaces. These cells are probably attracted to the lung by a variety of stimuli, particularly products of complement activation and chemotactic factors released by alveolar macrophages.

The eventual movement of PMNs out of the vasculature and into the lung parenchyma depends on the initial adherence of PMNs to the vascular endothelium. A variety of factors have been identified that mediate this process of adhesion, including integrins (on the surface of the PMNs) and adhesion molecules (on the surface of the vascular endothelial cells).

When PMNs are involved, they play a crucial role in phagocytosis and killing of the population of invading and proliferating bacteria. The neutrophil granules contain several antimicrobial substances, including defensins, lysozyme, and lactoferrin. In addition, the neutrophil is capable of generating products of oxidative metabolism that are toxic to microbes.

IMMUNE RESPONSES

A third major category of defense mechanisms for the respiratory system is the immune response, which involves recognizing and responding to specific antigenic material. Bacteria, viruses, and other microorganisms are perhaps the most important antigens to which the respiratory tract is repetitively exposed. Presumably, immune defense mechanisms are particularly important in protecting the individual against these agents. Although it is possible to provide only a superficial discussion here of the complicated immune system, the general principles should serve as a basis for understanding immune responses in the lung. For more detailed information, the reader is referred to specialized texts and review articles on immunology.

The two major components of the immune system are humoral, or B lymphocyte related, and cellular, or T lymphocyte related. Humoral immunity involves the activation of B lymphocytes (which do not require the thymus for differentiation) and the production of antibodies by plasma cells (which are derived from B lymphocytes). Cellular immunity refers to the activation of T lymphocytes (which depend on the thymus for differentiation) and the execution of certain specific T lymphocyte functions, including the production of soluble mediators or cytokines. The two lymphocyte systems are not entirely independent of each other; in particular, T lymphocytes appear to have an important role in regulating immunoglobulin or antibody synthesis by the humoral immune system.

A third type of lymphocyte, which lacks surface markers characteristic of either the T or the B lymphocyte, is the *natural killer (NK) cell.* These cells are capable of killing microorganisms (or tumor cells) without prior sensitization, and they can be stimulated by certain cytokines produced by sensitized T lymphocytes.

Both humoral and cellular immunity are important in the protection of the respiratory system against microorganisms. For certain infectious agents, humoral immunity is the primary mode of protection; for other agents, cellular immunity appears to be paramount. In the lung and in the blood, T lymphocytes are more numerous than B lymphocytes, but both systems are essential for effective defense against the spectrum of potentially harmful microorganisms.

Lymphocytes can be found in many locations within the respiratory tract, extending from the nasopharynx down to distal regions of the lung parenchyma. True lymph nodes are present around the trachea, the carina, and at the hilum of each lung, in the region of the mainstem bronchi. These lymph nodes receive the lymphatic drainage from most of the airways and lung parenchyma. There is also lymphoid tissue in the nasopharynx, and collections of lymphocytes arranged in nodules are also found along medium to large bronchi. These latter collections are called *bronchus-associated lymphoid tissue* and may be responsible for intercepting and handling antigens deposited along the conducting airways. Smaller aggregates of lymphocytes can be found in more distal airways and even scattered throughout the pulmonary parenchyma.

Humoral Immune Mechanisms

Humoral immunity in the respiratory tract appears in the form of two major classes of immunoglobulins: IgA and IgG. Antibodies of the IgA class are particularly important in the nasopharynx and upper airways, where they constitute the primary antibody type. The form of IgA present in these areas is secretory IgA, which includes a pair of IgA molecules (joined by a polypeptide) plus an extra glycoprotein component termed the *secretory component*. Secretory IgA appears to be synthesized locally, and the quantities of IgA are much greater in the respiratory tract than in the serum.

Major components of the immune system operative in the respiratory tract are the following:

1. T lymphocytes
2. B lymphocytes
3. IgA
4. IgG

There is evidence to suggest that secretory IgA plays a role as part of the respiratory defense system. By virtue of its ability to bind to antigens, IgA may bind to viruses and bacteria, preventing their attachment to epithelial cells. In addition, IgA is efficient in agglutinating microorganisms; the agglutinated microbes are more easily cleared by the mucociliary transport system. Finally, IgA appears to have the ability to neutralize a variety of respiratory viruses, as well as some bacteria.

In contrast to IgA, IgG is particularly abundant in the lower respiratory tract. It is also synthesized locally to a large extent, although a fraction also originates from serum IgG. It has a number of biologic properties: agglutinating particles, neutralizing viruses and bacterial toxins, serving as an opsonin for macrophage handling of bacteria, activating complement, and causing lysis of gram-negative bacteria in the presence of complement.

As far as is known, the overall role of the humoral immune system in respiratory defenses includes protecting the lung against a variety of bacterial and, to some extent, viral infections. Another section of this chapter deals with the clinical implications of this role and the consequences of impairment in the humoral immune system.

Cellular Immune Mechanisms

Cellular immune mechanisms, those mediated by thymus-dependent (T) lymphocytes, also operate as part of the lungs' overall defense system. Sensitized T lymphocytes produce a variety of soluble, biologically active mediators called *cytokines*, some of which (e.g., interferon-γ) have the ability to attract or activate other protective cell types, particularly macrophages. T lymphocytes also are capable of interacting with the humoral immune system and modifying antibody production.

Two important types of T lymphocytes have been well characterized on the basis of specific cell surface markers and functional characteristics. One type consists of cells that are positive for the CD4 surface marker, commonly called CD4$^+$ or helper T cells. CD4$^+$ cells, in turn, are divided into T_H1 and T_H2 subsets, which mediate cellular immune defense and allergic inflammation, respectively. The other major type of T lymphocyte consists of cells that are positive for the CD8 surface marker; these CD8$^+$ cells include suppressor and cytotoxic T cells. On exposure to specific antigens, both CD4$^+$ and CD8$^+$ cells produce a variety of cytokines, which interact with other components of the immune system, particularly B lymphocytes and macrophages.

One important role for the cellular immune system is to protect against bacteria that have a pattern of intracellular growth, especially *M. tuberculosis* (see the discussion of tuberculosis in Chapter 24). In addition, the cellular immune system has a critical role in the handling of many viruses, fungi, and protozoa.

FAILURE OF RESPIRATORY DEFENSE MECHANISMS

For each of the three major categories of respiratory defense mechanisms, clinically important deficiencies have been recognized. As a result, respiratory infections may ensue, and analysis of the specific types of infections associated with each type of defect is both extremely informative and clinically useful.

Impairment of Physical Clearance

Within the category of physical or anatomic factors affecting deposition and clearance of particles, both genetic abnormalities and environmental factors may alter the normal process of particle clearance by the mucociliary transport system. Especially interesting information has been provided by a genetic abnormality termed the *dyskinetic cilia syndrome,* also sometimes called the *immotile cilia syndrome.* In this disorder, a defect in ciliary structure and function leads to absent or impaired ciliary motility and hence to ineffective mucociliary clearance. Although more than 20 types of defects are recognized, the most common is absence of dynein arms on the microtubules. Clinically, the impairment in mucociliary clearance is associated with chronic sinusitis, chronic bronchitis, and bronchiectasis. In males, the sperm tail, which has a structure similar to that of cilia, is also abnormal, resulting in poor sperm motility and infertility. As mentioned in Chapter 7, the disorder called Kartagener's syndrome, consisting of a triad of chronic sinusitis, bronchiectasis, and situs inversus, is a variant of the dyskinetic cilia syndrome. It is believed that normal ciliary motion in a specific direction is responsible for the proper rotation of the heart and positioning of intra-abdominal organs during embryogenesis. When ciliary function is significantly disturbed, the positioning of the heart and the intra-abdominal organs becomes random, accounting for the fact that approximately 50 percent of patients with dyskinetic cilia syndrome have situs inversus.

Viral respiratory tract infections frequently cause temporary structural damage to the tracheobronchial mucosa. Functionally, the alteration of the mucosa is associated with impaired mucociliary clearance, which may retard the transport of invading bacteria out of the tracheobronchial tree. This is only one of the mechanisms by which viral respiratory tract infections predispose the individual to complicating bacterial superinfections.

Environmental factors may also cause impairment of mucociliary clearance. Exposure to cigarette smoke is certainly the most important clinically and probably contributes to the predisposition of heavy smokers to recurrent respiratory tract infections. Some atmospheric pollutants, such as sulfur dioxide (SO_2), nitrogen dioxide (NO_2), and ozone (O_3), appear to depress mucociliary clearance, but the clinical consequences are not entirely clear. High concentrations of O_2, such as 90 to 100 percent, inhaled for more than several hours also appear to be associated with impaired mucociliary function; here the consequences are obviously limited to patients with respiratory failure who require these extremely high concentrations.

Finally, as will be described in Chapter 29, management of patients with respiratory failure often involves insertion of a tube into the trachea (an endotracheal tube) and support of gas-exchange with a mechanical ventilator. Endotracheal tubes pose a significant risk for bacterial infection of the lower respiratory tract, often called *ventilator-associated pneumonia*, in part through preventing glottic closure, a critical component of the sequence of events leading to an effective cough. In addition, the endotracheal tube provides a direct conduit into the trachea for any bacteria that have colonized or contaminated the ventilator tubing or the endotracheal tube itself.

Impairment of Phagocytic and Inflammatory Cells

Clinical problems can be seen with deficiencies in number or function of the two major phagocytic and inflammatory cell types—alveolar macrophages and polymorphonuclear leukocytes. One of the more important ways that macrophage function can be impaired is by viral respiratory tract infections. These infections may paralyze the ability of the macrophage to kill bacteria, an additional reason why patients with viral infections are more susceptible to superimposed bacterial bronchitis or pneumonia.

Cigarette smoking also depresses the ability of alveolar macrophages to take up and kill bacteria. Hypoxia, starvation, alcoholism, and cold exposure similarly appear to be conditions in which impaired bacterial killing is at least partly due to depressed macrophage function. Treatment with corticosteroids, given for a myriad of diseases, seems to alter migration and function of macrophages, which may compound additional adverse effects of steroids on lymphocytes and the immune system. Some data suggest that macrophage migration is impaired in the acquired immunodeficiency syndrome (AIDS), which may complicate the other host defense defects recognized in this disease (see Chapter 26).

PMNs are depressed in number in several clinical circumstances, generally as a result of an underlying disease of the bone marrow, such as leukemia, or as a result of treatment administered. Chemotherapeutic agents used to treat malignancy commonly destroy rapidly proliferating cells of the bone marrow, resulting in a temporary loss of PMN precursors and a marked depression in the number of circulating PMNs. When PMNs are present at less than 1000/mm³ of blood, the risk of bacterial infection begins to rise, becoming particularly marked when the count drops below 500/mm³. Although opportunistic fungal infections are generally associated with impairment of cellular immunity rather than with neutropenia, the fungus *Aspergillus* is an important respiratory pathogen in the neutropenic patient.

Causes of impaired mucociliary clearance are the following:

1. Dyskinetic (immotile) cilia syndrome
2. Viral respiratory tract infection
3. Cigarette smoking
4. High concentrations of O_2 for prolonged periods

Causes of problems with macrophage function are the following:

1. Viral respiratory tract infections
2. Cigarette smoking
3. Alcoholism
4. Starvation
5. Cold exposure
6. Hypoxia
7. Corticosteroid therapy
8. AIDS

Causes of decreased numbers of PMNs are the following:

1. Bone marrow replacement by tumor
2. Cancer chemotherapeutic agents

Defects in Immune System

The immune system is subject to defects in function that affect its humoral and cellular components. Deficiencies in the humoral immune system, such as decreased or absent immunoglobulin production (i.e., hypogammaglobulinemia or agammaglobulinemia), are associated with recurrent bacterial respiratory infections, often leading to bronchiectasis. The risk of infection is best defined for individuals with IgG or global immunoglobulin deficiency. Although some individuals with selective IgA deficiency seem to have an increased risk of respiratory infections, either viral or bacterial, this risk may be at least partly related to a coexisting deficiency of one of the four recognized IgG subclasses.

Cellular immunity is disturbed most frequently by treatment with corticosteroids, cytotoxic or other immunosuppressive drugs, and in some well-defined disease states, such as Hodgkin's disease and AIDS. Unlike most other deficits in respiratory defenses, problems with cell-mediated immunity may lead to infection with a special group of microorganisms, including intracellular bacteria (especially mycobacteria), fungi, *Pneumocystis*, and certain viruses, particularly cytomegalovirus. Some of these organisms, such as *Pneumocystis* and several of the fungi, rarely affect individuals with normal cellular immunity, whereas others, such as *M. tuberculosis,* can also affect individuals without any defined defects in cellular immunity.

Causes of immune deficiency are the following:
1. Humoral—decreased or absent immunoglobulins
2. Cellular—corticosteroids, cytotoxic drugs, Hodgkin's disease, AIDS

In summary, the defense mechanisms available to protect the respiratory tract from invading microorganisms are varied and complex. People are capable of thwarting these defenses by exposing themselves to such damaging influences as cigarette smoke and ethanol. Just as important, physicians often manage patients with pharmacologic agents or other modalities that disrupt host defense mechanisms, making it essential that physicians be aware of the potential infectious complications of therapy.

In the clinical setting, deficiencies in immunoglobulins and in PMNs are strongly associated with an increased risk of bacterial infections. Although problems with mucociliary clearance and with macrophage function are somewhat less well defined in terms of the specific infectious risk, bacterial infections also appear to be prominent in these settings. In contrast, disturbances in cellular immunity are characterized by an increased risk of a different subset of infections, especially infections due to mycobacteria, *Pneumocystis,* fungi, and certain viruses.

Because of the frequency and serious nature of respiratory infections in immunosuppressed patients, this chapter continues with a brief consideration of the problems posed by the immunocompromised patient with pulmonary infiltrates. More detailed discussions can be found in several articles listed in the references at the end of this chapter.

THE IMMUNOSUPPRESSED PATIENT WITH PULMONARY INFILTRATES

During the last several decades, physicians have been faced with increasing numbers of patients who have impaired host defense mechanisms, particularly granulocytopenia (decreased PMNs) and depressed cellular immunity; these occur frequently as a result of chemotherapy given for malignancy or immunosuppressive agents administered following organ transplantation. Since the early 1980s, an entirely new population of individuals at risk for opportunistic infections has also emerged. These patients have AIDS, with its devastating consequences on the cellular immune system. Because of the importance of AIDS, Chapter 26 is devoted to the respiratory complications associated with this particular form of immunodeficiency.

Immunocompromised patients are extremely susceptible to the development of respiratory tract infections with a variety of organisms, some of which rarely cause disease in the immunocompetent host. When the immunosuppressed patient has fever and new pulmonary infiltrates, the possibility of an "opportunistic" infection comes immediately to mind. However, patients with malignancy are also susceptible to noninfectious complications of their tumor or its treatment; thus, such complications must also be seriously considered in the differential diagnosis.

The spectrum of infectious and noninfectious causes of pulmonary infiltrates in the immunosuppressed host is shown in Table 22-1. Even though fungi and other relatively unusual types of organisms are commonly thought to be the major causes of infiltrates in patients receiving treatment for malignancy, bacterial pneumonia is actually the most frequent problem in this setting. Granulocytopenia is the primary predisposing factor for bacterial pneumonias, which are frequently due to gram-negative rods or to *Staphylococcus.*

Other bacteria, namely mycobacteria (either *M. tuberculosis* or nontuberculous mycobacteria) and *Nocardia,* cause problems mainly in the patient with impaired cellular immunity. Defective cellular immunity also predisposes the individual to infections with *Pneumocystis carinii,* fungi, and viruses. The fungus *Aspergillus,* which causes an invasive pneumonia in the immunosuppressed patient, seems to be most commonly found in the patient who is neutropenic (and also has impaired cellular immunity) from cytotoxic chemotherapy.

Common noninfectious diagnoses are the interstitial lung diseases resulting as a side effect from radiation therapy or a variety of chemotherapeutic agents (see Chapter 10). However, congestive heart failure (often secondary to cardiac toxicity from chemotherapeutic agents), pulmonary dissemination of the underlying malignancy, and hemorrhage into the pulmonary

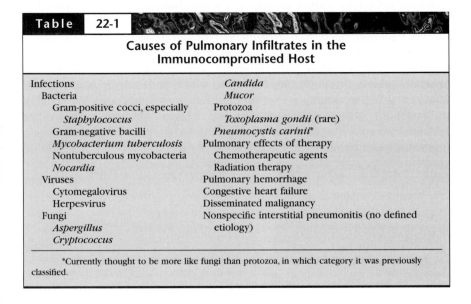

Table 22-1

Causes of Pulmonary Infiltrates in the Immunocompromised Host

Infections
  Bacteria
    Gram-positive cocci, especially
      Staphylococcus
    Gram-negative bacilli
    Mycobacterium tuberculosis
    Nontuberculous mycobacteria
    Nocardia
  Viruses
    Cytomegalovirus
    Herpesvirus
  Fungi
    Aspergillus
    Cryptococcus
    Candida
    Mucor
  Protozoa
    Toxoplasma gondii (rare)
    *Pneumocystis carinii**
Pulmonary effects of therapy
  Chemotherapeutic agents
  Radiation therapy
Pulmonary hemorrhage
Congestive heart failure
Disseminated malignancy
Nonspecific interstitial pneumonitis (no defined etiology)

*Currently thought to be more like fungi than protozoa, in which category it was previously classified.

parenchyma are additional causes of infiltrates that can closely mimic infectious etiologies. In many circumstances, an interstitial inflammatory process can be proved histologically, but no definite cause can be identified. These cases are often diagnosed as nonspecific interstitial pneumonitis, with the realization that neither the pathology nor the clinical history provides clues to an etiologic diagnosis.

The approach to the immunocompromised patient with pulmonary infiltrates revolves around trying to identify an infectious agent or a noninfectious etiology. Traditional methods have included examination of sputum and specimens obtained by bronchoscopy or thoracoscopic lung biopsy. There has been great recent interest in the use of newer, more rapid, and more sensitive techniques for identifying a variety of opportunistic pathogens. Improved methods of culture, molecular probes, and polymerase chain reaction technology are being investigated and sometimes used clinically in the diagnosis of specific opportunists. The particular procedure chosen is based on specific clinical features relevant to each patient, such as the nature of the underlying disease, the suspected cause of the pulmonary infiltrate, the presence or absence of other predisposing factors, and the potential risks of a diagnostic procedure. However, in some immunocompromised patients with pulmonary infiltrates, empiric treatment is given without a definitive diagnosis, particularly when the patients are at high risk for invasive procedures or when a specific diagnosis appears to be fairly likely.

AUGMENTATION OF RESPIRATORY DEFENSE MECHANISMS

Rather than ending this chapter with the negative aspects of what physicians and disease can do to impair normal lung defense mechanisms, we should keep in mind the progress that has been made in augmenting defense mechanisms and protecting against some forms of respiratory tract infection. Immunization against certain respiratory pathogens has induced production of antibodies against the organisms and has conferred either relative or complete protection against infection by these microbes. Perhaps the most notable examples are immunization against the bacteria that cause pertussis (whooping cough) and immunization against influenza virus and many subtypes of the common bacterium *Streptococcus pneumoniae* (pneumococcus). Whereas universal immunization against pertussis is recommended during childhood, immunization with influenza and pneumococcal vaccines is generally targeted to individuals believed to be at relatively high risk for contracting or developing complications from these infections. We look to the future for additional vaccines that will enhance immunity against other respiratory pathogens and allow us to approach these infections more from a preventive standpoint.

References

Fraser RS, Müller NL, Colman N, and Paré PD: Pulmonary defense and other nonrespiratory functions. *In:* Diagnosis of Diseases of the Chest, 4th ed. Philadelphia, WB Saunders, 1999, pp 126-135.

Hance AJ: Pulmonary immune cells in health and disease: dendritic cells and Langerhans' cells. Eur Respir J 6:1213-1220, 1993.

Harada RN and Repine JE: Pulmonary host defense mechanisms. Chest 87:247-252, 1985.

Johnston RB: Monocytes and macrophages. N Engl J Med 318:747-752, 1988.

Lambrecht BN, Prins J-B, and Hoogsteden HC: Lung dendritic cells and host immunity to infection. Eur Respir J 18:692-704, 2001.

Lipscomb MF: Lung defenses against opportunistic infections. Chest 96:1393-1399, 1989.

Mason CM and Nelson S: Pulmonary host defenses. Implications for therapy. Clin Chest Med 20:475-488, 1999.

Moore BB, Moore TA, and Toews GB: Role of T- and B-lymphocytes in pulmonary host defences. Eur Respir J 18:846-856, 2001.

Pilette C et al: Lung mucosal immunity: immunoglobulin-A revisited. Eur Respir J 18:571-588, 2001.

Reynolds HY: Host defense impairments that may lead to respiratory infections. Clin Chest Med 8:339-358, 1987.

Reynolds HY: Immunoglobulin G and its function in the human respiratory tract. Mayo Clin Proc 63:161-174, 1988.

Reynolds HY: Immunologic system in the respiratory tract. Physiol Rev 71:1117-1133, 1991.

Reynolds HY: Integrated host defense against infection. *In* Crystal RG, West JB, Weibel ER, and Barnes PJ (eds): The Lung: Scientific Foundations, 2nd ed. Philadelphia, Lippincott-Raven, 1997, pp 2353-2365.

Rose RM: The host defense network of the lungs: an overview. *In* Niederman MS, Sarosi GA, and Glassroth J (eds): Respiratory Infections: A Scientific Basis for Management. Philadelphia, WB Saunders Co., 1994, pp 3-15.

Pulmonary Disease Associated with Impaired Defense Mechanisms

Dukes RJ, Rosenow EC III, and Hermans PE: Pulmonary manifestations of hypogammaglobulinemia. Thorax 33:603-607, 1978.

Eliasson R, Mossberg B, Camner P, and Afzelius BA: The immotile cilia syndrome. N Engl J Med 297:1-6, 1977.

Fishman JA and Rubin RH: Infection in organ-transplant recipients. N Engl J Med 338:1741-1751, 1998.

Mayaud C and Cadranel J: A persistent challenge: the diagnosis of respiratory disease in the non-AIDS immunocompromised host. Thorax 55:511-517, 2000.

Niederman MS: Strategies for the prevention of pneumonia. Clin Chest Med 8:543-556, 1987.

Rosenow EC III, Wilson WR, and Cockerill FR III: Pulmonary disease in the immunocompromised host: I. Mayo Clin Proc 60:473-487, 1985.

Shelhamer JH et al: The laboratory evaluation of opportunistic pulmonary infections. Ann Intern Med 124:585-599, 1996.

Shelhamer JH et al: Respiratory disease in the immunosuppressed patient. Ann Intern Med 117:415-431, 1992.

Talbot EA and Hicks CB: Opportunistic thoracic infections. Bacteria, viruses, and protozoa. Chest Surg Clin N Am 9:167-192, 1999.

Walsh FW, Rolfe MW, and Rumbak MJ: The initial pulmonary evaluation of the immunocompromised patient. Chest Surg Clin N Am 9:19-38, 1999.

Wilson WR, Cockerill FR III, and Rosenow EC III: Pulmonary disease in the immunocompromised host. II. Mayo Clin Proc 60:610-631, 1985.

Augmentation of Respiratory Defense Mechanisms

Ahmed F, Singleton JA, and Franks AL: Influenza vaccination for healthy young adults. N Engl J Med 345:1543-1547, 2001.

Couch RB: Influenza: prospects for control. Ann Intern Med 133:992-998, 2000.

Couch RB: Prevention and treatment of influenza. N Engl J Med 343:1778-1787, 2000.

Fedson DS, Shapiro ED, La Force LM, et al: Pneumococcal vaccine after 15 years of use. Arch Intern Med 154:2531-2535, 1994.

Nguyen-Van-Tam JS and Neal KR: Clinical effectiveness, policies, and practices for influenza and pneumococcal vaccines. Semin Respir Infect 14:184-195, 1999.

Örtqvist A: Pneumococcal vaccination: current and future issues. Eur Respir J 18:184-195, 2001.

Pneumonia

By any of several criteria, pneumonia (infection of the pulmonary parenchyma) must be considered one of the most important categories of disease affecting the respiratory system. First, it is extraordinarily common, accounting for nearly 10 percent of admissions to many large general hospitals. Overall, it has been estimated that more than 5 million cases of pneumonia occur in the United States each year. Second, it is a significant cause of death; more than 80,000 Americans die of bacterial pneumonia each year, making it the sixth most common cause of death in the nation. It is no wonder that Sir William Osler referred to pneumonia as "the captain of the men of death," particularly as he spoke before the era of effective antibiotic therapy. For many types of pneumonia, medical therapy with antibiotics (along with supportive care) has great impact on the duration and outcome of the illness. Because of the effectiveness of treatment, the diseases discussed in this chapter are typically gratifying to treat for all involved medical personnel. Unfortunately, the emerging trend during the 1990s was the acquisition of antibiotic resistance by some of the organisms causing pneumonia, and the treatment of pneumonia has therefore been evolving to keep pace with patterns of antibiotic resistance.

Although many of the specific agents causing pneumonia are considered here, this chapter is organized primarily as a general discussion of the problem of pneumonia. As appropriate, the focus on individual etiologic agents will highlight some characteristic features of each that are particularly useful to the physician. Also covered is a commonly used categorization of pneumonia based on the clinical setting: community-acquired versus nosocomial (hospital-acquired) pneumonia. According to current clinical practice, the approach to evaluation and management of these two types of pneumonia is often quite different.

The chapter will conclude with a brief discussion of several infections that were uncommon or primarily of historical interest until September 11, 2001. After the terrorist attack on the World Trade Center and the Pentagon, the threat of bioterrorism became a reality when spores of *Bacillus anthracis* sent through the mail resulted in cases of cutaneous and inhalational anthrax. In addition to reviewing inhalational anthrax, we will also briefly describe two other organisms considered to be of concern as potential weapons of bioterrorism: *Yersinia pestis* (the cause of plague) and *Francisella tularensis* (the cause of tularemia).

ETIOLOGY AND PATHOGENESIS

As discussed in Chapter 22, the host defenses of the lung are constantly challenged by a variety of organisms, both viruses and bacteria. Viruses in particular are likely to avoid or to overwhelm some of the defenses of the upper respiratory tract, causing a transient, relatively mild clinical illness with symptoms limited to the upper respiratory tract. When host defense mechanisms of the upper and lower respiratory tracts are overwhelmed, microorganisms may establish residence, proliferate, and cause a frank infectious process within the pulmonary parenchyma. With particularly virulent organisms, there need not be any major impairment of host defense mechanisms, and pneumonia may be seen even in essentially normal individuals. At the other extreme, if host defense mechanisms are quite impaired, microorganisms that are not particularly virulent—that is, unlikely to cause disease in a normal host—may produce a life-threatening pneumonia.

In practice, there are several factors that frequently cause enough impairment of host defenses to contribute to the development of pneumonia, even though individuals with such impairment are not considered "immunosuppressed." Viral upper respiratory tract infections, ethanol abuse, cigarette smoking, and preexisting chronic obstructive pulmonary disease are just a few of these contributing factors. More severe impairment of host defenses is caused by diseases that are associated with immunosuppression (such as the acquired immunodeficiency syndrome), by various underlying malignancies (particularly leukemia and lymphoma), and by the use of corticosteroids and other immunosuppressive or cytotoxic drugs. In these cases associated with impairment of host defenses, individuals are susceptible both to bacterial and to more unusual nonbacterial infections, which will be covered in subsequent chapters.

There are two major ways that microorganisms, especially bacteria, find their way to the lower respiratory tract. The first is by inhalation, whereby organisms are usually carried in small droplet particles that are inhaled into the tracheobronchial tree. The second is by aspiration, whereby secretions from the oropharynx pass through the larynx and into the tracheobronchial tree. Aspiration is usually thought of as a process occurring in individuals unable to protect their airways from secretions by glottic closure and coughing. Although clinically significant aspiration is more likely to occur in such individuals, it is also true that everyone is subject to aspirating small amounts of oropharyngeal secretions, particularly during sleep. Defense mechanisms seem able to cope with this nightly onslaught of bacteria, and frequent bouts of aspiration pneumonia are not experienced.

Less commonly, bacteria may reach the pulmonary parenchyma through the blood stream rather than by the airways. This route is an important one

> Contributing factors for pneumonia in the immuno-competent host are the following:
>
> 1. Viral upper respiratory tract infection
> 2. Ethanol abuse
> 3. Cigarette smoking
> 4. Chronic obstructive pulmonary disease

for the spread of certain organisms, particularly *Staphylococcus.* When pneumonia results in this way from bacteremia, the implication is either that a distant, primary source of bacterial infection is present or that bacteria were introduced directly into the blood stream, for example, as a consequence of intravenous drug abuse.

Many individual infectious agents are associated with the development of pneumonia. The frequency with which each agent is involved is quite difficult to assess and depends to a large extent on the specific population studied. The largest single category of agents is probably bacteria; the other two major categories are viruses and mycoplasma. Of the bacteria, the organism most frequently associated with pneumonia is *Streptococcus pneumoniae,* in common parlance often called the pneumococcus. It has been estimated that approximately half of all pneumonias in adults serious enough to require hospitalization are pneumococcal in origin.

Streptococcus pneumoniae (pneumococcus) is the most common cause of bacterial pneumonia; the polysaccharide capsule is an important factor in its virulence.

Bacteria

S. pneumoniae, a normal inhabitant of the oropharynx in a large proportion of adults, is a gram-positive coccus seen in pairs or diplococci. Pneumococcal pneumonia is commonly acquired in the community, i.e., in nonhospitalized patients, and frequently occurs after a viral upper respiratory tract infection. The organism has a polysaccharide capsule, which protects the bacteria from phagocytosis and is therefore an important factor in its virulence. There are many antigenic types of capsular polysaccharide; in order for host defense cells to phagocytize the organism, antibody against the particular capsular type must be present. As discussed in Chapter 22, antibodies contributing in this way to the phagocytic process are called *opsonins.*

Staphylococcus aureus is another gram-positive coccus, usually appearing in clusters when examined microscopically. There are three major settings in which this organism is seen as a cause of pneumonia: (1) as a secondary complication of respiratory tract infection with the influenza virus, (2) in the hospitalized patient, who often has some impairment of host defense mechanisms, and whose oropharynx has been colonized by *Staphylococcus,* and (3) as a complication of widespread dissemination of staphylococcal organisms through the blood stream.

Factors predisposing to oropharyngeal colonization and pneumonia with gram-negative organisms are the following:

1. Hospitalization
2. Underlying disease and compromised host defenses
3. Recent antibiotic therapy

A variety of gram-negative organisms are potential causes of pneumonia, but only a few of the most important examples from this group of organisms are mentioned here. *Haemophilus influenzae,* which is a small coccobacillary gram-negative organism, is often found in the nasopharynx of normal individuals and in the lower airways of patients with chronic obstructive lung disease. It can cause pneumonia in children and adults, the latter often with underlying chronic obstructive lung disease as a predisposing factor. *Klebsiella pneumoniae,* a relatively large gram-negative rod that may normally be found in the gastrointestinal tract, has been best described as a cause of pneumonia in the setting of underlying alcoholism. *Pseudomonas aeruginosa,* which may be found in a variety of environmental sources (especially in the hospital environment), is seen primarily in patients who are debilitated, hospitalized, and often previously treated with antibiotics.

Anaerobes normally found in the oropharynx are the usual cause of aspiration pneumonia.

The bacterial flora normally present in the mouth are also potential etiologic agents in the development of pneumonia. A multitude of organisms (both gram-positive and gram-negative) that favor or require anaerobic conditions for growth are the major organisms comprising mouth flora. The most common predisposing factor for anaerobic pneumonia is aspiration of secretions from the oropharynx into the tracheobronchial tree. Patients with impaired consciousness (e.g., as a result of coma, alcohol ingestion, or seizures) and those with difficulty swallowing (e.g., as a result of diseases causing muscle weakness) are prone to aspirate and are at risk for pneumonia due to anaerobic mouth organisms.

In some settings, such as prolonged hospitalization or recent use of antibiotics, the type of bacteria residing in the oropharynx may change. Specifically, aerobic gram-negative bacilli and *S. aureus* are then more likely to colonize the oropharynx, and any subsequent pneumonia due to aspiration of oropharyngeal contents may include these aerobic organisms as part of the process.

The two final types of bacteria mentioned here are relative newcomers to the list of etiologic agents. The first of these organisms, *Legionella pneumophila,* was identified as the cause of a mysterious outbreak of pneumonia in 1976 affecting American Legion members at a convention in Philadelphia. Since then it has been recognized as an important cause of pneumonia occurring in epidemics as well as in isolated, sporadic cases. In addition, it seems to affect both previously normal individuals and those with prior impairment of respiratory defense mechanisms. In retrospect, several prior outbreaks of unexplained pneumonia have been shown to be due to this organism. Although the organism is a gram-negative bacillus, it stains very poorly and is generally not seen by conventional staining methods.

The other organism, *Chlamydia pneumoniae,* has been recognized in epidemiologic studies as the cause of approximately 5 to 10 percent of cases of pneumonia. It is an obligate intracellular parasite that appears more related to gram-negative bacteria than to viruses, the category in which it had previously been placed. Diagnosis is rarely made clinically, because there are no distinguishing clinical or radiographic features, and the organism is not readily cultured. As a result, serologic studies, which are not readily available, serve as the primary means of diagnosis.

Many other types of bacteria can certainly cause pneumonia. Because all of them cannot be covered in this chapter, the interested reader should consult some of the more detailed references listed at the end of this chapter.

Viruses

Although viruses are extremely common causes of upper respiratory tract infections, they are diagnosed relatively infrequently as a cause of frank pneumonia except in children. In adults, influenza virus is the most commonly diagnosed agent; outbreaks of pneumonia due to adenovirus are also well recognized, particularly in military recruits. A relatively rare cause of a fulminant and often lethal pneumonia was described in the southwest United States, but cases in other locations have also been recognized. The virus responsible for this pneumonia, called *hantavirus,* is found in rodents and was previously described as a cause of fever, hemorrhage, and acute renal failure in other parts of the world.

Mycoplasma

Mycoplasma appears to be a class of organisms intermediate between viruses and bacteria. Unlike bacteria, they have no rigid cell wall; unlike viruses, they do not require the intracellular machinery of a host cell to replicate and are capable of free-living growth. Similar in size to a large virus, mycoplasmas are the smallest free-living organisms that have yet been identified. These

Mycoplasma, the smallest known free-living organism, is a frequent cause of pneumonia in young adults.

organisms are now recognized as a common cause of pneumonia, perhaps responsible for a minimum of 10 to 20 percent of all cases of pneumonia. Although mycoplasmal pneumonia occurs most frequently in young adults, it is certainly not limited to this age group. The pneumonia is generally acquired in the community, i.e., in previously normal, nonhospitalized individuals, and may occur either in isolated cases or in localized outbreaks.

PATHOLOGY

The pathologic process common to all pneumonias is infection and inflammation of the distal pulmonary parenchyma. An influx of polymorphonuclear leukocytes (PMNs), edema fluid, erythrocytes, mononuclear cells, and fibrin is seen to a variable extent in all cases. The bacterial pneumonias, in particular, are characterized by an exuberant outpouring of PMNs into alveolar spaces as they attempt to limit proliferation of the invading bacteria.

The individual types of pneumonia may differ in the exact location and mode of spread of the infection. In the past, a distinction was often made between those pneumonias that follow a "lobar" distribution, those that behave more like a "bronchopneumonia," and those with the pattern of an "interstitial pneumonia." However, these distinctions are often difficult to make, because individual cases of pneumonia frequently do not adhere to any one particular pattern but have mixtures of the three in varying proportions. Given this limitation, a brief mention of the three major types follows.

Lobar Pneumonia. Lobar pneumonia has classically been described as a process not limited to segmental boundaries but rather tending to spread throughout an entire lobe of the lung. Spread of the infection is believed to occur from alveolus to alveolus and from acinus to acinus through interalveolar pores, known as the pores of Kohn. The classic example of a lobar pneumonia is that due to *S. pneumoniae,* although many cases of pneumonia recognized as being due to pneumococcus do not necessarily follow this typical pattern.

Bronchopneumonia. In bronchopneumonia, distal airway inflammation is prominent along with alveolar disease, and spread of the infection and the inflammatory process tends to occur through airways rather than through adjacent alveoli and acini. Whereas lobar pneumonias appear as dense consolidations involving part or all of a lobe, bronchopneumonias are more patchy in distribution, depending on where spread by airways has occurred. Many of the other bacteria, such as staphylococci and a variety of gram-negative bacilli, may produce this patchy pattern.

Interstitial Pneumonia. Interstitial pneumonias are characterized by an inflammatory process within the interstitial walls rather than the alveolar spaces. Although viral pneumonias classically start as interstitial pneumonias, severe cases generally show extension of the inflammatory process to alveolar spaces as well.

In some cases of pneumonia, the organisms are not highly destructive to lung tissue, even though an exuberant inflammatory process may be seen. Pneumococcal pneumonia classically (although not always) behaves in this way, and the healing process is associated with restoration of relatively normal parenchymal architecture. In other cases, when the organisms are more destructive, tissue necrosis can occur, with resulting abscess formation or scarring of the parenchyma. Many cases of staphylococcal and anaerobic pneumonias follow this more destructive course.

PATHOPHYSIOLOGY

Infections of the pulmonary parenchyma produce their clinical sequelae not only by altering the normal functioning of the lung parenchyma, but also by inducing a more generalized, systemic response to the invading microorganisms. The major pathophysiologic consequence of inflammation and infection involving the distal air spaces is a decrease in ventilation to the affected areas. If perfusion is relatively maintained, as it often is, ventilation-perfusion mismatch results, with low ventilation-perfusion ratios in the diseased regions. When alveoli are totally filled with inflammatory exudate, there may be no ventilation to these regions, and extreme ventilation-perfusion inequality (i.e., shunt) results.

This ventilation-perfusion inequality generally translates into an effect on gas-exchange, namely hypoxemia. Although frank shunting may explain part of the hypoxemia, ventilation-perfusion mismatch with areas of low ventilation-perfusion ratio is usually a more important factor. Carbon dioxide retention is not a feature of pneumonia unless the patient already has an extremely limited reserve, especially from underlying chronic obstructive lung disease. In fact, patients with pneumonia frequently hyperventilate and have a Pco_2 that is less than 40 torr.

> Pneumonia commonly results in ventilation-perfusion mismatch (with or without shunting) and hypoxemia.

The systemic response to pneumonia is certainly not unique but rather a reflection of the body's response to serious infection. Perhaps the most apparent aspects of this response are fever, an outpouring of PMNs into the circulation (particularly with bacterial pneumonia), and often a "toxic" appearance of the patient. These indirect systemic responses can be clues that an infectious process is the cause of a new pulmonary infiltrate.

CLINICAL FEATURES

In many ways the clinical manifestations of pneumonia are similar, even when different infectious agents are involved; in other ways the presentations and manifestations are quite different. Although recognition of subtle clinical differences sometimes allows the astute clinician to suggest an etiologic diagnosis, methods for identifying a specific infectious agent play an equally if not more important role in the final diagnosis. However, in many cases, a specific agent cannot be clearly identified, and patients are often managed in an empiric way based on the setting in which they present (as discussed later in this chapter).

Perhaps the most important constellation of symptoms in almost any type of pneumonia consists of fever, cough, and often shortness of breath. The cough is nonproductive in some cases, particularly in those pneumonias due to viruses or mycoplasma; in others, especially bacterial pneumonias, sputum production is a prominent feature. When the inflammatory process in the pulmonary parenchyma extends out to the pleural surface, the patient often reports pleuritic chest pain. If the fever is high and "spiking," patients frequently experience shaking chills associated with the rapid rise in body temperature.

> Frequent clinical features in patients with pneumonia are the following:
> 1. Fever (± chills)
> 2. Cough (± sputum)
> 3. Dyspnea
> 4. Pleuritic chest pain
> 5. Crackles overlying affected region
> 6. Dullness and bronchial breath sounds with frank consolidation
> 7. Polymorphonuclear leukocytosis

Physical examination reflects the systemic response to infection and the ongoing inflammatory process in the lung. Patients often have tachycardia, tachypnea, and fever. Examination of the chest typically reveals crackles or rales overlying the region of the pneumonia. If there is dense consolidation and the bronchus supplying the area is patent, then sound transmission is greatly increased through the consolidated, pneumonic area. As a result, breath sounds may be bronchial in quality, fremitus is increased, and egophony is present. The consolidated area is also characteristically dull to percussion of the overlying chest wall. Examination of the peripheral blood generally shows an increase in the white blood count (leukocytosis). Especially in patients with bacterial pneumonia, the leukocytosis is composed primarily of PMNs, and there may be a shift toward immature, younger neutrophils, i.e., bands.

In pneumococcal pneumonia, the onset of the clinical illness is often relatively abrupt, with shaking chills and high fever. Cough may be productive of yellow, green, or blood-tinged (rusty-colored) sputum. Before the development of pneumonia, patients often experience a viral upper respiratory tract infection, which presumably is an important predisposing feature.

Mycoplasmal pneumonia, in contrast to pneumococcal pneumonia, characteristically has a somewhat slower, more insidious onset. Cough is a particularly prominent symptom, but it is often nonproductive. Fever is not as high, and shaking chills are uncommon. Young adults are the individuals most likely to have mycoplasmal pneumonia, although the disease is not limited to this age group.

Patients with either staphylococcal or gram-negative bacillary pneumonias are often quite ill. Frequently, they are patients with complex underlying medical problems who have already been hospitalized, and many have impaired defense mechanisms or have recently received antibiotics. Staphylococcal pneumonia may also be seen as a secondary complication of influenza infection or as a result of dissemination of the organism through the blood stream.

Pneumonia with anaerobic organisms generally occurs in patients with impaired consciousness or difficulty swallowing, who cannot adequately protect the airway from aspiration of oropharyngeal secretions. Dentition is often poor, and patients frequently have gingivitis or periodontal abscesses. Clinical onset of the pneumonia tends to be gradual, and sputum may have a foul odor, suggesting anaerobic infection. Because the organisms are likely to cause substantial tissue destruction, necrosis of affected tissue and abscess formation are relatively common sequelae.

As mentioned earlier, pneumonia due to *L. pneumophila,* commonly called legionnaires' disease, can be seen as isolated cases or in the form of localized outbreaks. Otherwise normal hosts may be affected, but patients with impaired respiratory defense mechanisms also appear to be predisposed. Patients are often extremely ill, not only with respiratory compromise and even respiratory failure but also nonrespiratory manifestations; specifically, gastrointestinal, central nervous system, hepatic, and renal abnormalities may accompany the pneumonia.

DIAGNOSTIC APPROACH

As with other disorders affecting the pulmonary parenchyma, the single most useful tool for assessing pneumonia at a macroscopic level is the chest radiograph. The radiograph not only confirms the presence of a pneumonia; it also shows the distribution and extent of disease and sometimes gives clues about the nature of the etiologic agent. The classic pattern for *S. pneumoniae* (pneumococcus) and for *K. pneumoniae* is a lobar pneumonia (Fig. 23-1). Staphylococcal and many of the gram-negative pneumonias may be localized or extensive and often follow a patchy distribution (Fig. 23-2). *Mycoplasma*

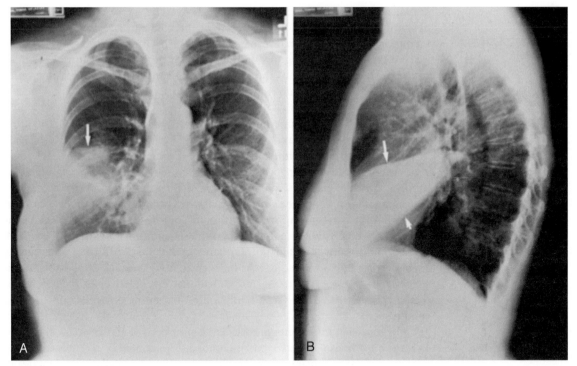

Figure 23-1 —— Posteroanterior (*A*) and lateral (*B*) chest radiographs show lobar pneumonia (probably due to *Streptococcus pneumoniae*) affecting right middle lobe. In *A*, arrow points to the minor fissure, which defines upper border of middle lobe. In *B*, long arrow points to the minor fissure; short arrow to the major fissure.

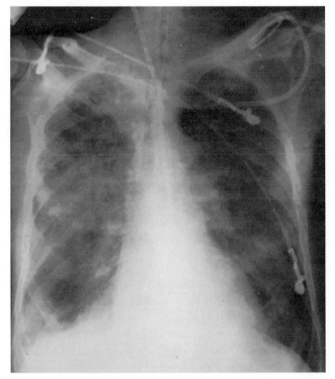

Figure 23-2 —— Chest radiograph of patient with extensive gram-negative pneumonia. Note patchy infiltrates throughout both lungs, more prominent on right.

organisms can produce a variety of radiographic presentations, classically described as being more impressive than the clinical picture would suggest. Pneumonias due to aspiration of oropharyngeal secretions characteristically involve the dependent regions of lung—the lower lobe in the upright patient or the posterior segment of the upper lobe or superior segment of the lower lobe in the supine patient (Fig. 23-3).

The chest radiograph is also useful for demonstrating pleural fluid, which frequently accompanies pneumonia, particularly of bacterial origin. As will be discussed later in the chapter, the pleural fluid can be either thin and serous or thick and purulent; in the latter case the term *empyema* is used.

Microscopic examination of the sputum may play an important role in the evaluation of patients with pneumonia. However, the importance of obtaining a sputum specimen and using it as a guide to treatment, as opposed to treating the patient empirically without a sputum specimen, is an issue that has generated substantial controversy. When a sputum specimen is obtained, it is also important to evaluate the quality of the specimen, as a poor-quality specimen may give inadequate or inaccurate information. In a good sputum specimen—one that contains few squamous epithelial cells picked up in transit through the upper respiratory tract—inflammatory cells and bacteria can be seen.

In most bacterial pneumonias, large numbers of PMNs are seen in the sputum; mycoplasmal and viral pneumonias, in contrast, have fewer PMNs and more mononuclear inflammatory cells. Pneumococcal, staphylococcal, and gram-negative bacillary pneumonias commonly demonstrate a relatively homogeneous population of the infecting bacteria. Anaerobic aspiration pneumonias, caused by a mixture of organisms from the oropharynx, show

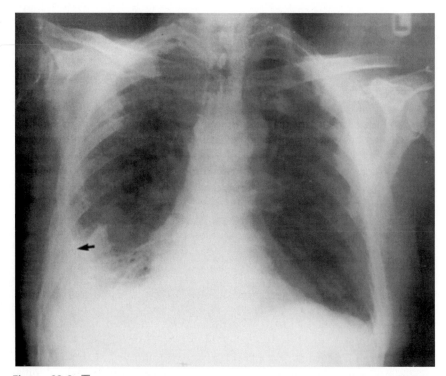

Figure 23-3 ▬— Chest radiograph of right lower lobe aspiration pneumonia. In addition to infiltrate at right base, note loculated pleural effusion, which represents empyema complicating pneumonia. Arrow points to edge of loculated effusion. (Courtesy of Dr. T. Scott Johnson.)

a mixed population of bacteria of many different morphologies. In legionnaires' disease, the bacterium does not stain well with the usual Gram's stain reagent and is therefore not seen with conventional staining techniques. In mycoplasmal and viral pneumonia, the infecting agent is not visualized at all, and only the predominantly mononuclear cell inflammatory response can be seen.

In conjunction with the initial Gram's stain and microscopic examination of sputum, the specimen is also cultured for bacteria. However, it is well recognized that some bacteria are relatively difficult to grow, and in many if not most cases the initial Gram's stain is just as important in making the etiologic diagnosis. Special culture media are available to facilitate the growth of *Legionella* species.

When sputum is not spontaneously expectorated by the patient, other methods for obtaining respiratory secretions (or even material directly from the lung parenchyma) may be necessary. The techniques that have been used, including fiberoptic bronchoscopy, needle aspiration of the lung, and occasionally even thoracoscopic or open lung biopsy, are described in more detail in Chapter 3.

For three of the important causes of pneumonia—*Mycoplasma*, *Chlamydia*, and *Legionella*—routine stains and cultures of sputum are not useful. The diagnosis can sometimes be confirmed by a variety of serologic techniques that demonstrate a rise in antibody titer against the organism, but these techniques provide a retrospective diagnosis and are not useful clinically. Several newer methods are now being used and have had increasing clinical utility over time. For example, direct fluorescent antibody staining can be performed for *Legionella*, especially on tissue specimens, but more recent methods include culture on special supplemented media and a commonly used urinary antigen radioimmunoassay (only for *L. pneumophila* serotype 1). Polymerase chain reaction methods are also being investigated for all three organisms and may have an important role in the future.

The functional assessment of patients with acute infectious pneumonia is usually limited to evaluation of gas-exchange. Arterial blood gas values characteristically demonstrate hypoxemia, accompanied by a normal or decreased PCO_2. Pulmonary function tests have little usefulness in this setting except in the patient with previously compromised lung function, for whom it may be important to assess the extent of further acute compromise.

THERAPEUTIC APPROACH: GENERAL PRINCIPLES AND ANTIBIOTIC SUSCEPTIBILITY

The cornerstone of treatment of bacterial pneumonia is antibiotic therapy directed at the infecting organism. However, because the causative organism is often not known when the pneumonia is first diagnosed—and, in fact, is frequently not identified at any point during the clinical course—initial treatment strategies have been developed based on the clinical setting (e.g., community-acquired vs. hospital-acquired pneumonia). These initial treatment strategies are outlined in the next section. If and when an organism is identified, the regimen may be changed to allow for more focused or more effective antibiotic coverage. Because knowledge of antibiotic susceptibility of specific organisms helps with an understanding of the rationale behind initial treatment strategies, we will first consider some of the general patterns of antibiotic susceptibility for the major organisms causing pneumonia.

Frequently used antibiotics for common pneumonias are the following:

1. *S. pneumoniae* (penicillin, macrolide, selected quinolones)
2. *Staphylococcus* (oxacillin, nafcillin, vancomycin)
3. *Haemophilus influenzae* (second- or third-generation cephalosporins, trimethoprim-sulfamethoxazole)
4. Gram-negative rods (aminoglycosides, third-generation cephalosporins)
5. Anaerobes (penicillin, clindamycin)
6. *Mycoplasma* organisms (macrolide, quinolone)
7. *Legionella* (macrolide, quinolone)
8. *Chlamydia pneumoniae* (tetracycline, macrolide)

In the case of pneumococcal pneumonia, penicillin has traditionally been the most appropriate agent, assuming the patient is not allergic to penicillin, although cases with various degrees of resistance to penicillin are now being encountered with increasing frequency. In addition, because penicillin is not effective against some of the other common causes of community-acquired pneumonia, such as *Mycoplasma pneumoniae* or *Chlamydia pneumoniae*, other classes of antibiotics with a broader spectrum against agents causing community-acquired pneumonia are typically used when antibiotics are initiated. These include the macrolides (erythromycin or a derivative, e.g., azithromycin) or quinolones (e.g., levofloxacin). When high-level resistance of pneumococcus to penicillin is found, then either a quinolone or vancomycin is typically necessary.

Staphylococci that are now identified generally produce penicillinase, which requires that a penicillinase-resistant derivative of penicillin, such as oxacillin or nafcillin, be used. Some staphylococci are also resistant to these derivatives, in which case vancomycin is the antibiotic of choice. *H. influenzae* may be sensitive to ampicillin, but the increasing frequency of organisms resistant to this antibiotic generally justifies alternative coverage, such as a second- or third-generation cephalosporin or trimethoprim-sulfamethoxazole. Many of the other gram-negative bacillary pneumonias often display resistance to a variety of antibiotics; aminoglycosides (such as gentamicin and tobramycin), third-generation cephalosporins, or a quinolone may be used initially while antibiotic sensitivity testing is performed. Pneumonia due to anaerobes is treated most commonly with either penicillin or clindamycin. A macrolide or a quinolone is the antibiotic of choice for pneumonias due either to *Legionella* or to *Mycoplasma*. Finally, there are no definitive forms of therapy for viral pneumonias, although rapid advances in this field may lead to development of clinically useful therapeutic agents. Influenza vaccine (discussed in Chapter 22) is effective for preventing influenza in the majority of individuals who receive it, while antiviral agents (amantadine or rimantadine for influenza A, a neuraminidase inhibitor such as zanamivir or oseltamivir for influenza A or B) may reduce the duration of the illness if given soon after the onset of clinical symptoms.

Other modalities of therapy are mainly supportive. Chest physical therapy and other measures to assist clearance of respiratory secretions are useful for some patients with pneumonia. If patients have inadequate gas-exchange, as demonstrated by significant hypoxemia, administration of supplemental O_2 is beneficial. Occasionally, frank respiratory failure develops, in which case the therapeutic measures discussed in Chapter 29 are utilized.

INITIAL MANAGEMENT STRATEGIES BASED ON CLINICAL SETTING OF PNEUMONIA

During the last decade, greater emphasis on the cost-effective use of medical resources has spurred the development of algorithms and guidelines for the clinician when approaching common clinical problems. Pneumonia is a particularly good example of an important clinical problem for which such management strategies have been developed, relating both to diagnostic evaluation and to initiation of therapy. Separate strategies are being promulgated for two distinct groups of patients with pneumonia, depending on the setting in which the pneumonia developed, i.e., *community-acquired pneumonia* and *nosocomial (hospital-acquired) pneumonia*. The patients in these categories to whom the guidelines apply are those who do not have significant underlying impairment of systemic host defense mechanisms, such as patients with acquired immunodeficiency syndrome or those receiving immunosuppressive drugs or cancer chemotherapy.

Community-Acquired Pneumonia

Community-acquired pneumonia refers to pneumonia that develops in the community setting, i.e., in an individual who is not hospitalized. Although this category is not meant to include patients with significant impairment of systemic host defense mechanisms, it can include patients with other coexisting illnesses or risk factors that alter the profile of organisms likely to be responsible for pneumonia.

Perhaps surprisingly, the cause of community-acquired pneumonia is never identified in a high proportion of patients, estimated to be up to 50 percent. It is believed that the likelihood of particular agents is influenced by a number of modifying factors—the presence of coexisting illness, recent treatment with antibiotics, residence in a nursing home, and the severity of illness at initial presentation. One issue that has sparked controversy is whether patients with community-acquired pneumonia should have an attempt made at identifying a specific etiologic agent, using Gram's staining and culture, or whether empiric therapy should be used based on the patient's risk factors and clinical characteristics. If a specific pathogen is identified, then it is often appropriate to modify the initial antibiotic regimen, particularly to avoid an overly broad spectrum of coverage.

Four subcategories of patients with community-acquired pneumonia have been defined, as summarized in Table 23-1.

The first group comprises patients who do not have coexisting cardiopulmonary disease or other modifying risk factors, and who do not require hospitalization. The most common pathogens in this group of patients include *S. pneumoniae*, *Mycoplasma pneumoniae*, *Chlamydia pneumoniae*, respiratory viruses, and, in smokers, *H. influenzae*. The preferred therapeutic regimen is one of the newer (advanced-generation) macrolide antibiotics, such as azithromycin or clarithromycin.

The second group of patients includes those who have coexistent cardiopulmonary disease or other modifying risk factors, but can still be treated in an outpatient setting. In these patients, age greater than 65 years is considered a modifying factor that increases the likelihood of drug-resistant *S. pneumoniae*, while residence in a nursing home increases the risk of pneumonia due to a gram-negative organism. Poor dentition (leading to an increased burden of anaerobic organisms in the mouth), problems with swallowing, or impaired consciousness increases the risk of an anaerobic aspiration pneumonia. Recommended options for management of this group have included either an oral quinolone (used as a single agent), or a β-lactam antibiotic (such as a second- or third-generation cephalosporin) given in combination with a macrolide (particularly an advanced-generation macrolide such as azithromycin or clarithromycin).

The third and fourth groups differ from the first two based on the severity of the pneumonia. The third group is defined by a need for hospitalization, whereas the fourth group includes those patients with the most severe disease, necessitating admission to an intensive care unit. Although these patients still commonly have pneumonia due to *S. pneumoniae* or the other organisms found in outpatients, there is the additional concern for

In community-acquired pneumonia, factors influencing the likelihood of certain organisms and therefore the therapeutic approach include age, the presence of coexisting illness, and the severity of the pneumonia at initial presentation.

Table 23-1

Etiology and Initial Management of Community-Acquired Pneumonia[1]

Patient Category	Common Organisms	Other Miscellaneous Organisms	Initial Therapy
Outpatient, no cardiopulmonary disease or other modifying risk factors	S. pneumoniae M. pneumoniae C. pneumoniae Respiratory viruses H. influenzae (in smokers)	Legionella M. tuberculosis Endemic fungi	Advanced generation macrolide (e.g., azithromycin or clarithromycin) or Doxycycline
Outpatient, with cardiopulmonary disease and/or other modifying factors	S. pneumoniae M. pneumoniae H. influenzae Aerobic gram-negative bacilli Respiratory viruses Anaerobes C. pneumoniae	Moraxella catarrhalis Legionella M. tuberculosis Endemic fungi	Oral quinolone (with activity against pneumococcus) or β-lactam plus macrolide or doxycycline
Hospitalized	S. pneumoniae H. influenzae Polymicrobial (including anaerobes) Aerobic gram-negative bacilli Legionella C. pneumoniae Respiratory viruses	M. pneumoniae M. catarrhalis M. tuberculosis Endemic fungi	IV β-lactam plus IV or oral macrolide or doxycycline or IV quinolone*
Hospitalized, severe pneumonia	S. pneumoniae Legionella H. influenzae Aerobic gram-negative bacilli M. pneumoniae Respiratory viruses S. aureus	M. tuberculosis C. pneumoniae Endemic fungi	IV β-lactam plus either IV macrolide (azithromycin) or IV quinolone†

[1]Excludes patients with HIV infection.
*If no cardiopulmonary disease and no modifying factors, IV azithromycin or an IV antipneumococcal quinolone is sufficient.
†If high risk for Pseudomonas, adjust regimen to include two antipseudomonal agents.
Adapted from American Thoracic Society: Am J Respir Crit Care Med 163:1730-1754, 2001.

gram-negative bacilli, *Legionella,* and sometimes *Staphylococcus aureus,* and therapy is adjusted accordingly, as outlined in Table 23-1. Intravenous antibiotics, such as a quinolone or an advanced-generation macrolide, often with a β-lactam (particularly a third-generation cephalosporin), are typically used in these settings.

Nosocomial (Hospital-Acquired) Pneumonia

In contrast to community-acquired pneumonia, nosocomial pneumonia is acquired by hospitalized patients, generally after more than 48 hours of hospitalization. Patients in intensive care units, especially those who are receiving mechanical ventilation, are at particularly high risk for developing this form of pneumonia. Perhaps the most common problem leading to nosocomial pneumonia is colonization of the oropharynx by organisms not usually present in this site, which is then followed by microaspiration of oropharyngeal secretions into the tracheobronchial tree. The patients at risk often have other underlying medical problems, have been receiving antibiotics, or have an endotracheal tube in their airway that bypasses some of the normal protective mechanisms of the respiratory tract.

Organisms of particular concern in patients who develop hospital-acquired pneumonia are enteric gram-negative bacilli and *S. aureus,* but other organisms such as *Pseudomonas aeruginosa* and *Legionella* can also be involved. Diagnostic evaluation is difficult and often complicated by the need to distinguish bacterial colonization of the tracheobronchial tree from true bacterial pneumonia. The clinical issues involved with diagnostic testing and optimal forms of therapy are beyond the scope of this discussion but can be found in the references at the end of this chapter.

> Organisms of particular concern in nosocomial pneumonia include *Staphylococcus aureus,* gram-negative bacilli, and *Legionella.*

INTRATHORACIC COMPLICATIONS OF PNEUMONIA

As part of our discussion of pneumonia, we will briefly consider two specific intrathoracic complications of pneumonia—lung abscess and empyema—because they represent important clinical sequelae.

Lung Abscess

A lung abscess, like an abscess elsewhere, represents a localized collection of pus. In the lung, abscesses generally result from tissue destruction complicating a pneumonia. The abscess contents are primarily PMNs, often with collections of bacterial organisms. When antibiotics have already been administered, organisms may no longer be obtainable from the abscess cavity.

Etiologic agents associated with formation of a lung abscess are generally those bacteria causing significant tissue necrosis. Most commonly, anaerobic organisms are responsible, suggesting that aspiration of oropharyngeal contents is the predisposing event. However, aerobic organisms, such as *Staphylococcus* or enteric gram-negative rods, can also cause significant tissue destruction, with excavation of a region of lung parenchyma and abscess formation.

> Anaerobic bacteria are the agents most frequently responsible for lung abscesses.

Treatment of a lung abscess involves antibiotic therapy, often given for a more prolonged duration than for an uncomplicated pneumonia. Although abscesses elsewhere in the body are drained by surgical incision, lung abscesses generally drain through the tracheobronchial tree, and surgical intervention is only rarely needed.

Empyema

When a pneumonia extends to the pleural surface, the inflammatory process may eventually lead to another intrathoracic complication of pneumonia—empyema. The term refers to pus in the pleural space; in its most florid form, an empyema represents thick, creamy, or yellow fluid within the pleural space. The fluid contains enormous numbers of leukocytes, primarily PMNs, often accompanied by bacterial organisms. With a frank empyema, or often even with other grossly inflammatory pleural effusions accompanying pneumonia (parapneumonic effusions), the pleural inflammation can result in formation of localized pockets of fluid or substantial scarring and limitation of mobility of the underlying lung.

Adequate drainage of pleural fluid is important in the management of empyema.

Several different bacterial organisms can be associated with development of an empyema. Anaerobes are particularly common, but staphylococci and other aerobic organisms are also potential causes. Once an empyema has been demonstrated, usually by thoracentesis and sampling of pleural fluid, drainage of the fluid is required. Most commonly, a relatively large tube is inserted into the pleural space. Alternative techniques are used in some specific clinical situations, especially when loculated regions of fluid or pus are present.

RESPIRATORY INFECTIONS ASSOCIATED WITH BIOTERRORISM

The magnitude of society's concerns about bioterrorism changed abruptly after September 11, 2001, following the terrorist attacks on the World Trade Center and the Pentagon. Subsequent recognition of cases of both cutaneous and inhalational anthrax contracted from handling mail containing anthrax spores illustrated all too vividly not only the danger posed by some previously uncommon biologic agents, but also the widespread fear that is elicited by the threat of bioterrorism. We will discuss briefly three biologic agents whose life-threatening effects can be mediated by infection involving the respiratory system: *Bacillus anthracis, Yersinia pestis,* and *Francisella tularensis.*

Anthrax

Bacillus anthracis, a gram-positive, spore-forming rod found in the soil, causes infection in farm and wild animals; human cases have occurred as a result of exposure to infected animals, contaminated animal products, or inhalation of aerosolized spores. The organism's virulence and potential lethality are related to elaboration of a toxin that causes prominent edema, inhibits neutrophil function, and alters the production of a number of cytokines. Whereas cutaneous anthrax results from spores introduced through a break in the skin, inhalational anthrax follows inhalation of spores into alveolar spaces and transport of viable spores via lymphatics to mediastinal lymph nodes. Germination of the spores in the mediastinum is associated with toxin release and with a hemorrhagic lymphadenitis and mediastinitis.

Clinically, patients with inhalational anthrax typically present with a flu-like illness, with symptoms of mild fever, myalgias, nonproductive cough, malaise, and chest discomfort. Several days later, patients become acutely and severely ill, with fever, dyspnea, cyanosis, septic shock, and often findings of meningitis. The most prominent abnormality on chest radiograph is mediastinal widening from the hemorrhagic lymphadenitis and mediastinitis. Despite treatment with ciprofloxacin or doxycycline, mortality is extremely high after the onset of clinical illness, and public health guidelines have focused on prophylaxis (with either of these antibiotics) to prevent inhalational anthrax following confirmed or suspected exposure to aerosolized spores.

> Inhalational anthrax characteristically produces a widened mediastinum on chest radiograph.

Plague

Despite its association with epidemics of devastating proportions, such as the Black Death of the 14th century, plague is now an uncommon disease in the United States, even though it is endemic in some parts of the world. However, plague is one of the conditions thought to be of major concern as a possible weapon of bioterrorism. The causative organism is *Yersinia pestis*, a gram-negative rod that is transmitted by fleas from rodents to humans. Infection through the skin disseminates to regional lymph nodes, leading to the clinical syndrome of *bubonic plague*. Infection of the lungs (*pneumonic plague*) can occur either secondary to bacteremic spread from skin or lymph nodes, or via airborne transmission of the organism from person to person.

Pulmonary involvement is characterized by a widespread bronchopneumonia, which can also have regions of homogeneous consolidation. Clinically, patients become acutely ill with high fever, malaise, myalgias, rigors, dyspnea, and cyanosis. Chest radiography demonstrates widespread bronchopneumonia, with a diffuse pattern that can resemble the acute respiratory distress syndrome (ARDS). Mortality is high unless antibiotic treatment is initiated soon after the onset of symptoms, with streptomycin or doxycycline being the agents of choice.

Tularemia

Tularemia is caused by *Francisella tularensis*, a gram-negative coccobacillary organism that infects small mammals and is transmitted to humans by insect vectors (such as ticks), exposure to contaminated animals, or inhalation of aerosolized organisms. Although several different forms of clinical presentation may occur with tularemia, depending upon the mechanism of transmission and the site of entry, pulmonary tularemia secondary to inhalation of *F. tularensis* is the primary concern for use of this organism as a bioterrorist weapon.

Pulmonary tularemia is characterized by patchy inflammation and consolidation of the lung parenchyma, sometimes with enlargement of hilar lymph nodes and development of pleural effusions. Patients develop fever, chills, malaise, and headache, with chest radiography showing patchy consolidation that may be accompanied by hilar lymphadenopathy and pleural effusions. Treatment is with streptomycin, and mortality is estimated to be approximately 35 percent without treatment.

References

General Reviews

American Thoracic Society: Guidelines for the initial management of adults with community-acquired pneumonia: diagnosis, assessment of severity, antimicrobial therapy, and prevention. Am J Respir Crit Care Med 163:1730-1754, 2001.

American Thoracic Society: Hospital-acquired pneumonia in adults: diagnosis, assessment of severity, initial antimicrobial therapy, and preventive strategies. Am J Respir Crit Care Med 153:1711-1725, 1996.

Bartlett JG et al: Practice guidelines for the management of community-acquired pneumonia in adults. Clin Infect Dis 31:347-382, 2000.

Bartlett JG and Mundy LM: Community-acquired pneumonia. N Engl J Med 333:1618-1624, 1995.

Bergogne-Bérézin E: Treatment and prevention of nosocomial pneumonia. Chest 108:26S-34S, 1995.

Chastre J and Fagon J-Y: Ventilator-associated pneumonia. Am J Respir Crit Care Med 165:867-903, 2002.

Craven DE and Steger KA: Epidemiology of nosocomial pneumonia. Chest 108:1S-16S, 1995.

Ewig S, Bauer T, and Torres A: Nosocomial pneumonia. Thorax 57:366-371, 2002.

Fine MJ et al: Prognosis and outcomes of patients with community-acquired pneumonia. JAMA 274:134-141, 1995.

Franquet T: Imaging of pneumonia: trends and algorithms. Eur Respir J 18:196-208, 2001.

Garrard CS and A'Court CD: The diagnosis of pneumonia in the critically ill. Chest 108:17S-25S, 1995.

Guthrie R: Community-acquired lower respiratory tract infections. Etiology and treatment. Chest 120:2021-2034, 2001.

Halm EA and Teirstein AS: Management of community-acquired pneumonia. N Engl J Med 347:2039-2045, 2002.

Kollef MH: The prevention of ventilator-associated pneumonia. N Engl J Med 340:627-634, 1999.

Mandell LA: Community-acquired pneumonia: etiology, epidemiology, and treatment. Chest 108:35S-42S, 1995.

Niederman MS (ed): Pneumonia. Clin Chest Med 20:475-691, 1999.

Shelhamer JH et al: The laboratory evaluation of opportunistic pulmonary infections. Ann Intern Med 124:585-599, 1996.

Vincent J-L: Prevention of nosocomial bacterial pneumonia. Thorax 54:544-549, 1999.

Pneumonia Due to Specific Organisms

Bartlett JG: Anaerobic bacterial infections of the lung. Chest 91:901-909, 1987.

Bourke SJ and Lightfoot NF: *Chlamydia pneumoniae*: defining the clinical spectrum of infection requires precise laboratory diagnosis. Thorax 50:S43-S48, 1995.

Catterall JR: *Streptococcus pneumoniae*. Thorax 54:929-937, 1999.

Grayston JT: *Chlamydia pneumoniae*, strain TWAR. Chest 95:664-669, 1989.

Hall CB: Respiratory syncytial virus and parainfluenza virus. N Engl J Med 344:1917-1928, 2001.

Hammerschlag MR: *Chlamydia pneumoniae* and the lung. Eur Respir J 16:1001-1007, 2000.

Harwell JI and Brown RB: The drug-resistant pneumococcus. Clinical relevance, therapy, and prevention. Chest 117:530-541, 2000.

Jakab GJ: Mechanisms of virus-induced bacterial superinfections of the lungs. Clin Chest Med 2:59-66, 1981.

Karned A, Alvarez S, and Berk SL: Pneumonia caused by gram-negative bacilli. Am J Med 79 (suppl 1A):61-67, 1985.

Kauppinen M and Saikku P: Pneumonia due to *Chlamydia pneumoniae*: prevalence, clinical features, diagnosis, and treatment. Clin Infect Dis 21:S244-S252, 1995.

Kaye MG et al: The clinical spectrum of *Staphylococcus aureus* pulmonary infection. Chest 97:788-792, 1990.

Levy H and Simpson SQ: Hantavirus pulmonary syndrome. Am J Respir Crit Care Med 149:1710-1713, 1994.

Mansel JK, Rosenow EC III, Smith TF, and Martin JW Jr: *Mycoplasma pneumoniae* pneumonia. Chest 95:639-646, 1989.

Marik PE: Aspiration pneumonitis and aspiration pneumonia. N Engl J Med 344:665-671, 2001.

Murray HW, Masur H, Senterfit LB, and Roberts RB: The protean manifestations of *Mycoplasma pneumoniae* infection in adults. Am J Med 58:229-242, 1975.

Musher DM, Kubitschek KR, Crennan J, and Baughn RE: Pneumonia and acute febrile tracheobronchitis due to *Haemophilus influenzae*. Ann Intern Med 99:444-450, 1983.

Pierce AK and Sanford JP: Aerobic gram-negative bacillary pneumonias. Am Rev Respir Dis 110:647-658, 1974.

Roig J, Domingo C, and Morera J: Legionnaires' disease. Chest 105:1817-1825, 1994.

Rose RM, Pinkston P, O'Donnell C, and Jensen WA: Viral infection of the lower respiratory tract. Clin Chest Med 8:405-418, 1987.

Sanders CV and Kamholz SL (eds): Pneumococcal disease: a symposium in honor of Robert Austrian, MD. Am J Med 107 (Suppl):1S-90S, 1999.

Stout JE and Yu VL: Legionellosis. N Engl J Med 337:682-687, 1997.

Straus WL et al: Risk factors for domestic acquisition of Legionnaires' disease. Arch Intern Med 156:1685-1692, 1996.

Tan MJ et al: The radiologic manifestations of Legionnaire's disease. Chest 116:398-403, 2000.

Tuomanen EI, Austrian R, and Masure HR: Pathogenesis of pneumococcal infection. N Engl J Med 332:1280-1284, 1995.

Whitney CG et al: Increasing prevalence of multidrug-resistant *Streptococcus pneumoniae* in the United States. N Engl J Med 343:1917-1924, 2000.

Wilson R and Dowling RB: *Pseudomonas aeruginosa* and other related species. Thorax 53:213-219, 1998.

Respiratory Infections Associated with Bioterrorism

Bellamy RJ and Freedman AR: Bioterrorism. QJM 94:227-234, 2001.

Borio L et al: Death due to bioterrorism-related inhalational anthrax. Report of 2 patients. JAMA 286:2554-2559, 2001.

Bush LM, Abrams BH, Beall A, and Johnson CC: Index case of fatal inhalational anthrax due to bioterrorism in the United States. N Engl J Med 345:1607-1610, 2001.

Centers for Disease Control. Recognition of illness associated with the intentional release of a biologic agent. MMWR 50:893-897, 2001.

Inglesby TV et al: Anthrax as a biological weapon, 2002. Updated recommendations for management. JAMA 287:2236-2252, 2002.

Mayer TA et al: Clinical presentation of inhalational anthrax following bioterrorism exposure. Report of 2 surviving patients. JAMA 286:2549-2553, 2001.

Swartz MN: Recognition and management of anthrax—an update. N Engl J Med 345:1621-1626, 2001.

chapter 24

Tuberculosis and Nontuberculous Mycobacteria

ETIOLOGY AND PATHOGENESIS	DIAGNOSTIC APPROACH
DEFINITIONS	PRINCIPLES OF THERAPY
PATHOLOGY	NONTUBERCULOUS
PATHOPHYSIOLOGY	MYCOBACTERIA
CLINICAL MANIFESTATIONS	

Throughout the centuries, few diseases have claimed so many lives, caused so much morbidity, and been so dreaded as tuberculosis. At the turn of the 20th century, tuberculosis was the single most common cause of death in the United States; more than 80 percent of the population was infected before the age of 20 years. However, since that time few diseases have declined so greatly in the frequency of cases and in mortality as has tuberculosis. Two main factors have been responsible: an overall improvement in living conditions and the development of effective chemotherapy, which has made tuberculosis a curable disease.

Now that more than 120 years have passed since the identification of the tubercle bacillus by Robert Koch in 1882, it is important not to become complacent about this disease. It has been estimated that approximately one-third of the world's population has been infected (i.e., has either latent or active infection) with the tubercle bacillus, and there are still 8 to 10 million new cases of active tuberculosis and approximately 2 to 3 million deaths worldwide each year. Although it is true that the overwhelming majority of cases of active tuberculosis occur in developing countries—approximately 70 million of the 88 million cases of tuberculosis during the 1990s were from Asia and sub-Saharan Africa—tuberculosis remains an important public health problem in the United States, particularly in indigent and immigrant populations and in patients with the acquired immunodeficiency syndrome (AIDS) (see Chapter 26). Reported cases of tuberculosis in the United States were decreasing until the mid-1980s, at which time the AIDS epidemic and immigration from countries with a high prevalence of tuberculosis combined to result in an increasing frequency of cases. Fortunately, since 1991 the number of cases reported annually in the United States has again begun decreasing. Perhaps most alarming, however, both in the United States and throughout the world, has been the relatively recent emergence of drug-resistant strains of the organism, some of which are resistant to multiple antituberculous drugs.

ETIOLOGY AND PATHOGENESIS

The etiologic agent that causes tuberculosis, *Mycobacterium tuberculosis,* is an aerobic rod-shaped bacterium. As will be discussed later, an important property of the tubercle bacillus is its ability to retain certain stains even after exposure to acid; thus mycobacteria are said to be *acid-fast.*

Transmission of the disease occurs by means of small aerosol droplets, generally from 1 to 5 μm in size, that contain the microorganism. The source of these droplets is an individual with tuberculosis who harbors the organism, often excreting tubercle bacilli in the sputum or in small droplets produced during such commonplace activities as speaking, coughing, singing, or laughing. Most commonly, transmission occurs with relatively close contact, often between related individuals or others living in the same household. The disease is not transmitted by fomites, i.e., articles of clothing, eating utensils, or the like; direct inhalation of droplets aerosolized by another individual is almost exclusively the mode of spread.

When droplets containing mycobacteria are inhaled and reach the distal pulmonary parenchyma, a small focus of *primary* infection develops, consisting of the organisms and an inflammatory process mounted by the host. Alveolar macrophages represent the primary initial defense against organisms reaching the parenchyma, and they are a particularly important component of the resulting inflammatory response. Organisms also frequently spread via lymphatic vessels to draining lymph nodes, as well as via the blood stream to distant organs and to other regions of lung, particularly the apices. In the majority of cases, even though lymphatic and hematogenous spread may occur, the body's defense mechanisms (in the lung and elsewhere) are capable of controlling and limiting the primary infection. An important component of the body's acquired defense against *M. tuberculosis* is the development of cell-mediated immunity—delayed hypersensitivity—against the mycobacterial organisms. This sensitization and development of a cell-mediated immune response generally occur within several weeks of initial exposure.

The patient is usually unaware of the primary infection, and the only tracks left by the organism are those related to the host's response to the bacillus: either the local tissue response or evidence that the host has become sensitized to the tubercle bacillus, i.e., a positive delayed hypersensitivity skin test reaction. In a few patients, probably 5 percent or fewer, the defense mechanisms are unable to control the primary infection, and clinically apparent primary tuberculosis results.

Even when the primary infection has been apparently controlled, the tubercle bacillus may not be completely eliminated from the host. Rather, a small number of organisms often remain in a dormant or latent state, not killed but also not proliferating or causing any apparent active disease. The majority of such patients will never have any further difficulty with development of clinically active tuberculosis. In some patients, however, the delicate balance between the organism and host defense mechanisms eventually breaks down, often after many years, and a dormant focus of infection becomes active. These patients with active disease occurring at a time removed from the primary infection are said to have *reactivation* tuberculosis. For both primary and reactivation disease, the lungs are the most commonly affected site. However, with either type of disease, distant organ systems may be involved as a result of hematogenous spread during the primary phase of the infection. In addition, there may be disseminated disease, known as

Transmission of tuberculosis is by inhalation of small aerosol droplets containing the organism.

The majority of active tuberculosis cases involve reactivation of a previously dormant focus within the lungs.

miliary tuberculosis, resulting from hematogenous dissemination of the organisms.

Over the course of a lifetime, it is estimated that approximately 10 percent of individuals with a normal immune system who have been infected with *M. tuberculosis* (and have not received "preventive" treatment to eradicate dormant organisms) will develop active disease. The risk of developing active tuberculosis is particularly notable within the first two years following the initial infection; approximately half of the patients who develop active disease do so within this time frame. The other half of patients who develop active disease do so at some later point in life. The above estimates of risk apply to patients with normal host defenses; the risk of developing active tuberculosis is dramatically higher in patients with defective cellular immunity as a consequence of human immunodeficiency virus (HIV) infection and low CD4$^+$ counts.

DEFINITIONS

Based on our understanding of disease pathogenesis, as just described, a few additional terms are worth defining. First is the distinction between tuberculous infection and tuberculous disease. *Tuberculous infection* (or *latent tuberculous infection*) is defined by a positive tuberculin skin test but no evidence of active disease. Patients with latent tuberculous infection have therefore been exposed to the organism, but the initial infection was controlled by the body's host defense mechanisms and can subsequently only be traced by the positive delayed hypersensitivity skin test response. The small number of remaining organisms are in a dormant or latent state, but they do pose a risk for reactivation at a later time, especially with any impairment in the host's cellular immunity. *Tuberculous disease* (or *active tuberculosis*), on the other hand, is defined by the presence of clinically active disease in one or more organ systems, ideally with confirmation of the diagnosis by isolation of the organism *M. tuberculosis.*

The other set of terms worth defining are those that describe different subsets of tuberculous disease. Most common are the terms *primary* and *reactivation tuberculosis,* referring respectively to disease following the initial exposure and disease that reactivates after a period of latency. Several other terms are sometimes used to describe clinical disease based on the presumed pathogenesis. The term *progressive primary tuberculosis* reflects primary disease that has not been controlled by host defense mechanisms and has continued to be active beyond the point at which delayed hypersensitivity has developed. As a general rule, cellular immunity develops from 2 to 10 weeks after the initial infection, and continuing active disease beyond this time has many of the features of reactivation tuberculosis. The term *postprimary tuberculosis* refers to disease beyond the initial primary infection. Although this term usually refers to reactivation disease, it sometimes is also used to include cases of progressive primary tuberculosis.

Finally, the term *reinfection tuberculosis* refers to disease in a previously infected person that results not from reactivation of dormant tubercle bacilli but rather from new exposure to another source of organisms. This type of infection has traditionally been considered uncommon; it is believed that individuals with prior exposure to tuberculosis, who manifest delayed hypersensitivity to the organism, are relatively resistant to exogenous reinfection from another source. However, studies using DNA fingerprinting techniques suggest that reinfection with another organism is more common than previously thought, particularly in patients who are infected with human immunodeficiency virus.

PATHOLOGY

The pathologic features of pulmonary tuberculosis vary according to the stage of infection. The primary infection in the lung consists of organisms along with a relatively nonspecific inflammatory response in the involved region of parenchyma. Regional lymph nodes often become involved by local spread of the organism, and the combination of the primary area in the lung (the *Ghon lesion*) and involved lymph nodes is termed a *Ranke complex*.

When delayed hypersensitivity is present, either weeks after the primary infection or during a period of reactivation disease, a different pathologic pattern emerges. The hallmarks are the presence of (1) granulomas—collections of phagocytic cells termed *epithelioid histiocytes*, and (2) caseous necrosis—foci of necrosis and softening at the center of a granuloma. Within the region of caseous necrosis, the contents can liquefy and slough, leaving behind a cavity, another hallmark of tuberculosis. Other features of the granulomas include multinucleated giant cells and often the presence of tubercle bacilli.

> After development of delayed hypersensitivity, the pathologic hallmarks of tuberculosis are granulomas and caseous necrosis, often with cavity formation.

A process of healing also tends to occur at the sites of disease. Fibrosis or scarring ensues, often associated with contraction of the affected area and deposition of calcium. With full-blown tuberculosis, there is extensive destruction of lung tissue, resulting from large areas of inflammation, granuloma formation, caseous necrosis, and cavitation, along with fibrosis, contraction, and foci of calcification.

As mentioned earlier, tuberculosis is capable of spread, and spread of organisms through the blood stream at the time of primary infection is probably the rule rather than the exception. When defense mechanisms break down, disease can become apparent at other sites—for example, in the liver, kidney, adrenal glands, bones, or central nervous system. Spread also occurs to other regions of the lung, either as a result of hematogenous seeding during the primary infection or because of spilling of infected secretions or caseous material into the bronchi and into other regions of the lung.

Within the lung, characteristic locations for reactivation tuberculosis are the apical regions of the upper lobes and, to a lesser extent, the superior segment of the lower lobes. It is believed that these are not the sites of the primary infection but rather the favored location for organisms to become implanted after hematogenous spread. These regions have a high P_{O_2} and are thus particularly suitable for survival of the aerobic tubercle bacilli.

PATHOPHYSIOLOGY

Most of the clinical features of pulmonary tuberculosis can be attributed to either of two aspects of the disease: the presence of a poorly controlled chronic infection, or a chronic destructive process within the lung parenchyma. A variety of other manifestations result from extrapulmonary spread of tuberculosis, but these consequences are not considered here.

Why the chronic infection within the lung produces systemic manifestations is not entirely clear. However, as implied by the term "consumption," used so frequently in the past, tuberculosis is a disease in which systemic manifestations such as weight loss, wasting, and loss of appetite are prominent features. These and other systemic effects of tuberculosis are discussed in the next section.

The chronic destructive process involving the pulmonary parenchyma entails progressive scarring and loss of lung tissue. However, respiratory function is generally preserved more than would be expected, perhaps because the disease is often limited to the apical and posterior regions of the upper lobes as well as to the superior segment of the lower lobes. Oxygenation also tends to be surprisingly preserved, presumably because ventilation and perfusion are destroyed simultaneously in the affected lung. Consequently, ventilation-perfusion mismatch is not nearly so great as in many other parenchymal and airway diseases.

CLINICAL MANIFESTATIONS

As was mentioned earlier, there is an important distinction—and thus there are important clinical differences—between tuberculous infection and tuberculous disease (active tuberculosis). Tuberculous infection is the consequence of primary exposure, by which the bacilli have become established in the patient; however, host defense mechanisms have prevented any clinically apparent disease. Specific immunity to the tubercle bacillus can be demonstrated by a positive reaction to a skin test for delayed hypersensitivity; otherwise, there is no evidence for proliferation of bacteria or for tissue involvement by disease. In contrast, the disease tuberculosis is associated with proliferation of organisms, accompanied by a tissue response and generally (although not always) clinical problems of which the patient is aware.

Patients with pulmonary tuberculosis can manifest (1) systemic symptoms, (2) symptoms referable to the respiratory tract, or (3) an abnormal finding on chest radiograph but no clinical symptoms. When symptoms occur, they are generally insidious rather than acute in onset.

The systemic symptoms are often relatively nonspecific—for example, weight loss, anorexia, fatigue, low-grade fever, and night sweats. The most common symptoms resulting from pulmonary involvement are cough, sputum production, and hemoptysis; chest pain is also occasionally present. Many patients have neither systemic nor pulmonary symptoms and come to the attention of a physician because of an abnormal finding on chest radiograph, often performed for an unrelated reason.

Patients with extrapulmonary involvement frequently have pulmonary tuberculosis as well, but occasional cases are limited to an extrapulmonary site. The pericardium, pleura, kidney, peritoneum, adrenal glands, and central nervous system may each be involved, with symptoms resulting from the particular organ or region that is affected. With miliary tuberculosis, the disease is disseminated, and the patients are usually systemically quite ill.

Physical examination of the patient with pulmonary tuberculosis may show the ravages of a chronic infection, with evidence of wasting and weight loss. Although this was a common occurrence in the past, it is now seen in only a minority of patients. Findings on chest examination also tend to be relatively insignificant, although there is sometimes evidence of crackles or rales over affected areas. If a tuberculous pleural effusion is present, the physical findings characteristic of an effusion may be found.

Common presenting problems with tuberculosis are the following:

1. Systemic symptoms: weight loss, fever, night sweats
2. Pulmonary symptoms: cough, sputum production, hemoptysis
3. Abnormal chest radiographic findings

DIAGNOSTIC APPROACH

One of the most commonly used diagnostic tools, the tuberculin skin test, documents tuberculous infection rather than active disease. A small amount of protein derived from the tubercle bacillus (purified protein derivative [PPD]) is injected intradermally. Individuals who have been exposed to *M. tuberculosis* and have acquired cellular immunity to the organism demonstrate a positive test reaction: induration or swelling at the site of injection after 48 to 72 hours. The criteria for determining a positive skin test reaction vary according to the clinical setting, based on the presence or absence of immunosuppression and/or epidemiologic risk factors affecting the likelihood of previous exposure to tuberculosis. The test does not distinguish between individuals who have active tuberculosis and those who merely have acquired delayed hypersensitivity from previous exposure. However, because reactivation tuberculosis occurs in patients with previous exposure and tuberculous infection, a positive skin test reaction does identify individuals at higher risk for subsequent development of active disease.

As is true of most diagnostic tests, false-negative results can occur with the tuberculin skin test. Faulty administration, an inactive batch of skin-testing material, and underlying diseases that depress cellular immunity are a few of the causes of a false-negative skin test reaction. On the other hand, not all patients who react to tuberculoprotein have been exposed to *M. tuberculosis*. Exposure to, or disease resulting from, nontuberculous mycobacteria, often called *atypical mycobacteria*, is also sometimes associated with a positive or a borderline positive skin test reaction.

In order to diagnose tuberculosis—i.e., actual tuberculous disease—an important initial diagnostic tool is the chest radiograph. In primary disease the chest radiograph may simply show a nonspecific infiltrate, often but certainly not exclusively in the lower lobes (contrast this with the upper-lobe predominance of reactivation disease). There may be hilar (and sometimes paratracheal) lymph node enlargement, reflecting involvement of the draining node by the organism and by the primary infection. Pleural involvement may also be seen, with development of a pleural effusion.

When the primary disease heals, the chest radiograph frequently shows some residua of the healing process. Most common are small calcified lesions within the pulmonary parenchyma, reflecting calcified granulomas. There may also be calcification within hilar or paratracheal lymph nodes.

With reactivation tuberculosis, the most common sites of disease are the apical and posterior segments of the upper lobes and, to a lesser extent, the superior segment of the lower lobes. A variety of patterns can be seen: infiltrates, cavities, nodules, and scarring and contraction (Fig. 24-1). The presence of abnormal findings on a chest radiograph, however, does not necessarily indicate active disease. The disease may be old, stable, and currently inactive; it is quite difficult if not impossible to gauge activity on the basis of the radiographic appearance.

Definitive diagnosis of tuberculosis rests upon culturing the organism, either from secretions (e.g., sputum) or from tissue. However, the organisms are slow growing, and 6 weeks may be required for growth and final identification of the organism. Culture of the organism is important not only for confirmation of the diagnosis, but also for testing of sensitivity to antituberculous drugs, particularly in light of recent concerns about resistance to some of the commonly used antituberculous agents.

Common features of the chest radiograph in primary tuberculosis are the following:

1. Nonspecific infiltrate (often lower lobe)
2. Hilar (and paratracheal) node enlargement
3. Pleural effusion

Radiographic location of reactivation tuberculosis: most commonly apical and posterior segments of upper lobe(s), superior segment of lower lobe(s).

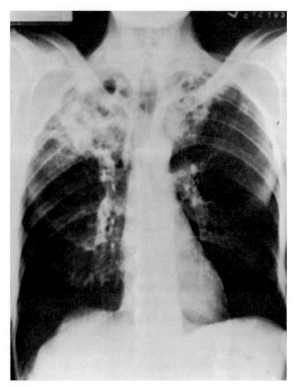

Figure 24-1 ▪— Chest radiograph of patient with reactivation tuberculosis. Note infiltrates with cavitation at both apices, more prominent on right.

Another extremely useful procedure, for which results are available almost immediately, is staining of material obtained from the tracheobronchial tree. The specimens obtained can be sputum, expectorated either spontaneously or following inhalation of an irritating aerosol (sputum induction), or washings or biopsy samples obtained by fiberoptic bronchoscopy. As mentioned earlier, a hallmark of mycobacterial organisms is their ability to retain certain dyes even after exposure to acid. This property of being acid-fast is generally demonstrated with Ziehl-Neelsen or Kinyoun's stains or with a fluorescent stain that utilizes auramine-rhodamine. Even the finding of only one acid-fast bacillus from sputum or from tracheobronchial washings is clinically significant in the majority of cases. One qualification is that nontuberculous mycobacteria, which either cause disease or are sometimes present as colonizing organisms or contaminants, also have the same staining properties. It therefore becomes critical to determine whether acid-fast bacilli seen on smear represent *M. tuberculosis* or nontuberculous mycobacteria; this distinction can be made either by certain growth characteristics on culture, or more recently by molecular biologic techniques.

In order for even one tubercle bacillus to be seen on smear, large numbers of organisms must be present in the lungs. Therefore, if fewer organisms are present, even if they are causing disease, the smear results may be negative, whereas culture findings often will be positive in this setting. In general, the infectiousness of a patient with tuberculosis correlates with the number of organisms the patient is harboring and with the presence of organisms on smear. Patients whose sputum is positive by smear tend to be much more infectious than those whose sputum is positive by culture but negative by smear.

Because of the insensitivity of sputum smears and the time required for *M. tuberculosis* to grow in culture, there has been significant interest in the development of rapid and more sensitive methods for establishing the diagnosis of tuberculosis. One technique involves detection of radiolabeled CO_2 following incubation of the specimen with radiolabeled palmitic acid, a metabolic substrate for mycobacteria. Results can be obtained much more quickly with this technique (called the BACTEC system) than with traditional culture techniques. Alternatively, newer methods employing molecular biologic techniques provide the opportunity to make a diagnosis in the presence of minute quantities of genetic material from the organism. Examples of these techniques include amplification of DNA with polymerase chain reaction technology, and use of DNA probes to detect ribosomal RNA. These genetic techniques are often applied following identification of acid-fast bacilli on a sputum smear, and are used as a rapid method for distinguishing whether the organisms represent *M. tuberculosis* or nontuberculous mycobacteria.

Functional assessment of the patient with tuberculosis often shows surprisingly little impairment of pulmonary function. Such testing is useful primarily for the patient who already has compromised pulmonary function, when there is concern about how much of the patient's reserve has been lost. Similarly, arterial blood gases are often relatively preserved, with Po_2 being either normal or decreased, depending on the amount of ventilation-perfusion mismatch that has resulted.

PRINCIPLES OF THERAPY

Effective chemotherapy is available for most cases of tuberculosis. Whereas treatment for tuberculosis used to be essentially ineffective, involving prolonged hospitalization (usually in a sanatorium) or a variety of surgical procedures, the majority of cases are now curable with appropriate drug therapy. Patients are treated for a prolonged period, generally with a minimum of two effective antituberculous agents. Therapy for as few as 6 months with two very effective antituberculous agents, isoniazid and rifampin, supplemented during the first 2 months by a third agent, pyrazinamide, is commonly used in cases of pulmonary tuberculosis, with excellent results. However, because of concern for organisms resistant to one or more antituberculous agents, a fourth drug (ethambutol) is typically added at the initiation of therapy until drug sensitivity results become available. When resistance to one or more of the usual antituberculous agents is documented, the specific regimen and the duration of therapy need to be adjusted accordingly.

Treatment can be administered in an outpatient setting, unless the patient is sufficiently ill to require hospitalization. Patients whose sputum smears were initially positive are generally considered no longer infectious after they have demonstrated a clinical response to antituberculous therapy, and after their sputum has become smear-negative on three successive samples. A critical issue determining the success of antituberculous therapy is the patient's compliance with the medical regimen. With erratic or incomplete therapy, there is a risk of treatment failure and a risk of emergence of resistant organisms, with potentially disastrous consequences. As a result, use of directly observed therapy, in which the drugs are given in a supervised outpatient setting, has become an important component of treatment for many cases of tuberculosis, and it is essential when there are concerns regarding patient compliance.

A common treatment for pulmonary tuberculosis is isoniazid and rifampin given for 6 months, supplemented by pyrazinamide for the first 2 months and ethambutol until the organism's antimicrobial sensitivity is known.

Isoniazid alone for 9 months is indicated for selected patients with a positive PPD (i.e., tuberculous infection) but no evidence for active disease.

In addition to multiple drug therapy administered for active tuberculosis, therapy with isoniazid alone (typically for 9 months) is generally administered to household members of patients with recently diagnosed tuberculosis and to newly infected persons (documented by recent conversion to a positive skin test reaction). Such therapy substantially decreases the chances of active tuberculosis developing in these individuals, who are at particularly high risk.

Certain other patients with latent tuberculous infection, documented by a positive tuberculin skin test reaction but no evidence for active disease, are also considered candidates for 9 months of treatment with isoniazid alone (or an alternative regimen). Specifically, this category includes patients who satisfy additional criteria (besides a positive PPD reaction) that put them at high risk for reactivation of a dormant infection. Examples include the presence of stable radiographic findings of old tuberculosis but no prior therapy, or the presence of underlying diseases or treatment that impairs host defense mechanisms. Although this form of single-drug therapy was often called "prophylactic" or "preventive," it actually represents treatment aimed at eradicating a small number of dormant but viable organisms. It has been shown to be effective in achieving its goal: substantially decreasing the eventual risk for reactivation tuberculosis.

One of the recent major public health issues has been the development of organisms that are resistant to one or more of the commonly used antituberculous agents. In a survey performed by the Centers for Disease Control and Prevention, approximately 14 percent of cases of tuberculosis were due to an organism that was resistant to one or more antituberculous agents, and 3.5 percent of all cases were resistant to both isoniazid and rifampin, the two most effective antituberculous agents. This problem underscores the importance of public health measures to limit person-to-person transmission of tuberculosis as well as efforts to improve patient compliance with antituberculous medication.

The goal of developing an effective vaccine against *M. tuberculosis* remains an important step toward achieving worldwide eradication of tuberculosis. Vaccination with Bacille Calmette-Guérin (BCG), a live, attenuated strain of *M. bovis,* has been used for many years in various countries around the world, but it has not been recommended for use in the United States except in selected, rare circumstances. Although BCG vaccination does appear to decrease the risk of serious and potentially life-threatening forms of tuberculosis in children, its efficacy in preventing pulmonary tuberculosis in adults is questionable.

NONTUBERCULOUS MYCOBACTERIA

A variety of nontuberculous mycobacteria, sometimes called *atypical mycobacteria,* are recognized as potential pulmonary pathogens. They are generally found in water and soil, which appear to be the sources of exposure rather than person-to-person transmission. The most common organisms within this group are classified as belonging to *Mycobacterium avium* complex (MAC), formerly called *Mycobacterium avium-intracellulare;* other organisms include *M. kansasii, M. xenopi,* and *M. fortuitum,* to name a few.

The nontuberculous mycobacteria are responsible for disease primarily in either of two settings: (1) the patient with underlying lung disease, in whom local host defense mechanisms are presumably impaired, and (2) the patient with a defect in systemic immunity, particularly AIDS (see Chapter 26). Nevertheless, there are a small number of patients without either of these risk factors in whom disease develops as a result of these organisms. Overall, the recognition of disease from nontuberculous mycobacteria has certainly increased over the past 10 to 20 years, in large measure due to its occurrence in patients with AIDS.

Disease caused by nontuberculous mycobacteria can be localized to the lung, where it can mimic tuberculosis, or it can be found after hematogenous dissemination throughout the body, particularly in AIDS. Diagnosis of disease caused by these organisms is often quite difficult. They can be found as laboratory contaminants and, in patients with other underlying lung diseases, can colonize the respiratory system without being responsible for invasive disease.

When these organisms cause disease, treatment typically involves multiple agents. The organisms are frequently resistant to some of the standard antimycobacterial drugs, so that treatment regimens were traditionally complicated and often unsuccessful. Fortunately, the newer macrolide antibiotics, such as clarithromycin or azithromycin, are often effective, and they become particularly useful components of the therapeutic regimen for many of the nontuberculous mycobacteria.

> Atypical mycobacteria are most frequently pathogens in patients with underlying lung disease or AIDS.

References

General Reviews

American Thoracic Society: Diagnostic standards and classification of tuberculosis in adults and children. Am J Respir Crit Care Med 161:1376-1395, 2000.
Iseman MD and Huitt GA (eds): Tuberculosis. Clin Chest Med 18:1-168, 1997.
Lauzardo M and Ashkin D: Phthisiology at the dawn of the new century. Chest 117:1455-1473, 2000.
Raviglione MC, Snider DE Jr, and Kochi A: Global epidemiology of tuberculosis. JAMA 273:220-226, 1995.

Pathogenesis

Alland D et al: Transmission of tuberculosis in New York City. N Engl J Med 330:1710-1716, 1994.
Schluger NW and Rom WN: The host immune response to tuberculosis. Am J Respir Crit Care Med. 157:679-691, 1998.
Stead WW: Pathogenesis of tuberculosis: clinical and epidemiologic perspective. Rev Infect Dis 11 (suppl 2):366-368, 1989.

Clinical Manifestations and Diagnostic Approach

Alvarez S and McCabe WR: Extrapulmonary tuberculosis revisited: a review of experience at Boston City and other hospitals. Medicine 63:25-55, 1984.
American Thoracic Society: Diagnostic standards and classification of tuberculosis in adults and children. Am J Respir Crit Care Med 161:1376-1395, 2000.
American Thoracic Society: Targeted tuberculin testing and treatment of latent tuberculosis infection. Am J Respir Crit Care Med 161:S221-S247, 2000.
Antoniskis D, Amin K, and Barnes PF: Pleuritis as a manifestation of reactivation tuberculosis. Am J Med 89:447-450, 1990.
Berger HW and Mejia E: Tuberculous pleurisy. Chest 63:88-92, 1973.
Khan MA et al: Clinical and roentgenographic spectrum of pulmonary tuberculosis in the adult. Am J Med 62:31-38, 1977.
Sahn SA and Neff TA: Miliary tuberculosis. Am J Med 56:495-505, 1974.
Schluger NW: Changing approaches to the diagnosis of tuberculosis. Am J Respir Crit Care Med 164:2020-2024, 2001.
Weir MR and Thornton GF: Extrapulmonary tuberculosis. Am J Med 79:467-478, 1985.

Treatment

American Thoracic Society: Targeted tuberculin testing and treatment of latent tuberculosis infection. Am J Respir Crit Care Med 161:S221-S247, 2000.
American Thoracic Society, Centers for Disease Control and Prevention, and Infectious Diseases Society of America: Treatment of tuberculosis. Am J Respir Crit Care Med 167:603-662, 2003.

Bloch AB et al: Nationwide survey of drug-resistant tuberculosis in the United States. JAMA 271:665-671, 1994.

Chaulk CP, Kazandjian VA, and the Public Health Tuberculosis Guidelines Panel: Directly observed therapy for treatment completion of pulmonary tuberculosis. JAMA 279:943-948, 1998.

European Respiratory Society Task Force: Tuberculosis management in Europe. Eur Respir J 14:978-992, 1999.

Horsburgh CR Jr, Feldman S, and Ridzon R: Practice guidelines for the treatment of tuberculosis. Clin Infect Dis 31:633-639, 2000.

Jasmer RM, Nahid P, and Hopewell PC: Latent tuberculosis infection. N Engl J Med 347:1860-1866, 2002.

Small PM and Fujiwara PI: Management of tuberculosis in the United States. N Engl J Med 345:189-200, 2001.

Van Scoy RE and Wilkowske CJ: Antimycobacterial therapy. Mayo Clin Proc 74:1038-1048, 1999.

Nontuberculous Mycobacteria

American Thoracic Society: Diagnosis and treatment of disease caused by nontuberculous mycobacteria. Am J Respir Crit Care Med 156:S1-S25, 1997.

Davidson PT: The diagnosis and management of disease caused by *M. avium* complex, *M. kansasii,* and other mycobacteria. Clin Chest Med 10:431-443, 1989.

Holland SM: Nontuberculous mycobacteria. Am J Med Sci 321:49-55, 2001.

O'Brien RJ: The epidemiology of nontuberculous mycobacterial disease. Clin Chest Med 10:407-418, 1989.

Phair JP and Young LS (eds): Clinical challenges of *Mycobacterium avium.* Am J Med 102 (suppl):1-55, 1997.

Sprince DS et al: Infection with *Mycobacterium avium* complex in patients without predisposing conditions. N Engl J Med 321:863-868, 1989.

Wallace RJ: Diagnosis and treatment of disease caused by nontuberculous mycobacteria. Am Rev Respir Dis 142:940-953, 1990.

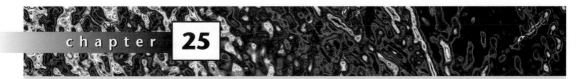

chapter 25

Miscellaneous Infections Due to Fungi and *Pneumocystis*

FUNGAL INFECTIONS
  Histoplasmosis
  Coccidioidomycosis
  Blastomycosis
  Aspergillosis
  Other Fungi
PNEUMOCYSTIS **INFECTION**

This chapter, which continues the discussion of infectious diseases involving the lungs, considers miscellaneous infections due to fungi and to *Pneumocystis.* For some of the organisms to be discussed, infection is clearly a potential problem for the relatively normal host, i.e., the individual with intact host defense mechanisms. Histoplasmosis, coccidioidomycosis, and blastomycosis are the major fungal infections in this category; yet even for these diseases, impairment of normal defense mechanisms may substantially alter the presentation, clinical consequences, and natural history of the illness.

For many other fungi and for *Pneumocystis,* the normal host is essentially protected from the organism, and disease occurs almost exclusively as a consequence of an underlying illness or a breakdown of normal defense mechanisms. *Aspergillus* is perhaps the most important fungus of this sort and is the main one considered in this chapter. *Pneumocystis,* which has a debatable taxonomic status, is considered both in this chapter and in the discussion of acquired immunodeficiency syndrome (AIDS) in Chapter 26. The less common fungi (e.g., *Cryptococcus, Mucor,* and *Candida*) and protozoa (e.g., *Toxoplasma*) affecting the immunosuppressed host are not considered in detail here, but further information can be obtained from the references listed at the end of this chapter.

FUNGAL INFECTIONS

Histoplasmosis

Histoplasmosis is caused by the fungus *Histoplasma capsulatum,* found primarily in the soil of river valleys in temperate zones of the world. The central United States, for example, in the Mississippi and Ohio river valleys, is particularly notable as a region in which this organism is endemic. *Histoplasma* is a dimorphic fungus, meaning that it exhibits two types of morphology, depending on the conditions for growth. In the soil the organism takes the form of branching hyphae; in the body at 37°C, it appears as a round or oval yeast.

Features of *Histoplasma capsulatum* are the following:

1. Common in river valleys of central United States
2. Found in soil contaminated by bird droppings
3. Present in yeast form in tissue
4. Elicits granulomatous response in tissue

Histoplasma organisms flourish best in soil that has been contaminated by bird droppings. When the soil becomes dry or disrupted (e.g., with bulldozing), the infectious spores become airborne, are inhaled by humans, and eventually reach the distal regions of the lung. Contact with chicken houses, bat caves, and starling, blackbird, and pigeon roosts often provides exposure for individuals or groups working in the contaminated area.

After an individual has been exposed and *H. capsulatum* has entered the lung, the organism (at body temperature) undergoes conversion to the yeast phase. An inflammatory response ensues in the lung parenchyma, with recruitment of phagocytic cells (macrophages). Commonly, there is also spread of the organism to regional lymph nodes and via the blood stream to other organs, such as the spleen. Within 3 weeks, delayed hypersensitivity against *Histoplasma* generally has developed, and the pathologic response becomes granulomatous in nature. Central areas of caseation necrosis often occur within the granulomas, making the pathologic response similar to that of tuberculosis.

When the initial or primary lesions heal, residua are absent or take the form of small, fibrotic pulmonary nodules, which may contain areas of calcification. Similarly, small foci of calcification within the spleen also may provide evidence of prior infection. However, there are alternatives to this benign pathologic course after exposure. In some cases, particularly in the immunosuppressed host or in the infant or young child, the dissemination of the organism to other organs is not controlled by host defense mechanisms, and the patient is said to have *progressive disseminated histoplasmosis*. In other cases, particularly in patients with significant underlying airways disease or emphysema, progressive parenchymal inflammation, destruction, and cavity formation occur in the lung, often called *progressive* or *chronic pulmonary histoplasmosis*.

Types of Infection

Clinical syndromes with histoplasmosis are the following:

1. Acute (primary) histoplasmosis
2. Progressive disseminated histoplasmosis
3. Chronic pulmonary histoplasmosis

Three main clinical syndromes are associated with histoplasmosis, corresponding to the three types of pathologic response just mentioned. In the normal, immunocompetent host a benign, self-limited infection called *acute* or *primary histoplasmosis* generally develops, with relatively few, if any, clinical sequelae. Often the affected person is symptom-free during the acute infection, particularly when the level of exposure has been relatively low. Other individuals have a variety of nonspecific symptoms, ranging from cough, fever, chills, and chest pain to headache, malaise, myalgias, and weight loss. The chest radiograph can reveal several types of patterns, commonly a pulmonary infiltrate with or without hilar adenopathy. The typical clinical syndrome resolves within a few weeks, even without therapy. The only clues remaining from the acute infection are often one or several pulmonary nodules (which can be calcified) seen on chest radiograph. Immunologic testing, by means of skin tests or serologic studies, may also indicate prior exposure to the organism. Relatively rarely and if the acute exposure has been particularly intense, however, patients may become quite ill and may even die as a result of acute histoplasmosis.

The syndrome of *progressive disseminated histoplasmosis* usually occurs in immunocompromised hosts or in infants or young children. What these patients appear to have in common that predisposes them to progressive disseminated histoplasmosis is impairment of cell-mediated immunity. In this potentially life-threatening illness, there is often widespread pulmonary involvement, accompanied by prominent systemic symptoms and infection of other organ systems.

Finally, *chronic pulmonary histoplasmosis* is generally seen in individuals with preexisting structural abnormalities of the lung, primarily chronic obstructive lung disease with emphysema. The clinical and radiographic patterns often resemble those of tuberculosis. Patients may have cough, sputum production, fever, fatigue, and weight loss. The chest radiograph also shows disease localized mainly to the upper lobes, with parenchymal infiltrates, often streaky in appearance, and cavity formation.

Diagnosis of histoplasmosis depends on the type of infection: acute, disseminated, or chronic. The options available to the clinician are culture of the organism, identification in tissue, detection of *Histoplasma* antigen in the urine, or documentation of an immunologic response by serologic studies. In order to identify the organism microscopically, special stains, such as methenamine silver, are required. The specific usefulness and limitations of each of these methods can be found in the references listed at the end of this chapter.

Treatment of pulmonary histoplasmosis also depends on the particular type of infection. Acute histoplasmosis generally requires no therapy and is a self-limited illness. Disseminated histoplasmosis requires treatment with a regimen using amphotericin B, typically followed by itraconazole. Chronic pulmonary histoplasmosis is generally treated with itraconazole alone or with amphotericin B followed by itraconazole, depending upon the severity of the disease.

Coccidioidomycosis

Like histoplasmosis, *coccidioidomycosis* also affects normal hosts but may have its clinical consequences altered in special categories of patients, especially those with impairment of host defense mechanisms. The causative organism, *Coccidioides immitis,* is also a dimorphic fungus. Mycelia are present in soil, whereas staining of tissue specimens shows characteristic round, thick-walled structures called *spherules,* which often contain multiple endospores.

Unlike *Histoplasma* organisms, the organisms of *Coccidioides* are limited to the Western hemisphere, particularly to the San Joaquin Valley region of California. Other areas in which the organism is endemic include parts of New Mexico, Nevada, Texas, and Arizona, as well as regions of Mexico and South America.

Features of *Coccidioides immitis* are the following:

1. Present in yeast form in tissue
2. Endemic in western and southwestern United States
3. Elicits granulomatous response in tissue

After the host inhales the infectious spore, primary disease develops. Pathologically, the inflammatory response to the organism is also a granulomatous one, once delayed hypersensitivity to *Coccidioides* has developed. The normal host generally has a relatively self-limited illness resulting from the primary infection. When dissemination occurs, it is usually in specific groups of predisposed individuals: immunosuppressed patients, pregnant women and, for unclear reasons, certain ethnic groups, particularly Filipinos and blacks. Chronic pulmonary coccidioidomycosis is found in some patients as a sequel to primary disease, perhaps related either to underlying lung disease or to immune impairment.

Primary infection with *Coccidioides immitis* may be subclinical and unassociated with symptoms, or it may produce respiratory tract symptoms or manifestations of hypersensitivity to the organism. When symptoms occur, they often include fever, cough, headache, and chest pain. Skin manifestations, presumably representing a form of hypersensitivity, are also common. One of these, erythema nodosum, consists of tender, red nodules on the anterior surface of the lower legs. The chest radiograph during the primary infection frequently shows a pulmonary infiltrate, often with associated hilar adenopathy and sometimes a pleural effusion.

The acute (primary) infection is usually self-limited, resolving within a few weeks. Residual findings on chest radiograph may be absent or may consist of one or more pulmonary nodules (with or without calcification) or thin-walled cavities.

Disseminated disease, resulting from hematogenous spread of the organism, is often associated with an ominous prognosis. As mentioned earlier, certain ethnic groups are at high risk for this complication, as are immunosuppressed patients and pregnant women.

Chronic pulmonary involvement by coccidioidomycosis can take several forms, including one or more chronic cavities, or upper lobe disease with streaky infiltrates and/or nodules resembling tuberculosis. Patients often have fever, cough (sometimes with hemoptysis), malaise, and weight loss and may appear subacutely or chronically ill.

As with histoplasmosis, diagnosis of coccidioidomycosis depends on the type of clinical presentation and rests upon culture, demonstration in tissue (e.g., with methenamine silver staining), and evidence of an immune response to the organism. The specific uses and interpretation of skin testing and serologic techniques for diagnosis are discussed in the more detailed references at the end of this chapter.

Treatment considerations are similar to those for histoplasmosis. Primary infections generally do not require therapy, although patients at high risk for dissemination are commonly treated with an oral azole antifungal agent (such as fluconazole) or amphotericin B. Chronic pulmonary disease frequently requires therapy with amphotericin B or an oral azole, but occasionally surgery plays a role in specific clinical settings. Disseminated coccidioidomycosis is treated with amphotericin B, and if patients are subject to prolonged immunosuppression, they then commonly receive prolonged suppressive therapy with an oral azole.

Blastomycosis

Blastomycosis, due to the soil-dwelling fungus *Blastomyces dermatitidis,* occurs primarily in the midwestern and southeastern United States, often overlapping the areas in which histoplasmosis is seen. Infection is initiated by inhalation of spores that have become airborne. The primary inflammatory response in the lung consists largely of neutrophils, with the subsequent response also including macrophages and T lymphocytes. As a result, the findings on histopathology show a combination of granulomas and a pyogenic (neutrophilic) response; if the latter is prominent, the response may mimic a bacterial infection. The organism can disseminate, especially to skin, but the frequency of dissemination is unknown.

Acute pulmonary infection with *Blastomyces* often resembles a bacterial pneumonia. Patients frequently have a relatively abrupt onset of symptoms, including fever, chills, and cough accompanied by purulent sputum production. However, subacute or chronic cases can be seen. It appears that there are also asymptomatic cases of blastomycosis, but their relative frequency compared with symptomatic cases is unknown. Patients with

Clinical syndromes with coccidioidomycosis are the following:
1. Acute (primary) coccidioidomycosis
2. Disseminated coccidioidomycosis
3. Chronic pulmonary coccidioidomycosis

Acute infection with *Blastomyces* may resemble a bacterial pneumonia.

impaired cellular immunity commonly develop more rapidly progressive or severe disease.

The chest radiograph of patients with blastomycosis shows unilateral or bilateral pulmonary infiltrates, which can resemble bacterial pneumonia, or localized densities, which can resemble carcinoma. Diagnosis can often be confirmed by demonstrating the characteristic yeast forms in sputum or tissue, or by culture of sputum.

Blastomycosis is generally treated with itraconazole (for less severe disease) or amphotericin B (for more severe disease). However, many cases of blastomycosis may be self-limited, and it is not clear whether all cases need treatment, particularly if the diagnosis is made as the disease seems to be resolving.

Aspergillosis

Of all the fungi, *Aspergillus* is particularly notable for the variety of clinical presentations seen and the types of individuals predisposed. Unlike *Histoplasma, Coccidioides,* and *Blastomyces, Aspergillus* species are widespread throughout nature and are not limited to particular geographic areas. Also unlike these other types of fungi, *Aspergillus* species are not dimorphic in appearance but always occur as mycelia, i.e., branching hyphal forms. Since virtually everyone is exposed to the organism, it is clear that disease must be associated with certain predisposing factors, which are now quite well defined.

Considered here are four major clinical forms of disease due to *Aspergillus* and the different settings in which these diseases occur. The first of these, *allergic bronchopulmonary aspergillosis,* is a hypersensitivity reaction to airway colonization with *Aspergillus,* seen almost exclusively in patients with underlying asthma. The second, *aspergilloma,* is a saprophytic colonization of a preexisting cavity in the lung by a mycetoma ("fungus ball") composed of a mass of *Aspergillus* hyphae. The third form, *invasive aspergillosis,* involves tissue invasion by the organism and is seen in patients who have significant impairment of their immune defense mechanisms. The fourth and least well-recognized form, *chronic necrotizing pulmonary aspergillosis,* involves a subacute to chronic invasion and destruction of the pulmonary parenchyma by *Aspergillus,* often complicated by cavity formation and secondary development of a mycetoma.

> Features of *Aspergillus* infection are the following:
> 1. Widespread distribution
> 2. Present as branching hyphae in tissue

> Clinical syndromes with aspergillosis are the following:
> 1. Allergic bronchopulmonary aspergillosis
> 2. Aspergilloma
> 3. Invasive aspergillosis
> 4. Chronic necrotizing pulmonary aspergillosis

Allergic Bronchopulmonary Aspergillosis

The presence of underlying reactive airways disease—asthma—appears to be the important predisposing factor for development of allergic bronchopulmonary aspergillosis. In this condition the organism resides in the patient's airways, where it appears to be important as an antigen rather than as an infectious, invasive fungus. Both type I (immediate, immunoglobulin E–mediated) and type III (immune complex, immunoglobulin G–mediated) immune reactions to the organism develop in affected persons.

Clinically, patients with allergic bronchopulmonary aspergillosis have manifestations of asthma (wheezing, dyspnea, and cough) and often low-grade fever and production of characteristic brownish plugs of sputum. *Aspergillus* species can frequently be cultured from these plugs of sputum. The chest radiograph may show transient pulmonary infiltrates, which can be a consequence of bronchial obstruction by the plugs or a result of eosinophilic infiltration of lung tissue. In addition, bronchiectasis of proximal airways can be present, and these dilated airways may also be filled with mucous plugs.

Diagnosis is made in the proper clinical setting of underlying asthma, and it is based on culturing the organism or demonstrating the host's immune response to the fungus, or both. For example, skin tests against *Aspergillus* antigen show a positive immediate reaction (reflecting type I immunity), often accompanied by a delayed reaction (called an Arthus reaction) after several hours (reflecting type III immunity). Precipitins in the blood and specific immunoglobulin E against the organism can also frequently be identified.

Treatment of allergic bronchopulmonary aspergillosis is not aimed at the fungus but rather at the host's immunologic response to the organism. Therefore, corticosteroids are the treatment for this syndrome, not the antifungal agent amphotericin B.

Aspergilloma

The second type of clinical problem resulting from *Aspergillus* is the aspergilloma, or fungus ball. The major predisposing feature for this entity is the presence of a preexisting cavity within the pulmonary parenchyma. Tuberculosis, sarcoidosis, and other fungal infections are a few examples of diseases in which cavities may be seen and therefore in which an aspergilloma may be a complicating problem. In these cases the organism is essentially a saprophyte or colonizer of the cavity, with little tissue invasion. The fungus ball itself represents a mass of fungal mycelia lying within the cavity proper.

Clinically, patients with an aspergilloma present either with hemoptysis or with no symptoms but suggestive findings on chest radiograph. Classically, the radiograph demonstrates an apparent mass surrounded by a lucent rim, representing air in the cavity around the fungus ball (Fig. 25-1). When the

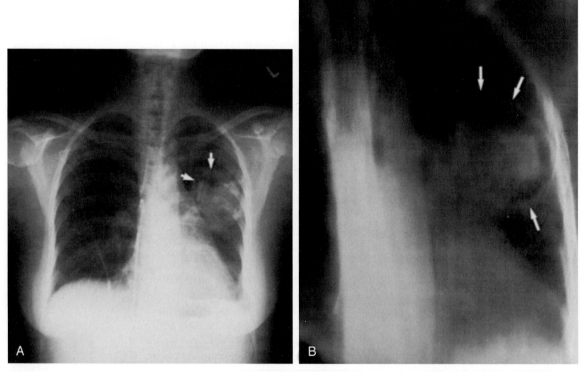

Figure 25-1 ◼— Posteroanterior radiograph (*A*) and tomogram (*B*) show aspergilloma in left lung. Fungus ball appears as mass sitting within radiolucent, thin-walled cavity. Arrows outline cavity wall. (Courtesy of Dr. Ferris Hall.)

patient changes position, the fungus ball often can be shown to change position within the cavity, according to the effects of gravity.

Diagnosis of an aspergilloma is generally suggested by the characteristic radiographic appearance and is confirmed by a culture of the organism or by a demonstration of the presence of precipitins against *Aspergillus* species. Treatment is often unnecessary inasmuch as the clinical sequelae are frequently inconsequential. In some cases, particularly those with significant amounts of hemoptysis, surgery is performed to remove the diseased area containing the fungus ball. Intravenous administration of amphotericin B is not effective in treatment of this syndrome, although direct instillation of amphotericin into the cavity has been performed in some cases.

Invasive Aspergillosis

Invasive aspergillosis is the third clinical presentation of *Aspergillus* infection in the lung. This is certainly the most life-threatening manifestation of *Aspergillus* infection, occurring almost exclusively in patients with marked impairment of host immune defense mechanisms. The most important risk factor is neutropenia—insufficient numbers of polymorphonuclear leukocytes—but patients often also have impairment of cellular immunity as a consequence of treatment with chemotherapeutic agents.

Pathologically, the organism invades and spreads through lung tissue, but it also tends to invade blood vessels within the lung. As a result of vascular involvement by the fungus, vessels can become occluded, and areas of pulmonary infarction can develop.

Clinically, patients are extremely ill, with fever, cough, dyspnea, and often pleuritic chest pain. The chest radiograph may show localized or diffuse pulmonary infiltrates, reflecting either tissue invasion and a fungal pneumonia or pulmonary infarction secondary to vascular occlusion.

Diagnosis of invasive aspergillosis generally requires identification of the organism—for example, by methenamine silver staining, on a biopsy specimen of lung tissue. Treatment consists of amphotericin B, but even with appropriate use of this agent the mortality rate is extremely high. Oral itraconazole is a potential alternative for selected patients, and is often used after initial intravenous therapy with amphotericin.

Chronic Necrotizing Pulmonary Aspergillosis

The final type of *Aspergillus* infection involving the lung has been called *chronic necrotizing pulmonary aspergillosis*. In this form, patients frequently have underlying lung disease or some impairment of either pulmonary or systemic host defense mechanisms. The name of this disorder describes the clinical process, which is characterized by an indolent, localized invasion of pulmonary parenchyma by *Aspergillus* organisms. Necrosis of the involved tissue often results in cavity formation, which may become the site for a mycetoma. Because there is tissue invasion, the infection is treated with amphotericin B or oral itraconazole.

Other Fungi

The remaining fungi are less frequent causes of respiratory infection. *Candida albicans*, although an extraordinarily common contaminant of sputum (particularly in the patient treated with antibiotics), is an uncommon cause of pneumonia, even in immunosuppressed patients. *Cryptococcus neoformans* is found primarily in immunosuppressed patients, in whom it causes lung disease and meningitis. Finally, *Mucor* is an opportunistic fungus that may cause pulmonary infection in the immunocompromised host or in patients with underlying diabetes.

PNEUMOCYSTIS INFECTION

Although *Pneumocystis carinii* has been recognized for several decades as a cause of pneumonia in immunocompromised patients, its clinical importance as a major pathogen in AIDS sparked a substantial increase in interest in the organism, its treatment, and prevention of infection in the high-risk patient. With the current use of highly active antiretroviral therapy for treatment of HIV as well as preventive therapy for *Pneumocystis*, the number of cases of AIDS-related *Pneumocystis* has decreased considerably. Nevertheless, it remains an important pulmonary pathogen, not only in the HIV-infected patient, but also in a variety of other immunosuppressed patients.

The taxonomy of *Pneumocystis* has not been clearly established. For many years the organism was considered a protozoan; however, techniques involving sequencing of genetic information and study of enzyme structure suggest it is more closely related to fungi than to protozoa.

Pneumocystis appears to be widely distributed in nature. It can normally be found in the lungs of a variety of animals as well as humans. Yet the organisms do not cause disease in normal hosts, only in individuals with significant impairment in host defenses, specifically cellular immunity. The key cell appears to be the helper ($CD4^+$) T lymphocyte, whose numbers or function, or both, can be diminished by specific diseases or by immunosuppressive drugs. Before the recognition of AIDS, *P. carinii* pneumonia was seen most commonly in the patient with malignancy, organ transplantation, or other diseases requiring treatment with steroids or other immunosuppressive agents. However, after the identification of AIDS and before the introduction of highly active antiretroviral therapy, the majority of cases were seen in patients with AIDS with greatly reduced numbers of $CD4^+$ lymphocytes. The problem of *Pneumocystis* pneumonia as it occurs in AIDS is discussed in more detail in Chapter 26.

Pneumocystis cysts, which are seen in the lung tissue of infected patients, appear on light-microscopic examination as round or cup-shaped structures. They do not stain well with the routine hematoxylin and eosin stain and instead require special stains such as methenamine silver (Fig. 25-2). The tissue response to the organism, seen on microscopic examination of lung tissue, includes infiltration of mononuclear cells within the pulmonary interstitium and exudation of foamy fluid (containing cysts) into alveolar spaces.

Clinically, *Pneumocystis* pneumonia usually manifests in the immunocompromised patient with dyspnea and fever. In the patient for whom treatment with corticosteroids was the risk factor for developing *Pneumocystis* pneumonia, the symptoms frequently develop and the infection is recognized as the dose of steroids is being tapered. The chest radiograph commonly shows diffuse bilateral infiltrates, which can have the appearance of either an interstitial or an alveolar filling pattern (Fig. 25-3). Hypoxemia is often a particularly prominent clinical feature in these patients. Although the disease is often insidious in onset in patients with AIDS, it commonly manifests in other immunocompromised patients as a relatively acute onset pneumonia that, if untreated, can progress to respiratory failure and death within days.

Because the organism is extremely difficult to cultivate in the laboratory setting, diagnosis depends on demonstrating the organism on stains of tissue

---

Features of *Pneumocystis carinii* are the following:

1. Ubiquitous distribution
2. Seen on methenamine silver stain rather than routine tissue stain
3. Tissue response is primarily exudation of foamy fluid into alveoli

---

Clinical features of *Pneumocystis* pneumonia are the following:

1. Symptoms: dyspnea, fever
2. Chest radiograph: frequently diffuse interstitial or alveolar infiltrates
3. Hypoxemia

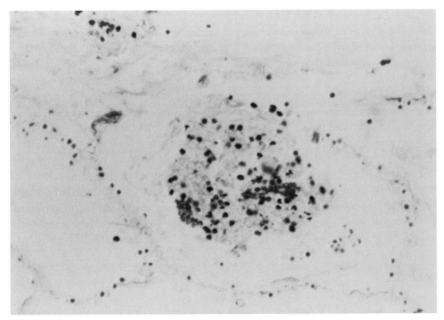

Figure 25-2 ■━ High-power photomicrograph of many *Pneumocystis* cysts, as seen with methenamine silver staining. Darkly staining cysts are within alveolar lumen. Note also foamy exudate in alveolar lumen. (Courtesy of Dr. Earl Kasdon.)

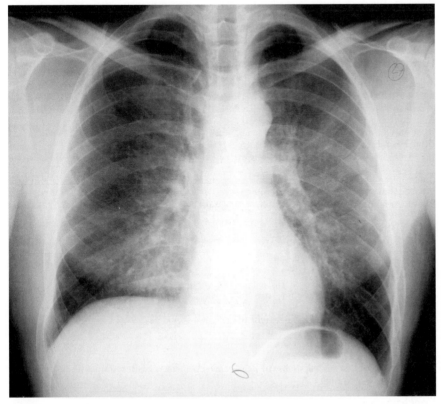

Figure 25-3 ■━ Chest radiograph of patient with AIDS and pneumonia due to *Pneumocystis carinii*. Infiltrates representing alveolar filling are most prominent at right base but are also seen in left midlung field as diffuse haziness.

sections, bronchoalveolar lavage fluid, or sputum that has been induced by having the patient inhale a hypertonic saline aerosol. The use of monoclonal antibodies (and, more recently, polymerase chain reaction [PCR] technology) as a means of detecting the organism in sputum or bronchoalveolar lavage fluid has improved the detection rate compared with the use of previous staining methods. No serologic or skin testing methods are available for diagnosis. In non-AIDS patients, the current treatment of choice for *Pneumocystis* infection is a combination of trimethoprim and sulfamethoxazole, which is effective in approximately 80 percent of patients. In high-risk patients, such as transplant recipients or children receiving chemotherapy for leukemia, low doses of the same agents are used prophylactically to prevent the infection. When patients with *Pneumocystis* pneumonia do not respond or are allergic to the trimethoprim-sulfamethoxazole regimen, an alternative drug, pentamidine, is also quite effective. Chapter 26 provides a discussion of some of the specific treatment and prophylaxis issues posed by patients with AIDS.

References

General

Baughman RP: The lung in the immunocompromised patient. Infectious complications (Part 1). Respiration 66:95-109, 1999.
Rosenow EC III, Wilson WR, and Cockerill FR III: Pulmonary disease in the immunocompromised host: I. Mayo Clin Proc 60:473-487, 1985.
Shelhamer JH et al: Laboratory evaluation of opportunistic pulmonary infections. Ann Intern Med 124:585-599, 1996.
Shelhamer JH et al: Respiratory disease in the immunosuppressed patient. Ann Intern Med 117:415-431, 1992.
Tamm M: The lung in the immunocompromised patient. Infectious complications (Part 2). Respiration 66:199-207, 1999.
Wilson WR, Cockerill FR III, and Rosenow EC III: Pulmonary disease in the immunocompromised host: II. Mayo Clin Proc 60:610-631, 1985.

Fungal Infections (General References)

American Thoracic Society: Chemotherapy of the pulmonary mycoses. Am Rev Respir Dis 138:1078-1081, 1988.
American Thoracic Society: Laboratory diagnosis of mycotic and specific fungal infections. Am Rev Respir Dis 132:1373-1379, 1985.
Davies SF: An overview of pulmonary fungal infections. Clin Chest Med 8:495-512, 1987.
Dismukes WE: Introduction to antifungal drugs. Clin Infect Dis 30:653-657, 2000.
Gold JWM: Opportunistic fungal infections in patients with neoplastic disease. Am J Med 76:458-463, 1984.
Goldman M, Johnson PC, and Sarosi GA: Fungal pneumonias. The endemic mycoses. Clin Chest Med 20:507-519, 1999.
Patel R: Antifungal agents. Part I. Amphotericin B preparations and flucytosine. Mayo Clin Proc 73:1205-1225, 1998.
Saubolle MA: Fungal pneumonias. Semin Respir Infect 15:162-177, 2000.
Terrell CL: Antifungal agents. Part II. The azoles. Mayo Clin Proc 74:78-100, 1999.

Histoplasmosis

Goodwin RA Jr and Des Prez RM: Histoplasmosis. Am Rev Respir Dis 117:929-956, 1978.
Goodwin RA, Loyd JE, and Des Prez RM: Histoplasmosis in normal hosts. Medicine 60:231-266, 1981.
Saag MS and Dismukes WE: Treatment of histoplasmosis and blastomycosis. Chest 93:848-851, 1988.
Wheat J: Histoplasmosis. Experience during outbreaks in Indianapolis and review of the literature. Medicine 76:339-354, 1997.
Wheat J et al: Practice guidelines for the management of patients with histoplasmosis. Clin Infect Dis 30:688-695, 2000.

Coccidioidomycosis

Bayer AS: Fungal pneumonias: pulmonary coccidioidal syndromes. Chest 79:575-583; 686-691, 1981.

Drutz DJ and Catanzaro A: Coccidioidomycosis. Am Rev Respir Dis 117:559-595; 727-771, 1978.
Galgiani JN: Coccidioidomycosis: a regional disease of national importance. Ann Intern Med 130:293-300, 1999.
Galgiani JN et al: Comparison of oral fluconazole and itraconazole for progressive, nonmeningeal coccidioidomycosis. A randomized, double-blind trial. Ann Intern Med 133:676-686, 2000.
Galgiani JN et al: Practice guidelines for the treatment of coccidioidomycosis. Clin Infect Dis 30:658-661, 2000.
Stevens DA: Coccidioidomycosis. N Engl J Med 332:1077-1082, 1995.

Blastomycosis

Chapman SW et al: Practice guidelines for the management of patients with blastomycosis. Clin Infect Dis 30:679-683, 2000.
Sarosi GA and Davies SF: Blastomycosis. Am Rev Respir Dis 120:911-938, 1979.

Aspergillosis

Binder RE et al: Chronic necrotizing pulmonary aspergillosis: a discrete clinical entity. Medicine 60:109-124, 1982.
Cockrill BA and Hales CA: Allergic bronchopulmonary aspergillosis. Annu Rev Med 50:303-316, 1999.
Glimp RA and Bayer AS: Fungal pneumonias—III: Allergic bronchopulmonary aspergillosis. Chest 80:85-94, 1981.
Glimp RA and Bayer AS: Pulmonary aspergilloma: diagnostic and therapeutic considerations. Arch Intern Med 143:303-308, 1983.
Herbert PA and Bayer AS: Fungal pneumonia—IV: Invasive pulmonary aspergillosis. Chest 80:220-225, 1981.
Horvath JA and Dummer S: The use of respiratory-tract cultures in the diagnosis of invasive pulmonary aspergillosis. Am J Med 100:171-178, 1996.
Paterson DL and Singh N: Invasive aspergillosis in transplant recipients. Medicine 78:123-138, 1999.
Reichenberger F, Habicht JM, Gratwohl A, and Tamm M: Diagnosis and treatment of invasive pulmonary aspergillosis in neutropenic patients. Eur Respir J 19:743-755, 2002.
Ricketti AJ, Greenberger PA, Mintzer RA, and Patterson R: Allergic bronchopulmonary aspergillosis. Chest 86:773-778, 1984.
Sharma OP and Chwogule R: Many faces of pulmonary aspergillosis. Eur Respir J 12:705-715, 1998.
Soubani AO and Chandrasekar PH: The clinical spectrum of pulmonary aspergillosis. Chest 121:1988-1999, 2002.
Stevens DA et al: Practice guidelines for diseases caused by *Aspergillus*. Clin Infect Dis 30:696-709, 2000.
Wardlaw A and Geddes DM: Allergic bronchopulmonary aspergillosis: a review. J R Soc Med 85:747-751, 1992.

Pneumocystis Infection

Arend SM, Kroon FP, and van't Wout JW: *Pneumocystis carinii* pneumonia in patients without AIDS, 1980 through 1993. Arch Intern Med 155:2436-2441, 1995.
Hughes WT et al: Successful intermittent chemoprophylaxis for *Pneumocystis carinii* pneumonitis. N Engl J Med 316:1627-1632, 1987.
Kovacs JA, Gill VJ, Meshnick S, and Masur H: New insights into transmission, diagnosis, and drug treatment of *Pneumocystis carinii* pneumonia. JAMA 286:2450-2460, 2001.
Masur H et al: *Pneumocystis* pneumonia: from bench to clinic. Ann Intern Med 111:813-826, 1989.
Peters SG and Prakash UBS: *Pneumocystis carinii* pneumonia. Ann Intern Med 82:73-78, 1987.
Russian DA and Levine SJ: *Pneumocystis carinii* pneumonia in patients without HIV infection. Am J Med Sci 321:56-65, 2001.
Yale SH and Limper AH: *Pneumocystis carinii* pneumonia in patients without acquired immunodeficiency syndrome: associated illness and prior corticosteroid therapy. Mayo Clin Proc 71:5-13, 1996.

chapter 26

Acquired Immunodeficiency Syndrome

ETIOLOGY AND PATHOGENESIS

INFECTIOUS COMPLICATIONS OF AIDS
  Pneumocystis carinii Pneumonia
  Mycobacterial Infections
  Other Bacterial Infections
  Viral Infection
  Fungal Infections

NONINFECTIOUS COMPLICATIONS OF AIDS
  Neoplastic Disease
  Inflammatory Disease
  Pulmonary Vascular Disease

DIAGNOSTIC EVALUATION OF PULMONARY INFILTRATES IN AIDS

In 1981, a number of cases of immunodeficiency of unknown cause were reported in homosexual males and in intravenous drug users. These patients had a variety of unusual infections, including *Pneumocystis carinii* pneumonia, mucosal candidiasis, and several types of viral infections; in some cases the unusual neoplasm Kaposi's sarcoma also occurred. Evaluation of these patients demonstrated a marked impairment of cellular immunity, characterized by anergy to skin tests for delayed hypersensitivity and decreased numbers of lymphocytes, specifically with loss of helper-inducer T lymphocytes and a reversal in the normal ratio of helper-to-suppressor T cells. This disease was subsequently given the name *acquired immunodeficiency syndrome* (AIDS).

What initially seemed to be an unusual problem that might be relegated to the realm of medical curiosities has since become one of the major worldwide public health problems confronting the medical profession at the turn of the 21st century. Approximately 40 million individuals around the world (including more than 900,000 in the United States) are currently infected with HIV, with approximately 5 million new infections occurring each year. It has been estimated that there are 3 million deaths worldwide per year from HIV/AIDS; in sub-Saharan Africa, HIV/AIDS is the leading cause of death.

During the last 20 years, an enormous amount of research has resulted in identification of the retrovirus responsible for this catastrophic attack on the cellular immune system. At the same time, there has been a wide and unexpected spectrum of clinical problems posed by a myriad of opportunistic infections and neoplasms resulting from the profound immunodeficiency in these patients. Fortunately, the recent development of highly active antiretroviral therapy (HAART) and the development of effective prophylactic regimens against several opportunistic infections have significantly decreased many of the clinical complications of the disease. Nevertheless, although substantial and rapid progress has been made in the therapy of the disease and in the prevention and treatment of secondary complications, management of

332

patients with AIDS continues to present a major challenge to the medical community. The most important challenge is at a worldwide level, primarily as a result of limited availability of therapeutic and prophylactic agents for the large number of affected individuals in developing nations.

In the United States the largest category of individuals affected by AIDS is homosexual and bisexual men, in whom the responsible virus is transmitted by sexual contact. Persons in the next largest group, intravenous drug users of either sex, introduce the virus into their circulation with infected needles or syringes. Recipients of contaminated blood products, including concentrates of factor VIII used for hemophilia, form another important group at risk for AIDS. Finally, there is a relatively small number of patients who have contracted AIDS by heterosexual contact, generally with an individual in one of the aforementioned risk groups. In other areas of the world, e.g., central Africa and Haiti, AIDS is common in both sexes and is transmitted primarily by heterosexual contact.

Although AIDS potentially leads to complications in almost any organ system, the lungs have been the organ system in which the largest number of complications has occurred. This chapter contains a brief overview of AIDS and focuses on the complications specifically affecting the respiratory system of these patients.

ETIOLOGY AND PATHOGENESIS

The etiologic agent responsible for AIDS is known to be a retrovirus formerly called human T-cell lymphotropic virus type III (HTLV-III) and now called *human immunodeficiency virus* (HIV). The virus appears to mediate its pathogenic effect by binding to the CD4 receptor on cells that carry this surface receptor. Although the most important cell type so affected is the helper-inducer subset of T lymphocytes, cells of the monocyte-macrophage series and certain neural cells may also be infected because they carry the CD4 receptor on their cell surface.

The immunodeficiency occurring with HIV infection results from the lysis and depletion of infected CD4$^+$ T lymphocytes. This loss of the helper-inducer cell population may also be complicated by altered macrophage function, which is probably secondary to direct effects of the virus and to impaired production of cytokines normally affecting macrophage activation and function.

> HIV binds to the CD4 receptor of helper-inducer T lymphocytes.

The major consequence of the immunodeficiency is opportunistic infection with organisms that normally are handled by an adequately functioning cellular immune system. The most common infection involving the lungs is pneumonia due to *Pneumocystis carinii* infection. Pulmonary infection also can result from a wide variety of other respiratory pathogens normally controlled by cell-mediated immune mechanisms, including cytomegalovirus, mycobacteria (*Mycobacterium tuberculosis* and nontuberculous or atypical mycobacteria), and fungi (especially *Cryptococcus*, *Histoplasma*, and *Coccidioides*). Surprisingly, it has been recognized that certain types of bacterial pneumonia, primarily due to *Streptococcus pneumoniae* (pneumococcus) and *Haemophilus influenzae*, are seen with increased frequency in AIDS. Whereas these types of bacterial pneumonia would not normally be predicted to result from the cellular immunodeficiency of AIDS, they probably can be explained by dysregulation of the humoral immune system and impaired antibody production against these organisms.

> Major pulmonary infections with AIDS are the following:
> 1. *Pneumocystis carinii*
> 2. Cytomegalovirus
> 3. Mycobacteria
> 4. Fungi (*Cryptococcus, Histoplasma, Coccidioides*)
> 5. Bacteria (*Streptococcus pneumoniae, Haemophilus influenzae*)

Even though the majority of pulmonary complications seen in patients with AIDS are infectious, a variety of noninfectious complications are also well recognized. This chapter divides the pulmonary complications of AIDS into these two broad categories—infectious and noninfectious—and concludes with a discussion of the diagnostic evaluation of the patient with AIDS and pulmonary infiltrates.

INFECTIOUS COMPLICATIONS OF AIDS

Pneumocystis carinii *Pneumonia*

Since the first identification of cases in 1981, *P. carinii* infection has been the most common respiratory complication in patients with AIDS, frequently representing the initial opportunistic infection that establishes the diagnosis of AIDS in the absence of other known causes of immunosuppression. It has been estimated that pneumonia due to *P. carinii* develops at least once during the illness of approximately three of every four patients with AIDS. The risk of developing this opportunistic infection is highly dependent upon the patient's peripheral blood $CD4^+$ count, with a level less than 200 cells per mm^3 being the cut-off below which patients are at high risk of infection. Fortunately, the availability of increasingly effective antiretroviral agents and the more frequent use of prophylaxis against *Pneumocystis* have significantly decreased the likelihood of infection and death due to this opportunistic infection.

Pneumocystis carinii pneumonia often has an indolent onset in AIDS.

A general discussion of *P. carinii* as a respiratory pathogen was presented in Chapter 25. In patients with AIDS, the onset of the disease is often more indolent than in immunosuppressed patients without AIDS. Fever, cough, and dyspnea are the usual symptoms bringing the patient to medical attention. The typical chest radiograph shows diffuse interstitial or alveolar infiltrates; often the lung fields look hazy, a pattern that may be difficult to characterize specifically as either interstitial or alveolar and is commonly described as looking like "ground glass" (see Fig. 25-3). However, atypical radiographic presentations are clearly recognized with documented *Pneumocystis* pneumonia, including even the finding of a normal chest radiograph. High-resolution CT scanning is particularly sensitive for demonstrating subtle changes associated with *Pneumocystis* pneumonia, and will generally be abnormal even in those patients with a normal chest radiograph.

Diagnosis of *Pneumocystis carinii* is made most commonly on samples obtained by induction of sputum or bronchoalveolar lavage.

Diagnosis is generally based on finding the organism in respiratory secretions by any number of techniques, especially immunofluorescent staining with a monoclonal antibody. Patients with AIDS often have a surprisingly large burden of organisms, making the organisms easier to obtain than from patients without AIDS. Inducing sputum by having the patient inhale a solution of hypertonic saline is frequently effective and is now often used as the initial diagnostic method when *P. carinii* is suspected. Fiberoptic bronchoscopy with bronchoalveolar lavage is another means for recovering the organism, having a positive yield of more than 85 percent in patients eventually proven to have *Pneumocystis* pneumonia.

Standard therapy for *Pneumocystis carinii* pneumonia is one of three options: trimethoprim-sulfamethoxazole, trimethoprim-dapsone, or pentamidine.

Treatment of pneumonia due to *Pneumocystis* organisms usually involves one of three agents—the combination antimicrobial trimethoprim-sulfamethoxazole, the combination of trimethoprim and dapsone, or pentamidine as a single agent given intravenously. These three regimens appear to be equally effective, each being successful in about 80 percent of cases. In patients without AIDS treated for *Pneumocystis* pneumonia, the combination trimethoprim-sulfamethoxazole is generally preferred because of fewer side effects. However, patients with AIDS have a peculiar predisposition to allergic reactions to sulfonamides, making the frequency of adverse side effects equivalent to that seen with pentamidine and making it necessary to switch to either trimethoprim-dapsone or to pentamidine in a relatively high proportion of patients. Other agents such as atovaquone or the combination of clindamycin and primaquine have also been used, especially in patients who fail or cannot tolerate one of the more standard agents.

In patients with moderate to severe disease caused by *Pneumocystis* pneumonia, adjunctive therapy with corticosteroids is often helpful in averting significant respiratory failure. Although steroid therapy would be expected to cause more immunosuppression and make the infection worse, this has not been the case, and the presumed benefit of reducing the inflammatory response in the lung outweighs any negative effects of the steroids.

In patients with AIDS, oral administration of trimethoprim-sulfamethoxazole (in low doses) or dapsone (either alone or with pyrimethamine) can be used with reasonable effectiveness to prevent *Pneumocystis* pneumonia. Alternatively, patients can receive aerosolized pentamidine once per month by inhalation. Such prophylactic therapy is routinely recommended in HIV-infected patients with a CD4$^+$ count below 200 cells per mm^3 and in selected other circumstances. Unfortunately, the propensity for development of allergic reactions to trimethoprim-sulfamethoxazole frequently makes this regimen difficult to use in AIDS, and therefore many patients are maintained on one of the other forms of prophylaxis. When *Pneumocystis* pneumonia develops despite the use of aerosolized pentamidine prophylaxis, the clinical presentation may be atypical. In particular, unusual radiographic patterns often develop in such patients, especially pulmonary infiltrates limited to the upper lung zones, rather than the more typical pattern of diffuse pulmonary infiltrates.

> Atypical presentations of *Pneumocystis carinii* infections commonly are seen in patients receiving aerosolized pentamidine.

Mycobacterial Infections

Mycobacterium tuberculosis has emerged as an important respiratory pathogen in patients with AIDS, not only because it is common but also because it is potentially treatable. Clinical disease may result from primary infection, reactivation of previous infection, or exogenous reinfection. Rather than occurring in all categories of patients with AIDS, disease due to *M. tuberculosis* is a particular problem in those groups of individuals with a high background prevalence of tuberculosis—for example, intravenous drug users and indigent and immigrant populations.

> Tuberculosis may be an early opportunistic infection in AIDS.

Because *M. tuberculosis* is a relatively virulent organism that does not require the same degree of immunosuppression to produce disease as do many of the other opportunistic infections, it is often seen early in the course of patients with AIDS. In this setting, its clinical presentation is similar to that seen in the typical patient with tuberculosis who does not have AIDS. However, it may also occur in those AIDS patients who are in a late stage of their disease with more severe immunosuppression, in which case the clinical manifestations are often atypical. In this latter circumstance, upper lobe cavitary disease is less frequent, and disseminated disease is more frequent than is usually seen in patients without AIDS. Interestingly, for patients with AIDS and tuberculosis (or, for that matter, with other opportunistic infections), it has also been recognized that improvement in the patient's overall immune status, particularly as a result of HAART, can be associated with a paradoxical clinical worsening of the opportunistic infection. In these cases, "reconstitution" of the immune system results in an augmented inflammatory reaction to the opportunistic infection, leading to the apparent clinical worsening.

Treatment considerations for tuberculosis in AIDS patients are generally similar to those in patients without AIDS, but there are also some differences. Because of the risk of disease with nontuberculous mycobacteria (as will be discussed shortly), an expanded list of drugs is sometimes given initially to AIDS patients until the organism is firmly identified. In addition, treatment may be given for a longer duration to AIDS patients, especially if the response to therapy appears slow. Patients with HIV infection who have positive tuberculin skin test reactions but no evidence for active disease should receive 9 months of treatment with isoniazid (or an alternative regimen), similar to the treatment of latent tuberculosis infection in individuals without HIV infection.

The other types of mycobacteria that frequently cause opportunistic infection in AIDS are members of *Mycobacterium avium* complex (MAC). What is surprising in patients with MAC infection is that the organism is associated primarily with disseminated disease, not with pulmonary disease. Even when disseminated disease is present, pulmonary involvement is not generally a significant part of the clinical picture. Because the risk of MAC infection is associated with extremely low CD4$^+$ counts, prophylactic treatment against MAC, typically with a newer macrolide antibiotic such as azithromycin or clarithromycin, is indicated when the CD4$^+$ count falls below 50 per mm^3.

Other Bacterial Infections

Patients with AIDS appear to have an increased frequency of bacterial pneumonia, primarily due to either *S. pneumoniae* or *H. influenzae*. The risk is increased at all levels of CD4$^+$ count, and it is highest when the count falls below 200 cells per mm^3. Intravenous drug users also appear to be at particularly high risk.

As mentioned earlier, one would not predict bacterial pneumonias to be a complication of AIDS, because impairment in cellular immunity should not by itself predispose an individual to bacterial pneumonia. However, there is dysregulation of the humoral immune system accompanying the impairment in cellular immunity. Patients frequently have polyclonal hyperglobulinemia at the same time they demonstrate a poor antibody response after antigen exposure. Presumably, loss of helper-inducer cells results in alteration of the normal interaction between helper-inducer cells and B lymphocytes that regulates antibody production.

Viral Infection

The most common virus afflicting patients with AIDS is cytomegalovirus (CMV), one of the viruses in the herpesvirus family. The most common sites of clinical involvement are the eye (CMV retinitis) and the gastrointestinal tract. Although CMV can frequently be cultured from lung tissue or bronchoalveolar fluid of patients with AIDS, its role as a clinically important respiratory pathogen is not clear. When patients with CMV in the lungs have clinical respiratory system disease, they almost always have a coexistent organism such as *Pneumocystis* that is thought to be the primary pathogen. Even when typical nuclear and cytoplasmic inclusions are present, the role played by CMV is uncertain in the presence of these other important pathogens.

Other viruses such as herpes simplex, varicella-zoster, and Epstein-Barr virus have been described as potential respiratory pathogens in AIDS, but they are distinctly uncommon and are not considered here.

Fungal Infections

Several fungi are recognized as causes of respiratory involvement in patients with AIDS, either as isolated respiratory system disease or as part of a disseminated infection. The most common of these fungal infections is due to *Cryptococcus neoformans,* which more commonly causes meningitis than respiratory disease. When respiratory involvement is present, the radiograph may show localized or diffuse disease, and sometimes there may be an associated pleural effusion or intrathoracic lymph node involvement. The lung may be the only organ involved, or its involvement may be accompanied by meningitis or disseminated disease. Treatment has traditionally been with amphotericin B, but fluconazole has also been used as an alternative agent.

Fungal infections that occur in specific endemic regions—histoplasmosis and coccidioidomycosis—are described in detail in Chapter 25. In patients with AIDS, pulmonary involvement with these organisms is most commonly a manifestation of disseminated disease, which has resulted either from reactivation of previous disease or from progressive primary infection. Consequently, histoplasmosis and coccidioidomycosis are seen primarily but not exclusively in their respective endemic areas. As is the case in patients without AIDS, amphotericin B (or an oral azole such as itraconazole) is the primary agent used for treatment of either of these infections.

Other fungal infections of the lung are much less common in AIDS. Surprisingly, even though oral candidiasis (thrush) is extremely common in AIDS, pulmonary infection with *Candida albicans* is extremely uncommon and rarely described except at autopsy. *Aspergillus* infection has also been described in AIDS, but generally in patients who have other predisposing factors for invasive aspergillosis, especially neutropenia.

NONINFECTIOUS COMPLICATIONS OF AIDS

Although infectious complications affecting the respiratory system are much more common, noninfectious complications are also recognized in patients with AIDS. These fall into the broad categories of neoplastic disease (which includes Kaposi's sarcoma and non-Hodgkin's lymphoma), inflammatory disease (which includes lymphocytic interstitial pneumonitis and nonspecific interstitial pneumonitis), and pulmonary vascular disease (i.e., pulmonary hypertension). A brief discussion of each of these potential complications follows.

Neoplastic Disease

Kaposi's sarcoma is the most common of the neoplastic diseases affecting AIDS patients. Formerly a rare diagnosis in the United States, characterized by slowly progressive cutaneous lesions of the lower extremities in elderly men, it was also seen in certain parts of Africa in a more aggressive form with frequent visceral involvement. In the early descriptions of AIDS patients in 1981, Kaposi's sarcoma was one of the peculiar clinical manifestations accompanying the profound cellular immunodeficiency. Since then, Kaposi's sarcoma has been recognized as one of the common manifestations, occurring generally with skin involvement but often complicated by dissemination to the lungs and to other organ systems. Recent data from a variety of studies, including

Kaposi's sarcoma in the thorax can manifest with parenchymal, airway, lymph node, and pleural involvement.

the identification of herpesvirus-like DNA sequences in patients with Kaposi's sarcoma (either with or without AIDS) but not in control subjects, indicate that human herpesvirus-8 is the causative agent responsible for Kaposi's sarcoma.

Kaposi's sarcoma is most commonly observed in patients with AIDS as violaceous, vascular-appearing skin lesions. Histologically, these lesions consist of spindle-shaped cells with intervening slit-like vascular spaces. When visceral involvement indicates the presence of dissemination, commonly involved organ systems include the gastrointestinal tract and the lungs. Pulmonary involvement has a variable presentation on chest radiograph; it can appear as diffuse infiltrates, localized disease, or pulmonary nodules. Pleural involvement with resulting pleural effusions can be present; this is often a helpful diagnostic point against *P. carinii* pneumonia, because pleural effusions are uncommon with the latter diagnosis. Involvement of the airways or mediastinal lymph nodes can also be seen with intrathoracic Kaposi's sarcoma.

Making a definitive diagnosis of Kaposi's sarcoma in the lung may be difficult, because bronchoalveolar lavage and even transbronchial biopsy provide infrequent diagnostic material. On the other hand, one prefers to avoid a more invasive lung biopsy, which does generally provide diagnostic material. When endobronchial involvement is present, the gross appearance of the lesions in the airways may be highly suggestive of the diagnosis. Another useful clinical clue may be provided by a gallium lung scan, which demonstrates pulmonary uptake in most opportunistic infections but not in Kaposi's sarcoma.

Unfortunately, therapy for Kaposi's sarcoma involving the lungs is palliative rather than curative. Patients may have progressive respiratory involvement, often complicated by pulmonary hemorrhage. Although they may die of disseminated Kaposi's sarcoma, these patients frequently succumb to coexisting opportunistic infections rather than to the neoplasm.

The next most common neoplasm in patients with AIDS is non-Hodgkin's lymphoma. Although extranodal involvement and disseminated disease are common when this malignancy occurs in patients with AIDS, intrathoracic involvement is uncommon.

Inflammatory Disease

An occasional patient with AIDS and diffuse pulmonary infiltrates has neither an opportunistic infection nor a neoplasm affecting the lung. Instead, the process is an inflammatory one without any known cause, although viral etiologies (especially Epstein-Barr virus and HIV) have been proposed. In some cases the microscopic appearance is notable for the prominence of lymphocytes and plasma cells infiltrating alveolar septa; in these cases a diagnosis of *lymphocytic interstitial pneumonitis* is made. This particular histologic pattern is a relatively common pulmonary complication seen in children with AIDS, but it is found infrequently in adults. When treatment is necessary, corticosteroids are used with variable success.

The other histologic pattern is a nonspecific one with a mixed inflammatory cell infiltrate. Patients with this pattern are diagnosed as having *nonspecific interstitial pneumonitis.* This is an uncommon complication of AIDS, about which relatively little is known.

> Lymphocytic interstitial pneumonitis is a common pulmonary complication of AIDS in children.

Pulmonary Vascular Disease

A number of cases of pulmonary hypertension in patients with HIV infection have now been reported. Although it is believed that this is a true rather than a coincidental relationship, there is no clear mechanistic or pathophysiologic explanation. The histopathology and clinical features are typically similar to those of primary pulmonary hypertension, but the disease may have a more rapid progression than is generally seen in patients without HIV infection. The prognosis is generally poor, without any consistent response to either vasodilator or antiretroviral therapy.

DIAGNOSTIC EVALUATION OF PULMONARY INFILTRATES IN AIDS

Pulmonary infiltrates, often accompanied by fever, dyspnea, and cough, present a common problem in the patient known to have either HIV infection or risk factors for exposure to HIV. Although typical radiographic presentations of some of the aforementioned diseases may suggest a particular diagnosis, often the findings are nonspecific. In addition, with the accumulation of experience with AIDS, more atypical presentations of many of these respiratory complications are being recognized. For example, with *Pneumocystis* infection, the use of aerosolized pentamidine decreases the likelihood of infection but increases the frequency of atypical radiographic presentations when the infection occurs despite the prophylactic therapy.

Frequently, the initial evaluation of patients with diffuse pulmonary infiltrates focuses on the diagnosis of *Pneumocystis* pneumonia, because it is the most common complication in AIDS. Induction of sputum accompanied by appropriate staining for *Pneumocystis* is often the first diagnostic procedure, because it is noninvasive. When sputum induction produces negative findings, fiberoptic bronchoscopy is often the next procedure performed, usually with bronchoalveolar lavage and sometimes with transbronchial biopsy. The yield for *Pneumocystis* is excellent on bronchoalveolar lavage, but making a diagnosis of some of the other infections, neoplasms, and inflammatory processes may require transbronchial biopsy. Thoracoscopic and open lung biopsy are the most invasive of the diagnostic procedures and are usually reserved for situations in which a diagnosis is crucial but not forthcoming by less invasive means.

Ancillary diagnostic techniques may sometimes be helpful. Although gallium scanning is not typically part of the diagnostic evaluation of patients with AIDS, it generally demonstrates uptake in the pulmonary parenchyma when an opportunistic infection is present. Therefore, a positive gallium scan may suggest an opportunistic infection in patients with fever and respiratory symptoms but with negative findings on a chest radiograph. Additionally, in patients with pulmonary infiltrates accompanying cutaneous Kaposi's sarcoma, a gallium scan may help distinguish an opportunistic infection from pulmonary involvement with the neoplasm, because the former is associated with a positive gallium scan whereas the latter is not.

Results of gallium scans are generally positive with opportunistic infections and negative with Kaposi's sarcoma.

References

Infectious Complications

American Thoracic Society: Fungal infection in HIV-infected persons. Am J Respir Crit Care Med 152:816-822, 1995.

Ampel NM, Dols CL, and Galgiani JN: Coccidioidomycosis during human immunodeficiency virus infection: results of a prospective study in a coccidioidal endemic area. Am J Med 94:235-240, 1993.

Baughman RP: Cytomegalovirus: the monster in the closet? Am J Respir Crit Care Med 156:1-2, 1997.

Baughman RP, Dohn MN, and Frame PT: The continuing utility of bronchoalveolar lavage to diagnose opportunistic infection in AIDS patients. Am J Med 97:515-522, 1994.

Beck JM, Rosen MJ, and Peavy HH: Pulmonary complications of HIV infection. Report of the fourth NHLBI workshop. Am J Respir Crit Care Med 164:2120-2126, 2001.

Boiselle PM, Crans CA, Kaplan MA, and Crans CA Jr: The changing face of *Pneumocystis carinii* pneumonia in AIDS patients. AJR Am J Roentgenol 172:1301-1309, 1999.

Bozzette SA et al: A randomized trial of three antipneumocystis agents in patients with advanced human immunodeficiency virus infection. N Engl J Med 332:693-699, 1995.

Burman WJ and Jones BE: Treatment of HIV-related tuberculosis in the era of effective antiretroviral therapy. Am J Respir Crit Care Med 164:7-12, 2001.

Girard P-M: Discontinuing *Pneumocystis carinii* prophylaxis. N Engl J Med 344:222-223, 2001.

Hajjeh RA: Disseminated histoplasmosis in persons infected with human immunodeficiency virus. Clin Infect Dis 21:S108-S110, 1995.

Havlir DV and Barnes PF: Tuberculosis in patients with human immunodeficiency virus infection. N Engl J Med 340:367-373, 1999.

Hirschtick RE et al: Bacterial pneumonia in persons infected with the human immunodeficiency virus. N Engl J Med 333:845-851, 1995.

Jules-Elysee KM et al: Aerosolized pentamidine: effect on diagnosis and presentation of *Pneumocystis carinii* pneumonia. Ann Intern Med 112:750-757, 1990.

Kovacs JA, Gill VJ, Meshnick S, and Masur H: New insights into transmission, diagnosis, and drug treatment of *Pneumocystis carinii* pneumonia. JAMA 286:2450-2460, 2001.

Kovacs JA and Masur H: Prophylaxis against opportunistic infections in patients with human immunodeficiency virus infection. N Engl J Med 342:1416-1429, 2000.

Masur H: Recommendations on prophylaxis and therapy for disseminated *Mycobacterium avium* complex disease in patients infected with the human immunodeficiency virus. N Engl J Med 329:898-904, 1993.

Masur H, Kaplan JE, and Holmes KK (eds): Guidelines for preventing opportunistic infections among HIV-infected persons—2002. Ann Intern Med 137:435-477, 2002.

Meyohas M-C et al: Pulmonary cryptococcosis: localized and disseminated infections in 27 patients with AIDS. Clin Infect Dis 21:628-633, 1995.

Murray JF and Mills J: Pulmonary infectious complications of human immunodeficiency virus infection. Am Rev Respir Dis 141:1356-1372; 1582-1598, 1990.

National Institutes of Health–University of California Expert Panel for Corticosteroids as Adjunctive Therapy for *Pneumocystis* Pneumonia: Consensus statement on the use of corticosteroids as adjunctive therapy for *Pneumocystis* pneumonia in the acquired immunodeficiency syndrome. N Engl J Med 323:1500-1504, 1990.

Rigsby MO and Curtis AM: Pulmonary disease from nontuberculous mycobacteria in patients with human immunodeficiency virus. Chest 106:913-919, 1994.

Stansell JD et al: Predictors of *Pneumocystis carinii* pneumonia in HIV-infected persons. Pulmonary Complications of HIV Infection Study Group. Am J Respir Crit Care Med 155:60-66, 1997.

USPHS/IDSA Prevention of Opportunistic Infections Working Group: 1999 USPHS/IDSA guidelines for the prevention of opportunistic infections in persons infected with human immunodeficiency virus. Ann Intern Med 131:873-908, 1999.

Wolff AJ and O'Donnell AE: Pulmonary manifestations of HIV infection in the era of highly active antiretroviral therapy. Chest 120:1888-1893, 2001.

Neoplastic, Inflammatory, and Pulmonary Vascular Complications

Bazot M et al: Primary pulmonary AIDS-related lymphoma. Radiographic and CT findings. Chest 116:1282-1286, 1999.

Cadranel J and Mayaud C: Intrathoracic Kaposi's sarcoma in patients with AIDS. Thorax 50:407-414, 1995.

Mehta NJ, Khan IA, Mehta RN, and Sepkowitz DA: HIV-related pulmonary hypertension. Analytic review of 131 cases. Chest 118:1133-1141, 2000.

Mesa RA, Edell ES, Dunn WF, and Edwards WD: Human immunodeficiency virus infection and pulmonary hypertension: two new cases and a review of 86 reported cases. Mayo Clin Proc 73:37-45, 1998.

Moore PS and Chang Y: Detection of herpesvirus-like DNA sequences in Kaposi's sarcoma in patients with and those without HIV infection. N Engl J Med 332:1181-1185, 1995.

Wallace JM: Mimics of infectious pneumonia in persons infected with human immunodeficiency virus. *In* Niederman MS, Sarosi GA, and Glassroth J (eds): Respiratory Infections: A Scientific Basis for Management. Philadelphia, WB Saunders Co., 1994, pp 217-223.

White DA and Matthay RA: Noninfectious pulmonary complications of infection with the human immunodeficiency virus. Am Rev Respir Dis 140:1763-1787, 1989.

chapter 27

Classification and Pathophysiologic Aspects of Respiratory Failure

DEFINITION OF RESPIRATORY
FAILURE

CLASSIFICATION OF ACUTE
RESPIRATORY FAILURE
   Hypoxemic Type
   Hypercapnic/Hypoxemic Type

PRESENTATION OF
GAS-EXCHANGE FAILURE

PATHOGENESIS OF
GAS-EXCHANGE ABNORMALITIES

Hypoxemic Respiratory Failure
Hypercapnic/Hypoxemic
   Respiratory Failure

CLINICAL AND THERAPEUTIC
ASPECTS OF
HYPERCAPNIC/HYPOXEMIC
RESPIRATORY FAILURE

Many types of respiratory disease are capable of impairing the lung's normal function as a gas-exchanging organ. In some cases, the degree of impairment is mild, and the patient suffers relatively few consequences. In other cases, dysfunction is marked, and the patient experiences disabling or life-threatening clinical sequelae. When the respiratory system can no longer function to keep gas-exchange at an acceptable level, the patient is said to be in *respiratory failure,* irrespective of the underlying cause.

The tempo for development of respiratory failure varies depending on the nature of the underlying problem. Many of the diseases discussed so far, such as chronic obstructive lung disease and interstitial lung disease, are characterized by a chronic clinical course, accompanied by relatively slow deterioration of pulmonary function and gas-exchange. However, because of their limited pulmonary reserve, patients with preexisting pulmonary disease are also susceptible to episodes of acute respiratory failure, either from an intercurrent illness or from transient worsening of their underlying disease. On the other hand, respiratory failure, generally acute or subacute in onset, also can develop in individuals without preexisting lung disease. The initiating problem in these patients is often a primary respiratory illness or a disorder of another organ system, complicated by major respiratory problems.

This chapter presents an overview of the problem of respiratory failure and discusses the different pathophysiologic types and consequences of respiratory insufficiency. Chapter 28 deals with a specific form of acute respiratory failure known as the acute respiratory distress syndrome, which does not require the presence of preexisting lung disease. Finally, Chapter 29 considers some principles of management of respiratory failure as well as specific modalities of current therapy.

DEFINITION OF RESPIRATORY FAILURE

Arterial blood gas criteria for respiratory failure: $Po_2 < 60$ torr or $Pco_2 > 50$ torr.

Respiratory failure is probably best defined as inability of the respiratory system to maintain adequate gas-exchange. Exactly where to draw the line for adequate gas-exchange is somewhat arbitrary, but in the previously normal individual an arterial Po_2 lower than 60 torr or a Pco_2 greater than 50 torr can be considered evidence for acute respiratory failure. In the individual with preexisting lung disease, the situation is even more complicated, because the patient chronically has impaired gas-exchange and abnormal blood gas values.

For example, it would not be unusual for a patient with significant chronic obstructive lung disease to perform daily activities with a Po_2 of perhaps 60 torr and a Pco_2 of 50 to 55 torr. By the blood gas criteria just mentioned, this patient is always in respiratory failure, but the condition is obviously chronic, not acute. A look at the patient's pH value shows that the kidneys have compensated for the CO_2 retention and that the pH is not far from the normal value of 7.40.

At what point is the condition called acute respiratory failure? Certainly, if an acute respiratory illness such as an acute pneumonia develops, the patient's gas-exchange becomes even worse. The Po_2 falls further and the Pco_2 may rise even higher. In this case, acute respiratory failure is defined as a significant change from the patient's base-line gas-exchange status. If the patient's usual arterial blood gases are known, the task is easier. If the blood gases are not known, the pH value can provide a clue about whether the patient's CO_2 retention is acute or chronic. When a patient is seen initially with a Pco_2 of 70 torr, the implications are quite different if the accompanying pH value is 7.15 as opposed to 7.36.

CLASSIFICATION OF ACUTE RESPIRATORY FAILURE

Hypoxemic Type

Categories of acute respiratory failure are the following:
1. Hypoxemic (with normal or low Pco_2)
2. Hypercapnic/hypoxemic

Examples of hypoxemic respiratory failure are the following:
1. Severe pneumonia
2. ARDS

In practice, it is most convenient to classify acute respiratory failure into two major categories, based on the pattern of gas-exchange abnormalities.

In the first category, hypoxemia is the major problem; the patient's Pco_2 is normal or even low. This condition is the hypoxemic variety of acute respiratory failure. As an example, localized diseases of the pulmonary parenchyma, such as pneumonia, can result in this type of respiratory failure, if the disease is sufficiently severe. However, an even broader group of etiologic factors causes hypoxemic respiratory failure by means of a generalized increase in fluid within the alveolar spaces, often as a result of leakage of fluid from pulmonary capillaries. The latter problem is frequently called the *acute respiratory distress syndrome* (ARDS) and can be the consequence of a wide variety of disorders that cause an increase in pulmonary capillary permeability.* Because of the importance of this syndrome as a major form of acute respiratory failure, the following chapter focuses entirely on this problem.

*The abbreviation ARDS was formerly used for *adult respiratory distress syndrome*, but "acute" has now generally replaced "adult," because the entity can occur in children as well.

Hypercapnic/Hypoxemic Type

In the second category, hypercapnia is present; for the respiratory failure to be considered acute, the pH must show that there is absent or incomplete metabolic compensation for the respiratory acidosis. From the discussion of alveolar gas composition and the alveolar gas equation in Chapter 1, it is apparent that hypercapnia is associated with a decreased arterial P_{O_2} because of an altered alveolar P_{O_2}. Therefore, even if ventilation and perfusion are relatively well matched and the fraction of blood shunted across the pulmonary vasculature is not increased, the arterial P_{O_2} falls in the presence of hypercapnia. In fact, many cases of hypercapnic respiratory failure have marked ventilation-perfusion mismatch occurring as well, which further accentuates the hypoxemia. With these concepts in mind, it is clear that the hypercapnic form of respiratory failure generally involves not just hypercapnia but rather may be more appropriately considered the hypercapnic/hypoxemic form of respiratory failure.

A number of types of respiratory disease are potentially associated with this second form of respiratory failure. A subsequent section of this chapter explains exactly how the various disorders result in hypercapnic/hypoxemic respiratory failure. These disorders primarily include: (1) depression of the neurologic system responsible for respiratory control, (2) disease of the respiratory bellows, either the chest wall or the neuromuscular apparatus responsible for thoracic expansion, and (3) chronic obstructive lung disease. It is also quite common for more than one of these three factors to be present, thus compounding the potential for respiratory insufficiency.

In the hypercapnic/hypoxemic form of respiratory failure, patients often have preexisting disease that is responsible either for chronic respiratory insufficiency or for limitations in respiratory reserve sufficient to make them much more susceptible to decompensation with an acute superimposed problem. In common parlance, this form of respiratory failure is called *acute on chronic respiratory failure,* obviously reflecting the prior problems or limitations with respiratory reserve. This expression has been used especially to describe the patient with chronic obstructive pulmonary disease in whom acute respiratory failure develops at the time of an infection or another acute respiratory insult.

> Causes of hypercapnic/ hypoxemic respiratory failure are the following:
> 1. Depression of central nervous system ventilatory control
> 2. Disease of the respiratory bellows
> 3. Chronic obstructive lung disease

PRESENTATION OF GAS-EXCHANGE FAILURE

When acute respiratory failure develops, the patient's symptom complex generally includes the manifestations of hypoxemia or hypercapnia, or both, accompanied by the specific symptoms related to the precipitating disorder. Dyspnea is also present in the majority of cases and is the symptom that often suggests to the physician the possibility of respiratory failure.

Impairment of mental abilities is a frequent result of either hypoxemia or hypercapnia. Patients may become disoriented, confused, and unable to conduct their normal level of activity. With profound hypercapnia, patients may become stuporous and eventually lapse into a frank coma. Headache is commonly found in patients with hypercapnia. Dilation of cerebral blood vessels as a consequence of increased P_{CO_2} probably is an important factor in the pathogenesis of the headache.

Physical findings associated with abnormal gas-exchange are relatively few. Patients may be tachypneic, tachycardic, and restless, findings that are

> Clinical presentation with respiratory failure consists of the following:
> 1. Dyspnea
> 2. Impaired mental status
> 3. Headache
> 4. Tachycardia
> 5. Papilledema (with ↑ P_{CO_2})
> 6. Variable findings on lung examination
> 7. Cyanosis (with severe hypoxemia)

relatively nonspecific. Examination of the optic fundus may show papilledema (an elevation of the optic disk) resulting from hypercapnia, cerebral vasodilation, and an increase in pressure at the back of the eye. Findings in the lung are related to the specific form of disease that is present—for example, wheezing and/or rhonchi in chronic obstructive lung disease, or crackles as a result of fluid in the small airways and alveolar spaces. When hypoxemia is severe, patients may become cyanotic, which is apparent as a dusky or bluish hue to the nail beds and the lips.

PATHOGENESIS OF GAS-EXCHANGE ABNORMALITIES

The basic principles of abnormal gas-exchange were discussed in Chapter 1; the focus here is on application of these principles to patients with respiratory failure. A discussion of hypoxemic respiratory failure is followed by a discussion of hypercapnic/hypoxemic failure.

Hypoxemic Respiratory Failure

In the patient with hypoxemic respiratory failure, two major pathophysiologic factors contribute to the lowering of arterial PO_2: ventilation-perfusion mismatch and shunting. In the patient with significant ventilation-perfusion mismatch, regions having a low ventilation-to-perfusion ratio contribute relatively desaturated blood to the systemic circulation. What sorts of problems cause ventilation to be decreased relative to perfusion in a particular region of lung? If an alveolus or a group of alveoli is partially filled with fluid, then a limited amount of ventilation reaches that particular area, whereas perfusion to the region may remain relatively preserved. Similarly, if an airway supplying a region of lung is diseased, either by pathology affecting the airway wall or by secretions occupying the lumen, then ventilation is again limited.

When these problems become extreme, ventilation to a region of lung may be totally absent, so that a true shunt exists. For example, alveoli may be completely filled with fluid, or an airway may be completely obstructed, preventing any ventilation to the involved area. Although the response of the pulmonary vasculature is to constrict and thereby limit perfusion to an underventilated or a nonventilated portion of the lung, this protective mechanism often cannot compensate fully for the loss of ventilation, and hypoxemia results.

As will be discussed in Chapter 28, alveolar filling with fluid and the collapse of small airways and alveoli seem to be the main pathogenetic features leading to ventilation-perfusion mismatch and shunting in ARDS. An earlier consideration of the ability of supplemental O_2 to raise the PO_2 in conditions of ventilation-perfusion mismatch versus shunt indicated that O_2 is unable to improve the PO_2 significantly for truly shunted blood (see Chapter 1). Therefore, when the shunt fraction of the cardiac output is quite high, oxygenation may be helped surprisingly little by the administration of supplemental O_2.

Despite the marked derangement of oxygenation in ARDS, CO_2 elimination typically remains adequate, because the patients are able to maintain alveolar ventilation at an acceptable level. Even when there are regions of lung that have a high ventilation-perfusion ratio and thus effectively act as dead space, the patients are generally able to compensate by increasing their overall minute ventilation.

Hypercapnic/Hypoxemic Respiratory Failure

In the hypercapnic form of respiratory failure, patients are unable to maintain a level of alveolar ventilation sufficient to eliminate CO_2 and to keep arterial P_{CO_2} within the normal range. Because ventilation is determined by a sequence of events ranging from the generation of impulses by the respiratory controller to the movement of air through the airways, there are several stages at which problems can adversely affect total minute ventilation. This sequence is shown in Figure 27-1, which also lists some of the disorders that can interfere at each level. Not only is the total ventilation per minute important; the "effectiveness" of the ventilation for CO_2 excretion—that is, the relative amount of alveolar versus dead space ventilation—is also important to ensure proper utilization of inspired gas. If the proportion of each breath going to dead space (i.e., the V_D/V_T ratio) increases substantially, then alveolar ventilation may fall to a level sufficient to cause an elevated P_{CO_2}, even if total minute ventilation is preserved.

In the hypercapnic form of respiratory failure, hypoventilation also leads to a decrease in alveolar P_{O_2}. Thus, arterial P_{O_2} may fall even if ventilation-perfusion matching and gas-exchange at the alveolar level are well maintained. In practice, however, many of the diseases associated with alveolar hypoventilation, ranging from neuromuscular and chest wall disease to chronic airflow obstruction, are accompanied by significant ventilation-perfusion mismatch. Therefore, these patients generally have two major reasons for hypoxemia—hypoventilation and ventilation-perfusion mismatch. Interestingly, true shunts usually play a very limited role in causing hypoxemia in these disorders, unlike the situation in ARDS.

Given the causes of hypoxemia in the hypercapnic/hypoxemic form of respiratory failure, patients frequently respond to supplemental O_2 with a substantial rise in arterial P_{O_2}. However, most of these patients have at least mild chronic CO_2 retention, with their acute respiratory failure due to some precipitating insult or to worsening of their underlying disease. As mentioned in Chapter 18, administration of supplemental O_2 to these chronically

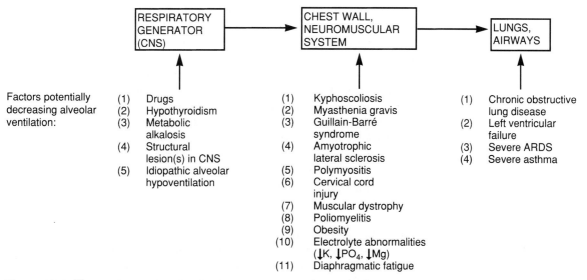

Figure 27-1 ▬— Levels at which there may be interference with normal ventilation, giving rise to alveolar hypoventilation. Factors contributing to decreased ventilation are listed under each level.

hypercapnic patients may lead to a further increase in arterial P_{CO_2}, based on a number of pathophysiologic reasons. With judicious use of supplemental O_2, substantial additional elevation of arterial P_{CO_2} can usually be avoided.

An elaboration of further features of the hypercapnic/hypoxemic form of respiratory failure follows.

CLINICAL AND THERAPEUTIC ASPECTS OF HYPERCAPNIC/HYPOXEMIC RESPIRATORY FAILURE

Whether the underlying disease is chest wall disease, such as kyphoscoliosis, or chronic obstructive lung disease, this type of respiratory failure often develops in patients who already have some degree of chronic respiratory insufficiency. This is not true of all cases, however, because there are certain neurologic problems, such as Guillain-Barré syndrome, in which hypercapnic respiratory failure occurs in a previously normal individual.

When the patient has chronic disease upon which acute respiratory failure is superimposed, the phrase "acute on chronic respiratory failure" is frequently used, as mentioned earlier. In such cases there is often a specific additional problem that precipitates the acute deterioration, and it is important to identify the problem if at all possible.

What are some of the intercurrent problems or factors that precipitate acute respiratory failure in these patients? Perhaps the most common is an acute respiratory tract infection, such as bronchitis, usually but not always due to a virus. Bacterial causes must always be investigated, however, because they are often amenable to specific therapy. Use of drugs that suppress the respiratory center, such as sedatives or narcotics, may also precipitate hypercapnic respiratory failure by virtue of depressing central respiratory drive in a person whose condition was previously marginal. Other intercurrent problems include congestive heart failure, pulmonary emboli, and exposure to environmental pollutants, each of which may be sufficient to induce further CO_2 retention in the patient with previously borderline compensation.

The general therapeutic approach to these patients involves three main areas: (1) support of gas-exchange, (2) treatment of the acute precipitating event, and (3) treatment of the underlying pulmonary disease. Support of gas-exchange involves maintaining adequate oxygenation and elimination of CO_2, problems to be discussed in more detail in Chapter 29. Briefly, supplemental O_2, generally in a concentration not much higher than that found in ambient air, is administered to raise the P_{O_2} to an acceptable level, i.e., greater than 60 torr. If CO_2 elimination deteriorates much beyond the usual level of P_{CO_2}, then an acute respiratory acidosis is superimposed on the patient's usual acid-base status. If significant acidemia develops or if the patient's mental status changes significantly as a result of CO_2 retention, then some form of ventilatory assistance, either intubation and mechanical ventilation or noninvasive assisted ventilation with a mask, may be required.

Treating the precipitating factor for acute respiratory failure is most successful when bacterial infection or congestive heart failure is responsible for the acute deterioration. Antibiotics for suspected bacterial infection, or diuretics and afterload reduction for congestive heart failure, are appropriate forms of therapy in these circumstances. For patients in whom respiratory secretions seem to be playing a role either chronically or in an acute exacerbation of their disease, attempts to assist in clearance of secretions may be

Frequent precipitants for acute on chronic respiratory failure are the following:

1. Respiratory tract infection
2. Drugs, e.g., sedatives, narcotics
3. Congestive heart failure
4. Less common: pulmonary emboli, exposure to environmental pollutants

beneficial. In particular, chest physical therapy, in which percussion and vibration of the chest are performed, followed by appropriate positioning to assist gravity in drainage of secretions, may sometimes be beneficial.

Treatment of the underlying pulmonary disease depends on the nature of the disease. For patients with obstructive lung disease, intensive therapy with bronchodilators and sometimes corticosteroids may be helpful in reversing whatever component of bronchoconstriction is present. If neuromuscular or chest wall disease is the underlying problem, then therapy is sometimes available, as is the case with myasthenia gravis. Unfortunately, for many neuromuscular or chest wall diseases, no specific form of therapy exists, and support of gas-exchange and treatment of any precipitating factors are the major modes of therapy.

When patients with irreversible chest wall or neuromuscular disease are in frank respiratory failure, they may require some form of ventilatory assistance on a chronic basis. Although the modalities for chronic ventilatory support are discussed in Chapter 29, it is important to realize here that the primary decision is whether chronic ventilatory support should be given to a patient with this type of irreversible disease. In many cases the joint decision of the patient, the family, and the physician is that life should not be prolonged with chronic ventilator support, given the projected poor quality of life and the irreversible nature of the process.

References

General

Bone RC (ed.): Symposium on respiratory failure. Med Clin North Am 67:55-746, 1983.
Greene KE and Peters JI: Pathophysiology of acute respiratory failure. Clin Chest Med 15:1-12, 1994.
Krachman S and Criner GJ: Hypoventilation syndromes. Clin Chest Med 19:139-155, 1998.
Weinberger SE, Schwartzstein RM, and Weiss JW: Hypercapnia. N Engl J Med 321:1223-1231, 1989.
Younes M: Mechanisms of ventilatory failure. *In* Tierney DF (ed): Current Pulmonology, vol. 14. St. Louis, Mosby-Year Book, 1993, pp 243-292.
Zwillich C, Kryger M, and Weil J: Hypoventilation: consequences and management. Adv Intern Med 23:287-306, 1978.

Respiratory Failure in Obstructive Lung Disease

Aubier M et al: Effects of the administration of O_2 on ventilation and blood gases in patients with chronic obstructive pulmonary disease during acute respiratory failure. Am Rev Respir Dis 122:747-754, 1980.
Bone RC, Pierce AK, and Johnson RL Jr: Controlled oxygen administration in acute respiratory failure in chronic obstructive pulmonary disease. Am J Med 65:896-902, 1978.
Davidson AC: Critical care management of respiratory failure resulting from COPD. Thorax 57:1079-1084, 2002.
Derenne J-P, Fleury B, and Pariente R: Acute respiratory failure of chronic obstructive pulmonary disease. Am Rev Respir Dis 138:1006-1033, 1988.
Phipps P and Garrard CS: Acute severe asthma in the intensive care unit. Thorax 58:81-88, 2003.

Respiratory Failure in Neuromuscular and Chest Wall Disease

Bergofsky EH: Respiratory failure in disorders of the thoracic cage. Am Rev Respir Dis 119:643-669, 1979.
Gracey DR, Divertie MB, and Howard FM Jr: Mechanical ventilation for respiratory failure in myasthenia gravis. Mayo Clin Proc 58:597-602, 1983.
Gracey DR, McMichan JC, Divertie MB, and Howard FM Jr: Respiratory failure in Guillain-Barré syndrome. Mayo Clin Proc 57:742-746, 1982.
Shneerson JM and Simonds AK: Noninvasive ventilation for chest wall and neuromuscular disorders. Eur Respir J 20:480-487, 2002.

Acute Respiratory Distress Syndrome

The continuation of our discussion of respiratory failure proceeds with more detailed consideration of one important type of acute respiratory failure—the *acute respiratory distress syndrome,* or *ARDS.* Although this entity has commonly been called the "adult respiratory distress syndrome," it is not limited to adults, and therefore "acute" is now considered preferable to "adult" in the naming of this syndrome. ARDS represents a major form of hypoxemic respiratory failure; its clinical and pathophysiologic features differ considerably from those noted for acute on chronic respiratory failure.

Rather than a specific disease, ARDS is truly a syndrome, resulting from any of a number of etiologic factors. It is perhaps simplest to consider this syndrome as the nonspecific result of acute injury to the lung, characterized by breakdown of the normal barrier that prevents leakage of fluid out of the pulmonary capillaries and into the interstitium and alveolar spaces. Another term, *acute lung injury* (ALI), is formally used to describe a similar process of lung injury in which the disturbance in oxygenation is less severe, whereas ARDS represents the more severe end of the spectrum. A number of other names have also been used to describe ARDS, including noncardiogenic pulmonary edema, shock lung, and post-traumatic pulmonary insufficiency, just to name a few.

In this chapter, the first consideration is the dynamics of fluid transfer between the pulmonary vessels and the alveolar interstitium, since an alteration in this process is so important in the pathogenesis of ARDS. Next, an outline of the many types of injury that can result in ARDS is accompanied by some of the theories proposed to explain how such a diverse group of disorders can produce this syndrome. A discussion of the pathologic, pathophysiologic, and clinical consequences then follows. Finally, a general approach to treatment concludes the chapter; however, more specific details about support of gas-exchange are presented in Chapter 29.

PHYSIOLOGY OF FLUID MOVEMENT IN THE ALVEOLAR INTERSTITIUM

Despite the diverse group of disorders that can cause ARDS, the net result of this syndrome is the same: a disturbance in the normal barrier that limits leakage of fluid out of the pulmonary capillaries and into the pulmonary parenchyma. Before a discussion of some of the theories explaining how this barrier is damaged, a brief consideration of the determinants of fluid transport between the pulmonary vessels, the interstitial space, and the alveolar lumen may be helpful. For this purpose, we can view the pulmonary parenchyma, as shown in Figure 28-1, consisting of (1) small vessels coursing through the alveolar walls, which for simplicity's sake we will refer to as the pulmonary capillaries; (2) the pulmonary capillary endothelium, the lining cells that normally limit but do not completely prevent fluid movement out of the capillaries; (3) the pulmonary interstitium, which for our purposes here refers to the alveolar wall exclusive of vessels and the epithelial cells lining the alveolar lumen; (4) lymphatic channels, which are found largely in perivascular connective tissue in the lung; (5) alveolar epithelial cells, lining the surface of the alveolar lumen; and (6) the alveolar lumen or alveolar space.

Movement of fluid out of the pulmonary capillaries and into the interstitial space is determined by a number of factors, including the hydrostatic pressures in the vessels and in the pulmonary interstitium, the colloid osmotic pressures in these same two compartments, and the permeability of the

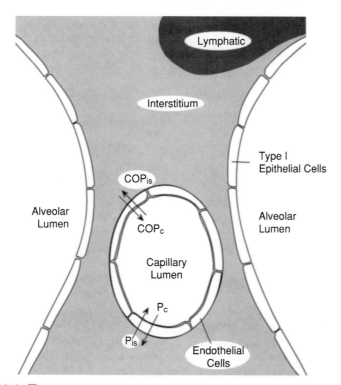

Figure 28-1 ■— Schematic diagram of lung's gas-exchanging region. Forces governing fluid movement between pulmonary capillary lumen and alveolar interstitium are shown. P_c = pulmonary capillary hydrostatic pressure; P_{is} = interstitial space hydrostatic pressure; COP_c = pulmonary capillary colloid osmotic pressure; COP_{is} = interstitial space colloid osmotic pressure. Arrows show direction of fluid movement favored by each of the important forces. Lymphatic vessels are located in perivascular connective tissue rather than within alveolar walls.

endothelium. The effect of these factors in determining fluid transport is summarized in the Starling equation, examined earlier in Chapter 15 with regard to fluid transport across the pleural space. This equation is reproduced again as Equation 28-1:

$$F = K[(P_c - P_{is}) - \sigma(COP_c - COP_{is})]$$

where F = fluid movement; P_c and P_{is} = pulmonary capillary and interstitial hydrostatic pressures; COP_c and COP_{is} = pulmonary capillary and interstitial colloid osmotic (oncotic) pressures; K = the filtration coefficient; and σ = the reflection coefficient (a measure of the permeability of the endothelium for protein).

Fluid normally moves from the pulmonary capillaries to the interstitial space; resorption by lymphatics prevents accumulation.

If we substitute an estimate of the actual numbers for normal hydrostatic and oncotic pressures in Equation 28-1, we find that F is a positive number, indicating that fluid normally moves out of the pulmonary capillaries and into the interstitial space. Even though the rate of fluid movement out of the pulmonary capillaries is estimated to be approximately 20 mL/hr, this fluid does not accumulate; the lymphatic vessels are quite effective in absorbing both protein and fluid that have left the vasculature and entered the interstitial space. However, if fluid movement into the interstitium increases substantially or if lymphatic drainage is impeded, then fluid accumulates within the interstitial space, resulting in interstitial edema. When sufficient fluid accumulates or when the alveolar epithelium is damaged, fluid also moves across the epithelial cell barrier and into the alveolar spaces, resulting in alveolar edema.

Two Mechanisms of Fluid Accumulation

In practice, the forces described in the Starling equation become altered in two main ways, producing interstitial and often alveolar edema (Table 28-1). The first occurs when hydrostatic pressure within the pulmonary capillaries (P_c) is increased, generally as a consequence of elevated left ventricular or left atrial pressures (e.g., in left ventricular failure or mitral stenosis). The resulting pulmonary edema is called *cardiogenic* or *hydrostatic* pulmonary edema, and the cause is essentially an imbalance between the hydrostatic and oncotic forces governing fluid movement. In this form of edema, the permeability barrier that limits movement of protein out of the intravascular space is intact, and the fluid that leaks out has a very low protein content.

In the second mechanism by which fluid accumulates, hydrostatic pressures are normal, but the permeability of the capillary endothelial and alveolar epithelial barriers is increased as a result of damage to one or both of these cell populations. Movement of proteins out of the intravascular space now occurs as a consequence of the increase in permeability. The fluid that leaks out has a relatively high protein content, often close to that found in plasma.

Table 28-1		
Categories of Pulmonary Edema		
Feature	**Cardiogenic**	**Noncardiogenic**
Major causes	Left ventricular failure, mitral stenosis	ARDS
Pulmonary capillary pressure	Increased	Normal
Pulmonary capillary permeability	Normal	Increased
Protein content of edema fluid	Low	High

This second mechanism is the one operative in ARDS. Since an elevation in pulmonary capillary pressure from cardiac disease is not involved, this form of edema is called *noncardiogenic* pulmonary edema.

Although cardiogenic and hydrostatic pulmonary edema are mentioned here, subsequent parts of this chapter focus on noncardiogenic edema, i.e., ARDS. However, it is important to remember that even patients with a permeability defect of their pulmonary capillary bed can simultaneously have high pulmonary capillary pressure as a result of coincidental left ventricular failure. In these cases, both a permeability defect and the elevated hydrostatic pressure contribute to leakage of fluid out of the pulmonary vasculature. Not only is the fluid leak compounded; when both factors are involved, it is often quite difficult to sort out the relative importance of each.

ETIOLOGY

As can be seen from Table 28-2, numerous and varied disorders are associated with the potential to produce ARDS. What these diverse etiologic factors in ARDS have in common is their ability to cause diffuse injury to the pulmonary parenchyma. Beyond that, it is difficult on the basis of our present knowledge to define other features linking the underlying causes. Even the route of injury varies. Some etiologic factors involve inhaled injurious agents; others appear to mediate their effects on the lung via the circulation rather than the airway.

Inhaled Injurious Agents

Numerous injurious agents that reach the pulmonary parenchyma through the airway have now been identified. In some cases, a liquid is responsible; examples include gastric contents, salt or fresh water, and hydrocarbons. With acid gastric contents, especially when the pH is lower than 2.5, patients sustain a "chemical burn" to the pulmonary parenchyma, resulting in damage to the

Table	28-2		
Causes of Diffuse Alveolar Damage and the Acute Respiratory Distress Syndrome			
Aspiration		Disseminated intravascular coagulation	
Gastric contents		Embolism	
Salt/fresh water (near drowning)		Fat embolism	
Hydrocarbons		Amniotic fluid embolism	
Toxic gas inhalation		Drugs	
Nitrogen dioxide (NO_2)		Narcotics	
Smoke		Sedatives	
Ammonia		Aspirin (rare)	
Phosgene		Thiazides (rare)	
Diffuse pneumonia		Multiple transfusions	
Viral		Pancreatitis	
Bacterial		Neurogenic	
Pneumocystis carinii		Head trauma	
Sepsis		Intracranial hemorrhage	
Shock (accompanied by other etiologic		Seizures	
factors)		*Mechanical ventilation (overdistention and/or	
Trauma		cyclic opening and closing of alveoli)	

*Generally not a primary cause of ARDS, but a potential secondary contributor to alveolar damage (see Chapter 29).

alveolar epithelium. In the case of near drowning, in either fresh or salt water, not only does the inhaled water fill alveolar spaces, but also secondary damage to the alveolar-capillary barrier causes fluid to leak from the pulmonary vasculature. Since salt water is hypertonic to plasma, it is capable of drawing fluid from the circulation as a result of an osmotic pressure gradient. Fresh water, on the other hand, is hypotonic to plasma and to cellular contents and thus may enter pulmonary parenchymal cells with resulting cellular edema. In addition, fresh water appears to inactivate surfactant, a complicating factor that will shortly be discussed in more detail. Finally, aspirated hydrocarbons can be quite toxic to the distal parenchyma, perhaps also in part because they inactivate surfactant and cause significant changes in surface tension.

A number of inhaled gases have been identified as potential acute toxins and precipitants of ARDS. Nitrogen dioxide is one example, as are some chemical products of combustion inhaled in smoke. High concentrations of oxygen, particularly when given for a prolonged period of time, have also been considered to contribute to alveolar injury. The mechanism of O_2 toxicity is believed to be generation of free radicals and superoxide anions, byproducts of oxidative metabolism that are toxic to pulmonary epithelial and endothelial cells. It is ironic that O_2 can contribute to lung injury, since it is so important in the supportive treatment of this syndrome. In patients requiring high concentrations of supplemental O_2 to maintain an adequate Po_2, the therapy itself may therefore compound the problem by furthering cellular damage and increasing alveolar-capillary permeability. In Chapter 29, we will discuss an additional way in which the treatment of ARDS may potentially worsen alveolar damage, through overdistention and/or cyclic opening and closing of alveoli induced by mechanical ventilation.

Infectious agents may also produce injury via airway access to the pulmonary parenchyma. Perhaps the most common and important example in recent years has been pneumonia due to *Pneumocystis carinii* in patients with AIDS. Another important example is viral pneumonia, which has the capability of damaging parenchymal cells and altering alveolar-capillary permeability.

Injury via the Pulmonary Circulation

For those causes of ARDS that do not involve inhaled agents or toxins, it has been presumed that the pulmonary circulation in some way initiates the injury. However, in most cases a specific circulating factor has not been identified with certainty, even though several possibilities have been proposed. One of the most common precipitants for ARDS is sepsis, in which microorganisms or their products (especially endotoxin) circulating through the blood stream can initiate a sequence of events resulting in toxicity to parenchymal cells.

Although the term *shock lung* has been used in the past for ARDS, the presence of hypotensive shock alone is probably not sufficient for the development of ARDS. Patients in whom ARDS develops seemingly as a result of hypotension usually have complicating potential etiologic factors (e.g., trauma, sepsis) or have received therapy (e.g., blood transfusions) also capable of cellular damage.

In patients with a coagulation disorder known as *disseminated intravascular coagulation* (DIC), there also appears to be the potential for development of ARDS. In DIC, patients have ongoing activation of both the clotting mechanism and the protective fibrinolytic system that prevents clot formation and propagation. Like ARDS, DIC is also a syndrome and can occur for a variety of primary or underlying reasons. However, it is not entirely clear how ARDS and DIC are related. Although there is frequently an association between these two problems, whether and exactly how one causes the other remain uncertain.

When fat or amniotic fluid enters the circulation, the material is transported to the lung, resulting in the clinical problems of fat embolism and amniotic fluid embolism, respectively. Presumably, these materials are directly toxic to endothelial cells of the pulmonary capillaries, and they certainly have been associated with the development of ARDS.

A variety of drugs, many of which fall into the class of narcotics, are potential causes of ARDS. In most cases an overdose of the drug has been taken, although this is not always the situation. One of the agents most frequently recognized has been heroin, and the name "heroin pulmonary edema" sometimes is used. In addition to heroin and other narcotics, several other drugs have been described as occasionally causing ARDS, including even aspirin and thiazide diuretics. Although the problem of drug-induced pulmonary edema has been well described, the mechanism by which it occurs is not at all certain.

In some patients with acute pancreatitis, a clinical picture consistent with noncardiogenic pulmonary edema develops. In this situation, it has been proposed that enzymes released into the circulation from the damaged pancreas may directly injure pulmonary parenchymal cells or initiate other indirect pathways, resulting in injury.

Finally, certain disorders of the central nervous system, particularly trauma or intracerebral bleeding associated with increased intracranial pressure, are known to be associated with development of ARDS. Similarly, ARDS occasionally occurs after generalized seizures. An interesting and commonly accepted hypothesis to explain this so-called *neurogenic pulmonary edema* is that intense sympathetic nervous system discharge in response to intracranial hypertension may produce extremely high pulmonary capillary pressures, resulting in mechanical damage to the endothelium.

PATHOGENESIS

How do these diverse clinical problems all result in the syndrome of increased pulmonary capillary permeability that we call ARDS? It appears that one important factor is the ability to produce injury to pulmonary capillary endothelial and alveolar epithelial cells (primarily type I epithelial cells, whose cytoplasmic processes provide most of the surface area lining the alveolar walls). Given the wide variety of insults that can damage these cell types, it seems unlikely that a single common mechanism is operative for all kinds of injury.

> The initial injury in ARDS affects alveolar epithelial (type I) or capillary endothelial cells, or both.

In the discussion of some of the specific causes of ARDS, brief mention was made of a few of the theories of pathogenesis for individual disorders. However, it is worthwhile now to consider more generalized theories proposed to explain how epithelial and endothelial cells become damaged, particularly during the course of sepsis. One popular theory revolves around the neutrophil and its potential for releasing products that are toxic to pulmonary parenchymal and capillary endothelial cells.

According to the neutrophil theory, an important role is played by the complement pathway. When complement is activated by sepsis, C5a is released and is responsible for aggregation of neutrophils within the

> Components of the neutrophil theory of ARDS induced by sepsis are the following:
>
> 1. Activation of complement
> 2. Aggregation of neutrophils in pulmonary vasculature
> 3. Release of toxic mediators from neutrophils

pulmonary vasculature. These neutrophils may then release a variety of substances potentially toxic to cellular and noncellular components of the alveolar wall. Superoxide radicals, other byproducts of oxidative metabolism, an array of cytokines, and various proteolytic enzymes can all be released by neutrophils and may be important pathogenetically in producing structural and functional injury to the alveolar wall.

However, several problems have arisen with this hypothesis. Data are available showing that the presence or absence of complement activation in patients with sepsis does not correlate well with subsequent development of lung injury. In addition, a number of cases of ARDS have been described in severely neutropenic patients, suggesting that other mechanisms must be operative. Despite these problems, the neutrophil theory is far from dead. Rather, it is believed to represent just one of many pathways by which acute lung injury may be produced.

Other cells have been implicated as well in the production of lung injury. Foremost among these are macrophages and platelets. A large number of chemical mediators have also been proposed to cause lung injury, either directly or indirectly by means of their effect on cells involved in the inflammatory process. Such mediators include endotoxin, products of arachidonic acid metabolism, and a variety of cytokines such as tumor necrosis factor-α, interleukin (IL)-8, endothelin, and transforming growth factor-β. An inflammatory response can also be augmented by a reduction in anti-inflammatory mediators, including cytokines such as IL-10 and IL-11.

Despite an extensive research effort over the past decade that has attempted to elucidate mechanisms of acute lung injury, we still have a long way to go before we really understand ARDS. Obviously, such an understanding is critical to our eventually being able to develop effective forms of prevention and therapy.

PATHOLOGY

Pathologic features of ARDS are the following:

1. Damage to alveolar type I epithelial cells
2. Interstitial and alveolar fluid
3. Areas of alveolar collapse
4. Inflammatory cell infiltrate
5. Hyperplasia of alveolar type II epithelial cells
6. Hyaline membranes
7. Fibrosis
8. Pulmonary vascular changes

Despite the number of etiologic factors in ARDS, the pathologic findings are relatively similar, no matter what the underlying cause. This pattern of injury accompanying ARDS, as observed by the pathologist, is frequently labeled *diffuse alveolar damage.*

As mentioned earlier, injury to the type I alveolar epithelial cell and the pulmonary capillary endothelial cell appears to be primary in the pathogenesis. Type I epithelial cells frequently appear necrotic and may slough from the surface of the alveolar wall. Damage to the capillary endothelial cells is generally more difficult, if not impossible, to recognize with light microscopy, and electron microscopy may be necessary to see the subtle ultrastructural changes.

Early in the course of ARDS, often called the *exudative phase,* fluid can be seen in the interstitial space of the alveolar septum, as well as in the alveolar lumen. One may see scattered bleeding as well as regions of alveolar collapse, which are at least partly related to inactivation of surfactant (by protein-rich alveolar exudates) and to decreased surfactant production due to injury to alveolar type II epithelial cells. The lung parenchyma also demonstrates an influx of inflammatory cells, both in the interstitial space and often in the alveolar lumen as well. The cellular response is relatively nonspecific, consisting of neutrophils and macrophages. In addition, one may see fibrin and cellular debris located in or around alveoli.

A characteristic finding in the pathology of ARDS is the presence of *hyaline membranes.* These membranes are believed to represent a combination of fibrin, cellular debris, and plasma proteins that are deposited or formed on the alveolar surface. Although they are nonspecific, their presence suggests that alveolar injury and a permeability problem, rather than elevated hydrostatic pressures, are the cause of pulmonary edema.

After approximately 1 to 2 weeks, the exudative phase evolves into a *proliferative phase.* As an important part of the reparative process that occurs during the proliferative phase, alveolar type II epithelial cells replicate in an attempt to replace the damaged type I epithelial cells. These hyperplastic type II epithelial cells often figure quite prominently in the pathologic picture of ARDS.

Another component of the proliferative phase is an accumulation of fibroblasts in the pulmonary parenchyma. In severe and prolonged cases of ARDS, this fibroblastic response becomes particularly important. The consequence is that, in some cases, the damaged lung parenchyma is not repaired but goes on to develop significant scar tissue (fibrosis). Accompanying the fibrosis are often changes in the pulmonary vasculature; these include extensive remodeling and compromise of the lumen of small vessels by intimal and medial proliferation and by microthrombi.

PATHOPHYSIOLOGY

Effects on Gas-Exchange

Most of the clinical consequences of ARDS follow in reasonably logical fashion from the presence of interstitial and alveolar edema. The most striking problem is alveolar flooding, which effectively prevents ventilation of affected alveoli even though perfusion may be relatively preserved. These alveoli, perfused but not ventilated, act as regions in which blood is shunted from the pulmonary arterial to pulmonary venous circulation without ever being oxygenated. As mentioned in Chapter 1, shunting is one of the mechanisms of hypoxemia, and there is perhaps no better example of shunting than in ARDS.

Not only are there regions of true shunting in ARDS, but also there are regions of ventilation-perfusion mismatch. To some extent, this phenomenon results from an uneven distribution of the pathologic process within the lungs. In areas where the interstitium is more edematous or where there is more fluid in alveoli, ventilation is more impaired (even though some ventilation remains) than in areas that have been relatively spared. Changes in blood flow do not necessarily follow the same distribution as do changes in ventilation, and ventilation-perfusion mismatch results.

In addition to the direct effects of interstitial and alveolar fluid on oxygenation, other changes also appear to be secondary to alterations in the production and effectiveness of surfactant. Chapter 8 refers to surfactant as a phospholipid that is responsible for decreasing surface tension and maintaining alveolar patency. When surfactant is absent, as is seen in the respiratory distress syndrome of neonates, there is extensive collapse of alveoli. In ARDS, surfactant production may be adversely affected by injury to alveolar type II epithelial cells. Additionally, evidence suggests that as a result of extensive fluid within the alveoli, surfactant is inactivated and therefore ineffective in preventing alveolar collapse.

In terms of oxygenation, both ventilation-perfusion mismatch (with regions of low ventilation-perfusion ratio) and true shunting (ventilation-

Pathophysiologic features of ARDS are the following:
1. Shunting and $\dot{V}/\dot{Q}$ mismatch
2. Secondary alterations in function of surfactant
3. Increased pulmonary vascular resistance
4. Decreased pulmonary compliance
5. Decreased FRC

perfusion ratio = 0) are responsible for hypoxemia. Insofar as shunting is responsible for the drop in P_{O_2}, supplemental O_2 alone may not be capable of restoring oxygenation to normal. In practice, the P_{O_2} does rise somewhat with administration of 100 percent O_2 but not nearly to the level expected after such high concentrations of O_2. Considering the nature of the problem of ARDS, this response to supplemental O_2 should not strike us as surprising. Oxygen improves whatever component of hypoxemia is due to ventilation-perfusion mismatch, but it is ineffective for true shunting.

On the other hand, the absolute level of ventilation in the patient with ARDS remains intact or even increases. As a result, patients do not typically have difficulty with CO_2 retention, except in terminal stages of the disease or if another underlying pulmonary process is present. Even though substantial amounts of what is effectively dead space may be present (as part of the overall ventilation-perfusion mismatch), the patient is able to increase total ventilation to compensate for the regions of maldistribution.

Changes in the Pulmonary Vasculature

The pulmonary vasculature is also subject to changes resulting from the overall pathologic process. Pulmonary vascular resistance increases, probably for a variety of reasons. Hypoxemia certainly produces vasoconstriction within the pulmonary arterial system, while fluid in the interstitium may increase interstitial pressure, resulting in a decrease in size and an increase in resistance of the small pulmonary vessels. As discussed earlier, the lumen of small vessels may be compromised by microthrombi and by proliferative changes in vessel walls.

One consequence of the pulmonary vascular changes is an alteration in the normal distribution of pulmonary blood flow. Naturally, blood flows preferentially to areas with lower resistance, which do not necessarily correspond to those regions receiving the most ventilation. Hence, ventilation-perfusion mismatch again results, with some areas having high and other areas low ventilation-perfusion ratios.

Effects on the Mechanical Properties of the Lungs

When considering the mechanical properties of the lung in ARDS, it is important for us to note that CT scanning has demonstrated that the distribution of disease is often more heterogeneous than would be expected based on the diffuse changes seen on a chest radiograph. Whereas some regions have been damaged and are quite abnormal, others appear to have been spared from injury. As a result, the alveoli are not diffusely and relatively homogeneously stiffened; rather, there are regions of the lung with significantly diseased alveoli that ventilate poorly or not at all, and other regions with relatively preserved and well-ventilated alveoli. The net result of having fewer effectively "functional" alveoli is that less volume enters the lung for any given inflation pressure, which by definition means that the compliance of the lung is decreased.

The decreased compliance and low FRC in ARDS are not associated with homogeneously affected alveoli, but rather with heterogeneous disease involvement.

The volume of gas contained within the lungs at functional residual capacity (FRC), i.e., the resting end-expiratory position of the lungs, is also significantly decreased. Again, based on the heterogeneity of the pathologic process, the decreased FRC is not due to a uniform decrease in volume over all alveoli, but rather to a group of alveoli containing little or no gas and another group containing a relatively normal volume of gas. The net result is that patients breathe at a much lower overall lung volume than normal, preferentially ventilating those alveoli that are relatively preserved. The typical breathing pattern resulting from these mechanical changes is characterized by rapid but shallow breaths. This type of breathing pattern is inefficient and demands increased energy expenditure by the patient, which probably contributes to the dyspnea that is so characteristic of patients with ARDS.

CLINICAL FEATURES

Since ARDS is a clinical syndrome with many different causes, the clinical picture reflects not only the presence of noncardiogenic pulmonary edema but also the presence of the underlying disease. Our concern here with the respiratory consequences of ARDS, irrespective of the cause, directs our focus to the clinical effects of the syndrome itself rather than to those of the underlying disorder.

After the initial insult, whatever it may be, there generally is a lag of several hours to a day or more before respiratory consequences ensue. In most cases, the first symptom experienced by the patient is dyspnea. At this time, examination often shows the patient to be tachypneic, although the chest radiograph may still not reveal significant findings. However, arterial blood gases reflect a disturbance of oxygenation, often with an increase in the alveolar-arterial O_2 difference ($AaDo_2$). Alveolar ventilation is either normal or more frequently increased, so that Pco_2 is generally low. In the most severe cases, however, alveolar ventilation cannot be maintained, and the Pco_2 rises.

As fluid and protein continue to leak from the vasculature into the interstitial and alveolar spaces, the clinical findings become even more florid. Patients may become extremely dyspneic and tachypneic, and chest examination may now show the presence of rales. Findings on the chest radiograph become grossly abnormal, revealing interstitial and alveolar edema that can be quite extensive. The radiographic aspects of ARDS are discussed further in the following section, Diagnostic Approach.

As a result of our improved ability over the past 30 years to provide respiratory support for these patients, death due to respiratory failure is now relatively uncommon. Rather, the high mortality seen with ARDS, currently estimated to be approximately 30 to 50 percent, is related to the underlying cause (particularly sepsis) or to failure of multiple organ systems in these critically ill patients. In those patients who are fortunate enough to recover, there may be surprisingly few respiratory sequelae that are both serious and permanent. Pulmonary function may return essentially to normal, although sophisticated assessment often shows some relatively subtle abnormalities.

Clinical features of ARDS are the following:
1. Dyspnea, tachypnea
2. Rales
3. ↓ Po_2, normal or ↓ Pco_2, ↑ $AaDo_2$
4. Radiography—interstitial and alveolar edema

DIAGNOSTIC APPROACH

The diagnosis of ARDS is generally based on a combination of clinical and radiographic information (assessment at a macroscopic level) and arterial blood gas values (assessment at a functional level). Although at one time some clinicians and investigators had advocated lung biopsy in patients with presumed ARDS, these procedures were performed primarily for research purposes and never achieved general clinical acceptance.

As mentioned earlier, the chest radiograph in patients with ARDS does not necessarily reveal abnormal findings at the onset of the clinical presentation. However, within a short period of time the evidence of interstitial and alveolar edema generally develops, the latter being the most prominent finding on the radiograph. The edema appears to be diffuse, affecting both lungs relatively symmetrically. As an indication that the fluid is filling alveolar spaces, air bronchograms often appear within the diffuse infiltrates. Unless the patient has prior heart disease and cardiac enlargement that is unrelated to the present problem, the heart size remains normal. A characteristic example of a chest radiograph in a patient with severe ARDS is shown in Figure 3-7.

Arterial blood gas values show hypoxemia and hypocapnia (respiratory alkalosis). If one calculates the AaDO$_2$, it is clear that gas-exchange actually is worse than it appears at first glance, since the alveolar PO$_2$ is elevated as a result of hyperventilation. As the amount of interstitial and alveolar edema increases, oxygenation becomes progressively more abnormal, and severe hypoxemia results. Because true shunting of blood across nonventilated alveoli is important in the pathogenesis of hypoxemia, the PO$_2$ may be relatively unresponsive to the administration of supplemental O$_2$. In order to allow a standardized method for interpreting the PO$_2$ in patients receiving different amounts of supplemental oxygen, it has been accepted that a ratio of PO$_2$ to fractional concentration of inspired oxygen (PaO$_2$/FIO$_2$) less than 200 mm Hg is an appropriate gas-exchange criterion for ARDS, whereas ALI is defined by less severe gas-exchange abnormalities and a PaO$_2$/FIO$_2$ ratio less than 300 mm Hg.

In many cases of ARDS, it has proved useful to obtain a direct measurement of pressures within the pulmonary circulation. This has been facilitated by use of a catheter inserted into a systemic vein and then passed through the right atrium and right ventricle into the pulmonary artery. The relatively easy passage of this catheter (commonly known as a Swan-Ganz catheter) results from a balloon at the tip, which can be inflated with air and then carried along with blood flow through the tricuspid and pulmonic valves into the pulmonary artery. The catheter is then positioned at a point in the pulmonary artery where inflation of the balloon occludes the lumen and prevents forward flow. Consequently, if pressure is measured at the tip of the catheter when forward flow has been prevented, the measured pressure is theoretically a reflection of pressure in the pulmonary capillaries. The pressure measured with the balloon inflated is commonly called the *pulmonary capillary wedge* (PCW) or *pulmonary artery occlusion pressure.*

A pulmonary artery (Swan-Ganz) catheter can measure pulmonary vascular pressures and cardiac output.

Using measurement of pressure within the pulmonary capillary system, we can distinguish whether the observed pulmonary edema is cardiogenic or noncardiogenic in origin. In cardiogenic pulmonary edema, the hydrostatic pressure within the pulmonary capillaries is high as a result of "back pressure" from the pulmonary veins and left atrium. On the other hand, in noncardiogenic pulmonary edema or ARDS, the pressure within the pulmonary capillary system, measured as the PCW pressure, is normal, indicating that the interstitial and alveolar fluid results from increased permeability of the pulmonary capillaries, not from high intravascular pressure.

Although use of these catheters in measurement of intravascular pressures is not essential to the diagnosis of ARDS, the information obtained may be useful for determining whether high intravascular pressures are contributing to the observed pulmonary edema. In addition, the catheters often provide helpful information during the course of the complicated management of these cases.

TREATMENT

Management of ARDS centers on three main issues: (1) treatment of the precipitating disorder; (2) interruption of, or interference with, the pathogenetic sequence of events involved in development of the capillary leak; and (3) support of gas-exchange until the pulmonary process improves. Although treatment of the precipitating disorder is not always possible or successful, the principle is relatively simple: as long as the underlying problem persists, the pulmonary capillary leak may remain. In the case of a disorder such as sepsis, management of the infection with appropriate antibiotics (and drainage, if necessary) is crucial in allowing the pulmonary vasculature to regain the normal permeability barrier for protein and fluid.

Approaches aimed at altering the pathogenetic sequence of events in ARDS have focused on developing agents to block the effect of various cytokines or other mediators, such as endotoxin, in patients with septic shock. However, to date, this approach has been unsuccessful, and no agents blocking the effect of a particular mediator have yet been found to be useful. A more nonspecific approach has been to use corticosteroids in an attempt to block a variety of mediators and to control or reverse the capillary permeability defect allowing fluid and protein to leak into the interstitium and alveolar spaces. This approach is based in part on experimental evidence suggesting that steroids inhibit aggregation of neutrophils induced by activated complement. However, because of disappointing clinical results and the potential for harmful effects, corticosteroids are now generally not considered appropriately indicated for treatment of ARDS, at least early in its course. Limited data have suggested that steroids may be useful if administered during the proliferative phase of ARDS, but further studies are needed to confirm their efficacy.

Meticulous supportive management, particularly support of gas-exchange, is critical for patients with ARDS to survive the acute illness. Given the life-threatening nature of ARDS, patients are typically intubated, ventilated with a mechanical ventilator, and managed in an intensive care unit. Failure of other organ systems besides the respiratory system is common, and these patients often present some of the most complex and challenging management problems handled in intensive care units. Because of the importance of mechanical ventilation and ventilatory support in the management of respiratory failure associated with ARDS and with other disorders, we have devoted the next and final chapter of this book, Chapter 29, to a more detailed consideration of mechanical ventilation in the management of respiratory failure.

Finally, since the mortality of ARDS remains considerable, a variety of newer and experimental forms of therapy have been tried. For example, one interesting approach has been the use of inhaled nitric oxide as a selective pulmonary vasodilator. By producing preferential vasodilation in those areas of the lung that are well ventilated (because these are the areas to which the gas is delivered), inhaled nitric oxide can facilitate better perfusion of well-ventilated areas, leading to better $\dot{V}/\dot{Q}$ matching and improved oxygenation. Unfortunately, however, beneficial physiologic effects on gas-exchange have not been accompanied by improved survival in clinical trials conducted to date. In contrast, administration of human recombinant activated protein C, which has both antithrombotic and anti-inflammatory effects, has been shown in at least one large study to improve survival of patients with severe sepsis, one of the common forerunners of ARDS, but more experience with its use is needed before its overall role in severe sepsis complicated by ARDS is fully established.

References

General Reviews

Atabai K and Matthay MA: Acute lung injury and the acute respiratory distress syndrome: definitions and epidemiology. Thorax 57:452-458, 2002.

Bernard GR et al: The American-European consensus conference on ARDS: definitions, mechanisms, relevant outcomes, and clinical trial coordination. Am J Respir Crit Care Med 149:818-824, 1994.

Fulkerson WF, MacIntyre N, Stamler J, and Crapo JD: Pathogenesis and treatment of the adult respiratory distress syndrome. Arch Intern Med 156:29-38, 1996.

Ware LB and Matthay MA: The acute respiratory distress syndrome. N Engl J Med 342:1334-1349, 2000.

Wiedemann HF and Matthay MA (eds): Acute respiratory distress syndrome. Clin Chest Med 21:401-616, 2000.

Wyncoll DLA and Evans TW: Acute respiratory distress syndrome. Lancet 354:497-501, 1999.

Pathogenesis

Bellingan GJ: The pathogenesis of ALI/ARDS. Thorax 57:540-546, 2002.

Canonico AE and Brigham KL: Biology of acute injury. In Crystal RG, West JB, Weibel ER, and Barnes PJ (eds): The Lung: Scientific Foundations, 2nd ed. Philadelphia, Lippincott-Raven, 1997, pp 2475-2498.

Gattinoni L et al: Lung structure and function in different stages of severe adult respiratory distress syndrome. JAMA 271:1772-1779, 1994.

Parsons PE: Mediators and mechanisms of acute lung injury. Clin Chest Med 21:467-476, 2000.

Pittet JF et al: Biological markers of acute lung injury: prognostic and pathogenetic significance. Am J Respir Crit Care Med 155:1187-1205, 1997.

Sassler CN, Bloomfield GL, and Fowler AA III: Current concepts of sepsis and acute lung injury. Clin Chest Med 17:213-235, 1996.

Swank DW and Moore SB: Roles of the neutrophil and other mediators in adult respiratory distress syndrome. Mayo Clin Proc 64:1118-1132, 1989.

Swensen ER et al: Pathogenesis of high-altitude pulmonary edema. Inflammation is not an etiologic factor. JAMA 287:2228-2235, 2002.

Treatment

Anzueto A et al: Aerosolized surfactant in adults with sepsis-induced acute respiratory distress syndrome. N Engl J Med 334:1417-1421, 1996.

Bernard GR et al: Efficacy and safety of recombinant human activated protein C for severe sepsis. N Engl J Med 344:699-709, 2001.

Brower RG, Ware LB, Berthiaume Y, and Matthay MA: Treatment of ARDS. Chest 120:1347-1367, 2001.

Cranshaw J, Griffiths MJD, and Evans TW: Non-ventilatory strategies in ARDS. Thorax 57:823-829, 2002.

Meduri GU et al: Corticosteroid rescue treatment of progressive fibroproliferation in late ARDS. Chest 105:1516-1527, 1994.

Rossaint R et al: Inhaled nitric oxide for the adult respiratory distress syndrome. N Engl J Med 328:399-405, 1993.

Management of Respiratory Failure

GOALS OF SUPPORTIVE THERAPY FOR GAS-EXCHANGE	Complications of Mechanical Ventilation
MAINTENANCE OF CARBON DIOXIDE ELIMINATION	Noninvasive Ventilatory Support for Acute Respiratory Failure
MAINTENANCE OF OXYGENATION	**SELECTED ASPECTS OF THERAPY FOR CHRONIC RESPIRATORY FAILURE**
REDUCING WORK OF BREATHING	Chronic Ventilatory Support
MECHANICAL VENTILATION	Lung Transplantation

Supportive therapy aimed at maintaining adequate gas-exchange is critical in the management of both acute respiratory failure and chronic respiratory insufficiency. In acute respiratory failure, survival depends on our ability to provide this support until the patient recovers from the acute illness. In patients with chronic respiratory insufficiency, the goal is to maximize the patient's function and to minimize symptoms and pulmonary hypertension on a long-term basis. This chapter outlines the goals of supportive therapy and then provides a discussion of the ways in which adequate gas-exchange can be maintained, focusing on patients with acute respiratory failure. Because the principles for supportive management differ considerably in the two main categories of acute respiratory failure—acute respiratory distress syndrome (ARDS) and acute on chronic respiratory failure—these differences are emphasized in the course of the discussion. The chapter concludes with a consideration of two specific topics applicable to patients with chronic respiratory insufficiency: chronic ventilatory assistance and lung transplantation.

GOALS OF SUPPORTIVE THERAPY FOR GAS-EXCHANGE

Adequate uptake of O_2 by the blood, delivery of O_2 to the tissues, and elimination of CO_2 are all parts of normal gas-exchange. In terms of O_2 uptake by the blood, we must remember that almost all the O_2 carried by blood is bound to hemoglobin and that only a small portion is dissolved in plasma. It is apparent from the oxyhemoglobin dissociation curve that elevating the Po_2 beyond the point at which hemoglobin is almost completely saturated does not significantly increase the O_2 content of blood. On the average, assuming that the dissociation curve is not shifted, hemoglobin is approximately 90 percent saturated at a Po_2 of 60 torr. Increasing the Po_2 to this level is important, but a Po_2 much beyond this level does not provide any particular benefit. In

Goals for optimizing O_2 transport to tissues:

1. Arterial O_2 saturation >90% (i.e., Po_2 >60 torr)
2. Acceptable hemoglobin level (e.g., >10 g/dL, corresponding to a hematocrit >30%)
3. Normal or near normal cardiac output

practice, patients with respiratory failure often are maintained at a P_{O_2} slightly higher than 60 torr to allow a "margin of safety" for fluctuations in P_{O_2}.

Oxygen delivery to the tissues, however, depends not only on the arterial P_{O_2} but also on the hemoglobin level and the cardiac output. In patients who are anemic, O_2 content and thus O_2 transport can be compromised as much by the low hemoglobin level as by hypoxemia (see Equation 1-3). In selected circumstances, blood transfusion may be useful in raising the hemoglobin and the O_2 content to a more desirable level.

Similarly, when cardiac output is impaired, tissue O_2 delivery also decreases, and measures to augment cardiac output may improve overall O_2 transport. Unfortunately, some of the measures used to improve arterial P_{O_2} may have a detrimental effect on cardiac output. As a result, tissue O_2 delivery may not improve (and may even worsen) despite an increase in P_{O_2}. The use of positive-pressure ventilation, particularly with positive end-expiratory pressure, is most important in this regard. This technique will be discussed shortly.

Elimination of CO_2 by the lungs is important for maintaining adequate acid-base homeostasis. However, achieving an acceptable value for pH, not a "normal" P_{CO_2}, is actually the primary goal in managing respiratory failure and impaired elimination of CO_2. In patients with chronic hypercapnia (and metabolic compensation), abruptly restoring the P_{CO_2} to normal (40 torr) may cause a significant alkalosis and thus risk precipitating either arrhythmias or seizures.

> CO_2 is eliminated to maintain an acceptable pH rather than a "normal" P_{CO_2}.

MAINTENANCE OF CARBON DIOXIDE ELIMINATION

As mentioned, there are several types of patients for whom CO_2 retention is an important aspect of respiratory failure. Most frequently, these patients have some degree of chronic CO_2 retention, and their acute problem is appropriately termed "acute on chronic" respiratory failure. Patients with chronic obstructive lung disease, chest wall disease, and neuromuscular disease are all subject to the development of hypercapnia. There is also a group of patients in whom hypercapnia may be acute—for example, individuals who have suppressed their respiratory drive with drugs ingested in a suicide attempt, or occasional patients with severe asthma and *status asthmaticus*.

If the degree of CO_2 retention is sufficiently great to cause a marked decrease in the patient's pH (less than 7.25 to 7.30), ventilatory assistance with a mechanical ventilator is often necessary.* Similarly, if marked CO_2 retention has resulted in impairment of the patient's mental status, ventilatory assistance is again indicated. For the patient in whom there is a good chance of rapid reversal of CO_2 retention with therapy (assuming the level of CO_2 retention is not life-threatening), this therapy is often attempted first with the hope of avoiding mechanical ventilation.

> Mechanical ventilation is often indicated when arterial P_{CO_2} has risen sufficiently to cause the following:
> 1. Lowered pH: to 7.25-7.30 or below
> 2. Impaired mental status

There are also measurements reflecting muscle strength and pulmonary function that may be useful for the patient with acute or impending respiratory failure. These measurements serve as an indirect guide to the patient's

---

*To initiate ventilatory support, the patient is generally intubated (i.e., a tube is placed through the nose or mouth, through the vocal cords, and into the trachea) and a mechanical ventilator is connected to the endotracheal tube. An alternative method of assisting ventilation, called noninvasive positive-pressure ventilation, will also be described later in the chapter.

ability to maintain adequate CO_2 elimination. Hence they too have been used as criteria for instituting ventilatory assistance or, conversely, for deciding when a patient aided by a mechanical ventilator might be weaned from ventilatory support. Perhaps the most commonly used measurements and the associated criteria for mechanical ventilation are (1) vital capacity: less than 10 mL/kg body weight; and (2) inspiratory force: less than 25 cm H_2O negative pressure. The latter measurement, which is also called the *maximal inspiratory pressure*, is performed by having the patient inspire as deeply as possible through tubing connected to a pressure gauge. This quantitates the maximum negative pressure that the patient can generate when the airway is occluded.

Although these and other specific measurements have sometimes been used to determine when a patient requires ventilatory assistance for eliminating CO_2, it is important to realize that none of the guidelines is absolute. Some of the many additional factors that enter into such decisions include the nature of the underlying disease, the tempo and direction of change of the patient's illness, and the presence of additional medical problems.

MAINTENANCE OF OXYGENATION

Although hypoxemia is a feature of virtually all patients with respiratory failure when breathing air (21 percent O_2), the ease of supporting the patient and restoring an adequate Po_2 depends to a great degree on the type of respiratory failure. In most cases of acute on chronic respiratory failure, ventilation-perfusion mismatch and hypoventilation are responsible for hypoxemia. For these mechanisms of hypoxemia, administration of supplemental O_2 is quite effective in improving the Po_2, and particularly high concentrations of inspired O_2 are not necessary. Frequently, O_2 can be administered by face mask or by nasal prongs to provide inhaled concentrations of O_2 not exceeding 40 percent, with which patients are able to achieve a Po_2 greater than 60 torr.

However, as discussed in Chapter 18, patients with chronic hypercapnia may be subject to further increases in their Pco_2 when they receive supplemental O_2. If the Pco_2 rises to an unacceptably high range, the patient may require intubation and assisted ventilation with a mechanical ventilator in order to maintain an acceptable Pco_2. Fortunately, this complication is infrequent with the judicious use of supplemental O_2.

In the patient with hypoxemic respiratory failure such as ARDS, ventilation-perfusion mismatch and shunting are responsible for hypoxemia. When a large fraction of the cardiac output is being shunted and does not achieve oxygenation during passage through the lungs, supplemental O_2 is relatively ineffective at raising the Po_2 to an acceptable level. In these cases, patients may require inspired O_2 concentrations in the range of 60 to 100 percent, and even then they may have difficulty in maintaining a Po_2 greater than 60 torr.

Such patients with ARDS also require ventilatory assistance but generally for a different reason than the patient with acute on chronic respiratory failure. In the latter patient, an unacceptable degree of CO_2 retention is generally the indication for intubation and mechanical ventilation. In the patient with ARDS, oxygenation is extremely difficult to support, CO_2 retention is much less frequent, and hypoxemia rather than hypercapnia is the primary indication for mechanical ventilation.

For patients with hypoxemic respiratory failure, inability to achieve a Po_2 of 60 torr or greater on supplemental O_2 readily administered by face mask

Mechanical ventilation is often indicated when Po_2 ≥60 torr cannot be achieved with inspired O_2 concentration ≤40-60%.

(generally in the range of 40 to 60 percent) is often considered reason for intubation and mechanical ventilation. However, such decisions for ventilatory support are not based on just one number. Rather, other factors are also taken into consideration, including the nature of the underlying problem and the likelihood of a rapid response to therapy.

In the setting of ARDS, intubation and mechanical ventilation serve several useful purposes. First, high concentrations of O_2 can be administered much more reliably through a tube inserted into the trachea than through a mask placed over the face. Second, administration of positive pressure by a ventilator relieves the patient of the high work of breathing (as described in the next section), allowing the patient to receive more reliable tidal volumes than he or she would spontaneously take, particularly since the poorly compliant lungs of ARDS promote shallow breathing and low tidal volumes. Finally, when a tube is in place in the trachea, positive pressure can be maintained in the airway throughout the respiratory cycle, not just during the inspiratory phase. In common usage, positive airway pressure maintained at the end of expiration in a mechanically ventilated patient is termed *positive end-expiratory pressure,* or *PEEP,* a modality to be discussed in more detail later in this chapter.

Why is positive pressure throughout the respiratory cycle beneficial in patients with ARDS? As mentioned earlier, patients with ARDS often have a great deal of microatelectasis, resulting from fluid occupying alveolar spaces, low tidal volumes, and probably both decreased production and inactivation of surfactant. The resting end-expiratory volume of the lung—i.e., functional residual capacity (FRC)—is quite low in these patients but can be increased substantially by the administration of PEEP. At the higher FRC, many small airways and alveoli that were formerly closed and received no ventilation are opened and capable of gas-exchange. Therefore, blood supplying these regions no longer courses through unventilated alveoli and can now be oxygenated. Indeed, measurement of the "shunt fraction" shows that PEEP is quite effective at decreasing the amount of blood that would otherwise not be oxygenated during passage through the lungs.

When the shunt fraction is decreased by PEEP, supplemental O_2 is much more effective at elevating the patient's Po_2 to an acceptable level. The concentration of inspired O_2 can then be lowered, and the patient is less likely to experience O_2 toxicity from extremely high concentrations of O_2.

REDUCING WORK OF BREATHING

One pathophysiologic feature that most patients with respiratory failure have in common is an imbalance in the work of breathing relative to the ability of the respiratory muscles to perform that work. In the case of acute on chronic respiratory failure in the patient with chronic obstructive lung disease, the flattened and mechanically disadvantaged diaphragm must cope with an increase in airway resistance. In neuromuscular disease, in either the purely acute or the acute on chronic setting, respiratory muscle strength may be insufficient to handle even a relatively normal work of breathing. In the patient with ARDS, the noncompliant—i.e., stiff—lungs require an inordinately high work of breathing even though respiratory muscle strength may be intact.

Consequently, ventilatory assistance in the patient with respiratory failure is important not only for the temporary support of gas-exchange but also for the mechanical support of inspiration, allowing the respiratory

Beneficial effects of ventilatory assistance in ARDS:
1. More reliable administration of high concentrations of inspired O_2
2. Delivery of more reliable tidal volumes than those achieved spontaneously by the patient
3. Use of PEEP

PEEP is effective in ARDS by increasing FRC and preventing closure of small airways and alveoli.

Reducing the work of breathing is a benefit of mechanical ventilation in all forms of acute respiratory failure.

muscles to rest. Dyspnea is often alleviated when such support is provided and the patient no longer has to expend so much energy on the act of breathing. Fatigued respiratory muscles are allowed to recover, and the relatively large amount of blood flow required by overworking respiratory muscles can be shifted to perfusion of other organ systems.

MECHANICAL VENTILATION

Mechanical ventilators, which have gained widespread use over the past several decades, are critical to the effective management of respiratory failure. By supporting gas-exchange and assisting with the work of ventilation for as long a period as necessary, mechanical ventilators can keep a patient alive and as comfortable as possible while the acute process precipitating respiratory failure is treated or allowed to resolve spontaneously. This section contains a brief description of the operation of mechanical ventilators, the available modes of ventilation, and the complications that can ensue from their use.

Ventilators currently used for the management of acute respiratory failure are positive-pressure devices—that is, they deliver gas under positive pressure to the patient during inspiration. Most commonly, the ventilator is used in a *volume-cycled* fashion, meaning that each inspiration is terminated (and passive expiration allowed to occur) after a specified volume has been delivered by the machine. In contrast, when *pressure-limited* ventilation is used, the assistance provided by the ventilator is targeted to reaching a specified level of positive airway pressure. Volume cycling is much more reliable in delivering constant, specifiable tidal volumes than is pressure-limited ventilation. With the latter, changes in either lung compliance or airway resistance alter the volume of gas delivered as the specified target pressure is reached.

With volume-cycled ventilation, inspiration terminates after a specified tidal volume has been delivered by the ventilator; with pressure-limited ventilation, inspiration terminates after the targeted airway pressure has been achieved.

Several ventilatory patterns or modes are available with most mechanical ventilators when used in a volume-cycled fashion (Fig. 29-1). *Controlled ventilation* provides for ventilation to be supplied entirely by the ventilator at a respiratory rate, tidal volume, and inspired O_2 concentration chosen by the physician. If the patient tries to take a spontaneous breath between the machine-delivered breaths, he or she does not receive any inspired gas. This type of ventilation is quite uncomfortable for the awake patient capable of initiating inspiration and can therefore only be used for patients who are comatose, anesthetized, or unable to make any inspiratory effort.

Common modes of mechanical ventilation are assist-control ventilation, synchronized intermittent mandatory ventilation (SIMV), and pressure support ventilation (PSV).

In the *assist-control* mode of ventilation, the ventilator is able to "sense" when the patient initiates inspiration, at which point the machine assists by delivering a specified tidal volume to the patient. Although the tidal volume is set by the machine, the respiratory rate is determined by the number of spontaneous inspiratory efforts made by the patient. However, should the patient's spontaneous respiratory rate fall below a specified level, the machine provides a backup by delivering at least this minimum number of breaths. For example, if the backup rate set on the machine is 10 breaths per minute, the ventilator will automatically deliver a breath if and when 6 seconds have elapsed from the previous breath. Since the respiratory rate with this mode of ventilation is determined by the patient (once the rate is higher than the specified minimum level), fluctuations in minute ventilation can occur if the patient's respiratory rate changes significantly.

A third ventilatory mode is known as *intermittent mandatory ventilation,* or *IMV.* With IMV, the machine delivers a preset number of breaths per minute at a specified tidal volume and inspired O_2 concentration. In between

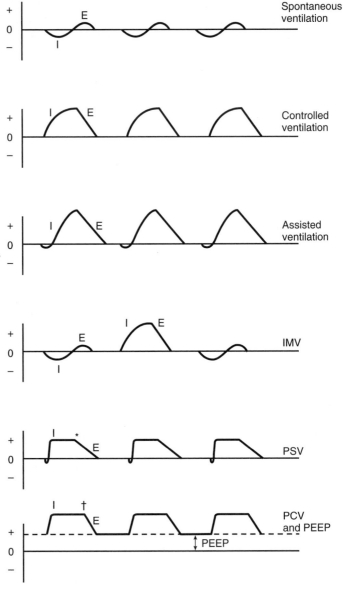

Figure 29-1 ▪— Airway pressure during spontaneous ventilation and during mechanical ventilation with several different ventilatory patterns. I = inspiration; E = expiration; IMV = intermittent mandatory ventilation; PEEP = positive end-expiratory pressure; PSV = pressure support ventilation; PCV = pressure-controlled ventilation.
*Inspiratory positive-pressure support ceases when the patient's flow rate falls below a threshold level.
†The relative timing of inspiration and expiration is controlled by the physician-determined ventilator settings.

the machine-delivered breaths, the patient is able to breathe spontaneously from a gas source providing the same inspired O_2 concentration given during the machine-delivered breaths. However, the machine does not assist these spontaneous breaths, and the tidal volume for these breaths is therefore determined by the patient. In a much more commonly used variant of IMV called *synchronized IMV*, or *SIMV*, each of the machine-delivered breaths is timed to coincide with and to assist a patient-initiated breath. If the patient being ventilated by IMV or SIMV modes changes his or her spontaneous respiratory rate significantly, the variation in minute ventilation is theoretically less than in the assist-control mode of ventilation, since each breath has not been supplemented by a comparatively large tidal volume delivered by the ventilator. In practice, both assist-control and SIMV are clinically useful and effective modes of ventilation, and there is little objective information to support the use of one over the other.

Finally, two types of pressure-limited ventilation are now used in some clinical settings. The first is called *pressure support ventilation,* or *PSV.* With PSV, the ventilator senses when the patient initiates a breath, at which time the ventilator assists the patient's efforts by providing a specified amount of positive pressure to the airway. This level of pressure support is reached rapidly and is maintained throughout most of inspiration. The ventilator stops providing inspiratory assistance when the patient's inspiratory flow rate falls below a specified target level, such as 25 percent of the peak inspiratory flow rate. The volume of each breath is potentially quite variable and is dependent upon the preset level of inspiratory pressure support, the patient's pattern of breathing, and the mechanical properties of the lungs. This type of ventilatory support is solely intended to assist a patient's own breathing efforts. If the patient stops making inspiratory efforts, no backup level of support is provided by the ventilator.

In *pressure-controlled ventilation,* or *PCV,* the targeted pressure level is set by the clinician and is achieved rapidly, as is the case with PSV. However, in PSV the patient's spontaneously initiated flow triggers the breath, and a decrease in flow terminates the breath. With PCV, in contrast, the initiation of the breath, the duration of inspiration, and the duration of expiration are determined by the clinician and set on the ventilator; the patient's breathing pattern does not influence the timing of the ventilatory assistance. Consequently, as was described above with volume-cycled controlled ventilation, PCV is quite uncomfortable for the patient, who must be heavily sedated to tolerate the imposed ventilatory pattern. PCV is used primarily in patients with ARDS in whom problems with oxygenation and decreased lung compliance are particularly severe. In these cases, the clinician's control of peak pressure and the relative timing of inspiration and expiration can facilitate improved oxygenation and minimize the risk of complications from high pressure delivered by the ventilator.

As mentioned in the discussion of ARDS, an important option available for the intubated patient with hypoxemic respiratory failure is the use of *positive end-expiratory pressure* (PEEP). When a patient is assisted by a mechanical ventilator without PEEP, airway (and alveolar) pressure falls during expiration from the positive level achieved at the height of inspiration down to zero. However, if the expiratory portion of the tubing is connected to a valve requiring a pressure of at least 10 cm H_2O, for example, to open it, then the valve closes and expiration ceases when the airway pressure falls to 10 cm H_2O. Consequently, airway pressure at the end of expiration does not fall to zero but remains at the level determined by the specifications of the expiratory valve. On the basis of the pressure required to open the expiratory valve, the level of PEEP can be set as desired.

A variation of PEEP that works on the same principle is called *continuous positive airway pressure,* or *CPAP.* The term CPAP is used when the patient is breathing spontaneously (without a mechanical ventilator) and expiratory tubing is connected to a PEEP valve. To use CPAP, the patient can either be intubated or given a tightly fitting face mask. Although no positive pressure is provided by a mechanical ventilator during inspiration, inspired gas is delivered from a reservoir bag under tension or at a high enough flow rate to keep airway pressure positive during inspiration as well as expiration.

With PEEP or CPAP, the benefit comes from the positive pressure within airways and alveoli at the end of expiration. FRC is increased by the positive pressure, and closure of airways and alveoli at the end of expiration is diminished.

In complicated cases of respiratory failure, such as in patients with ARDS, a variety of ventilatory strategies are now being used. Important goals of these particular strategies are to prevent closure of alveoli during expiration, and to avoid delivery of too high a level of pressure to the airways and the alveoli, with its attendant complications (see below). A particularly common strategy is called a *protective, open lung strategy,* in which sufficient PEEP is given to diminish airway closure during expiration, and relatively low tidal volumes (6 mL/kg) are used to protect the lung from inordinately high pressures during inspiration. Another strategy, used when oxygenation is particularly difficult, involves prolongation of inspiration relative to expiration, even to the point of having inspiration last longer than expiration. This pattern of breathing, which is the opposite of the normal pattern, is appropriately called *inverse ratio ventilation* (IRV). The rationale for its use is that oxygenation and inspiratory expansion of poorly ventilated alveoli are facilitated by prolongation of inspiration. Sometimes a strategy of *permissive hypercapnia* is used, in which PCO_2 is allowed to rise above normal levels. By minimizing the need for high levels of ventilation, this strategy theoretically decreases the risks of developing high alveolar pressures and overdistention of some alveolar units.

> A protective, open lung strategy (utilizing PEEP and avoiding excessive inspiratory inflation pressure) is commonly used in patients with ARDS.

When the underlying problem that precipitated the need for mechanical ventilation has improved, ventilatory support is discontinued, either rapidly (after a trial of spontaneous breathing) or more slowly (after a process of weaning). Measurements such as maximal inspiratory pressure and vital capacity were often used in the past as indirect guidelines to help predict the likelihood of successful weaning and discontinuation of ventilatory support. More recently, an indirect guideline that appears to have better predictive value is the *rapid shallow breathing index,* a ratio of the patient's respiratory rate divided by the tidal volume (expressed in L) when the patient is not receiving any assistance from the ventilator. An index less than 100 is predictive of successful weaning, whereas an index greater than 100 is associated with a much higher likelihood of weaning failure.

There are several commonly used methods of weaning. In the first, the patient is placed on an SIMV mode of ventilation (if not already used), and the number of breaths and thus the proportion of total minute ventilation provided by the ventilator are gradually decreased. In the second, mechanical ventilatory support is suspended and the patient's own spontaneous breathing must provide all the ventilatory requirements as tolerated for increasing periods of time. Finally, patients can be weaned with PSV, in which case the weaning process involves gradual reduction of the level of inspiratory pressure support provided by the ventilator. However, as rational as it seems to wean the patient gradually from ventilatory support, an alternative and probably superior strategy is to perform a single daily trial of spontaneous breathing. If the patient tolerates a two-hour trial, then the patient is extubated; if the trial is unsuccessful, the patient is given full ventilatory support for 24 hours until the time of the next daily trial.

> Mechanical ventilation can be discontinued after a successful trial of spontaneous breathing or following a weaning process with either SIMV or PSV.

Complications of Mechanical Ventilation

Unfortunately, intubation and mechanical ventilation of patients in respiratory failure are not entirely without risks or complications (Table 29-1). The procedure of intubation can be complicated acutely by such problems as arrhythmias, laryngospasm, and malposition of the endotracheal tube (either in the esophagus or in a mainstem bronchus). When a tube remains in the trachea for days to weeks, complications affecting the larynx and trachea can be seen. Vocal cord ulcerations and laryngeal stenosis and granulomas may develop, while the trachea is subject to ulcerations, stenosis, and tracheomalacia (degeneration of supporting tissues in the tracheal wall) resulting from pressure applied by the inflated balloon at the end of the tube. As a precaution to decrease tracheal complications, tubes are made with cuffs that minimize the pressure exerted on the tracheal wall and the resulting pressure necrosis. For prolonged ventilatory support (weeks to months), a tracheostomy tube, placed directly into the trachea through an incision in the neck, has some advantages over prolonged orotracheal or nasotracheal intubation, including patient comfort and prevention of further vocal cord injury.

The presence of an endotracheal tube also puts the patient at significant risk for pneumonia, usually called *ventilator-associated pneumonia.* Several factors appear to contribute to the patient's increased risk of developing pneumonia when intubated and receiving mechanical ventilation. These include bypassing of the normal anatomic barriers and upper airway clearance mechanisms that prevent organisms from reaching the lower respiratory tract, aspiration of oropharyngeal secretions around the endotracheal tube and into the lower respiratory tract, and bacterial contamination of the endotracheal tube or the ventilator circuitry connected to the endotracheal tube. Organisms causing ventilator-associated pneumonia are often relatively antibiotic-resistant bacteria, including gram-negative bacilli and *Staphylococcus aureus,*

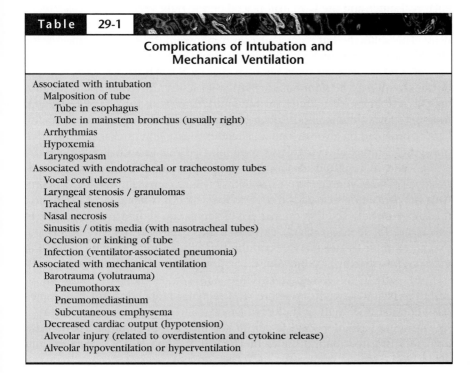

Table 29-1
Complications of Intubation and Mechanical Ventilation

Associated with intubation
  Malposition of tube
    Tube in esophagus
    Tube in mainstem bronchus (usually right)
  Arrhythmias
  Hypoxemia
  Laryngospasm
Associated with endotracheal or tracheostomy tubes
  Vocal cord ulcers
  Laryngeal stenosis / granulomas
  Tracheal stenosis
  Nasal necrosis
  Sinusitis / otitis media (with nasotracheal tubes)
  Occlusion or kinking of tube
  Infection (ventilator-associated pneumonia)
Associated with mechanical ventilation
  Barotrauma (volutrauma)
    Pneumothorax
    Pneumomediastinum
    Subcutaneous emphysema
  Decreased cardiac output (hypotension)
  Alveolar injury (related to overdistention and cytokine release)
  Alveolar hypoventilation or hyperventilation

leading to significant increases in both duration of hospitalization and mortality.

Barotrauma/volutrauma and impairment of systemic venous return to the heart are important adverse effects of positive-pressure ventilation.

The administration of positive pressure by a mechanical ventilator has its own attendant problems. Patients receiving positive-pressure ventilation are subject to barotrauma, i.e., traumatic changes such as pneumothorax or pneumomediastinum occurring as a result of high alveolar pressures. Because it is currently thought that alveolar overdistention with rupture is the cause of these complications, the term *volutrauma* is now often used instead of barotrauma. The development of a pneumothorax in patients receiving mechanical ventilation can have catastrophic consequences if not detected and treated quickly. The ventilator continues to deliver gas to the patient, and the pneumothorax can quickly be put under tension, thus severely diminishing venous return and cardiac output and causing rapid cardiovascular collapse. In such situations, a tube, catheter, or needle must be immediately inserted to decompress the pleural space, allow venous return to resume, and enable re-expansion of the lung.

Besides barotrauma, another major adverse effect of positive-pressure ventilation is impairment of cardiovascular function. At least two mechanisms are thought to play a role. The first of these involves a decrease in venous return to the heart. Whereas the normally negative intrathoracic pressure during inspiration promotes venous return from the periphery, positive inspiratory pressure from a ventilator impedes venous return. The hemodynamic consequences—low cardiac output and blood pressure—are even more likely when the patient is also receiving PEEP. In many cases, judicious administration of fluids can restore the effective intravascular volume and reverse the adverse hemodynamic consequences of positive-pressure ventilation.

The second mechanism involves an increase in pulmonary vascular resistance. When alveolar volume is increased with positive-pressure mechanical ventilation, alveolar vessels are compressed, compromising the overall cross-sectional area of the pulmonary vascular bed. As a result, pulmonary vascular resistance and the workload placed on the right ventricle increase. Right ventricular output is potentially compromised, and the right ventricle may dilate. This shifts the interventricular septum toward the left ventricular cavity, also impairing left ventricular filling and stroke volume.

Recently, there has been concern that high levels of pressure provided to the alveoli may be injurious to alveolar structures. Alveolar overdistention may be accompanied by microscopic injury to cells of the alveolar wall and to intercellular attachments, leading to disruption of the normal permeability barrier provided by alveolar epithelial and capillary endothelial cells. In addition, proinflammatory cytokines may be released, due to both alveolar overdistention and to repeated closure and opening of alveolar units. As a result, positive-pressure ventilation for respiratory failure, especially ARDS, can potentially perpetuate or worsen the process for which it is being used. Therefore, it is currently believed that the pattern of ventilation should avoid both alveolar closure (atelectasis) during expiration and overdistention during inspiration, the former by use of PEEP and the latter by keeping alveolar distending pressure less than approximately 30 to 35 cm H_2O.

In patients receiving positive-pressure ventilation, particularly those with hypoxemic respiratory failure who require PEEP, management becomes quite complicated. In these patients, many factors interact in a complex way—specifically oxygenation, cardiac output, and fluid status. Optimal care requires both sophisticated monitoring of the patient and substantial expertise from the team responsible for patient care. Such care is necessary not only for proper support of vital functions but also to keep complications of therapy at the minimum possible level.

Noninvasive Ventilatory Support for Acute Respiratory Failure

When patients with acute respiratory failure require mechanical ventilation, such support has traditionally been provided by positive pressure administered through a tube placed into the trachea, i.e., an endotracheal tube. However, there are risks and complications posed by the use of such tubes, including patient discomfort from the tube itself, injury to the airway mucosa, and development of lower respiratory tract infection (see Table 29-1). An alternative form of support for acute respiratory failure avoids use of an endotracheal tube, but instead provides positive pressure through a tightly fitting mask placed over the face. This approach has now been used for support of patients with a variety of types of acute respiratory failure, including patients with cardiogenic pulmonary edema, patients with acute exacerbation of chronic obstructive pulmonary disease, and those who are not thought to be suitable candidates for intubation. However, noninvasive ventilatory support is not appropriate if patients are unable to protect their airway, and conversely it is most useful when the respiratory failure is most likely to be readily reversible and therefore of relatively short duration.

SELECTED ASPECTS OF THERAPY FOR CHRONIC RESPIRATORY FAILURE

Chronic Ventilatory Support

A difficult problem is posed by patients with chronic, irreversible respiratory system disease who require continuous, long-term ventilatory support. The first question is whether the patient wishes "to be on a machine" for the rest of his or her life. Some patients clearly wish to prolong life even if it means permanent ventilatory support; others make the decision that life is not worth living if they must be dependent upon a ventilator for the remainder of their lives. When the patient chooses to be maintained on a ventilator, support is usually given by positive-pressure ventilation administered through a tracheostomy tube. The care of some patients can be handled at home with the proper support of family and visiting health care personnel; the management of other cases continues in chronic care hospitals or other facilities equipped to care for such patients.

A subgroup of patients with chronic respiratory insufficiency do not require continuous ventilatory support but benefit from nocturnal assistance with ventilation. These patients often have chronic neuromuscular or chest wall disease accompanied by chronic hypercapnia. Although it is not clear how much respiratory muscle fatigue contributes to the hypercapnia experienced by these patients, at least part of the rationale for using nocturnal ventilatory support is to afford these patients a number of hours each day when their inspiratory muscles are allowed to rest. After a period of nocturnal rest, the respiratory muscles are then presumably better able to handle the work of breathing during the day, and daytime hypercapnia may be improved.

Chronic ventilatory support can be provided by positive pressure administered to the airway or by a device that produces intermittent negative pressure around the chest wall.

When ventilatory support is needed only during the night, it is generally preferable to avoid a chronic tracheostomy. Instead, several options are available, the most appropriate one depending on the particular patient. Positive pressure can be administered at night through a mouthpiece or a mask (i.e., noninvasive positive pressure ventilation). Alternatively, inflation of the lungs can be achieved by negative-pressure ventilation—that is, intermittent negative pressure applied outside the chest wall, causing it to expand and the lungs to inflate. The original type of negative-pressure ventilator was the "iron lung," used for ventilatory support from the 1930s through the polio epidemics of the 1950s. Currently, other negative-pressure devices are used more frequently, the two most common types being called the "raincoat" (or "poncho") ventilator and the "cuirass" (or "chest shell") ventilator. Unlike the iron lung, which enclosed the entire body below the neck, the raincoat and cuirass ventilators do not enclose or limit movement of the lower half of the body. These negative-pressure ventilatory support devices have been used most frequently for patients with chronic respiratory failure due to neuromuscular disease such as muscular dystrophy.

Lung Transplantation

A relatively recent form of therapy available for management of severe and disabling chronic pulmonary disease is lung transplantation. However, the availability of this mode of therapy is limited, since only a relatively small number of medical centers have the experience and the capability to perform the procedure, and also because donor organs are scarce.

Several types of transplantation can be done, with the selection generally based on the underlying clinical problem. Single lung transplantation has been used effectively in patients with end-stage disease due to interstitial lung disease, severe emphysema, or pulmonary vascular disease. In patients with cystic fibrosis, in whom chronic bilateral pulmonary infection complicates their lung disease, bilateral lung transplantation has been performed to avoid infection of the new lung by spillover of infected secretions from a remaining diseased lung. When severe cardiac disease accompanies end-stage lung disease, combined heart-lung transplantation may be required. Finally, the most recent of the lung transplantation techniques is lobar transplantation from living donors. Used primarily in patients with cystic fibrosis, this technique involves the recipient's receiving bilateral implants of a lower lobe from each of two living donors.

The major complications following lung transplantation are rejection and infection.

The major potential complications of lung transplantation fall under the general categories of rejection and infection. Because of the risk of rejection, patients are routinely given immunosuppressive drugs, such as prednisone, azathioprine (or mycophenolate mofetil), and cyclosporine (or tacrolimus), as a regimen to prevent rejection. Nevertheless, either acute or chronic rejection can occur despite maintenance immunosuppression. *Acute rejection* is often characterized by fever, impairment of pulmonary function and gas-exchange, and pulmonary infiltrates on chest radiograph. Such episodes typically occur during the first several months after transplantation and are treated by an acute intensification of the immunosuppressive regimen, especially with increased doses of corticosteroids. *Chronic rejection* is usually manifested as bronchiolitis obliterans, which is characterized by progressive inflammation, fibrosis, and obstruction of small airways. The physiologic consequence of this process is progressive airflow obstruction, which unfortunately is typically unresponsive to augmentation of immunosuppressive therapy. As a result, bronchiolitis oblit-

Progressive airflow obstruction from bronchiolitis obliterans is thought to represent chronic transplant rejection.

erans is the major cause of graft failure and death occurring later in the course following lung transplantation. The main treatment option for post-transplant patients with severe bronchiolitis obliterans is repeat transplantation.

The other major complication of lung transplantation is infection, the risk of which is greatly increased by the need for immunosuppressive therapy. In some cases, organisms (such as bacteria or cytomegalovirus) accompanied the donor organ, and the development of a complicating infection is precipitated by immunosuppression and impairment of the recipient's defense mechanisms. Patients are also subject to the variety of opportunistic infections that are common to patients with impaired cell-mediated immunity, including other viruses, fungi, and *Pneumocystis*.

As experience with lung transplantation has accumulated over the past decade, there has been a modest improvement in survival. Survival at 1 and 3 years following transplantation is currently approximately 75 percent and 60 percent, respectively. It has become apparent that lung transplantation is now an important though expensive therapeutic option for a highly selected group of patients. As we gain more experience with this form of treatment and as technology and immunosuppressive therapy evolve, we continue to refine our thinking about where transplantation fits in the overall management of patients with severe lung disease.

References

Mechanical Ventilation

Brochard L, Mancebo J, and Elliott MW: Noninvasive ventilation for acute respiratory failure. Eur Respir J 19:712-721, 2002.

Brower RG, Ware LB, Berthiaume Y, and Matthay MA: Treatment of ARDS. Chest 120:1347-1367, 2001.

Chastre J and Fagon JY: Ventilator-associated pneumonia. Am J Respir Crit Care Med 165:867-903, 2002.

Cordingley JJ and Keogh BF: Ventilatory management of ALI/ARDS. Thorax 57:729-734, 2002.

Dekel B, Segal E, and Perel A: Pressure support ventilation. Arch Intern Med 156:369-373, 1996.

Hess D: Ventilator modes used in weaning. Chest 120 (Suppl):474S-476S, 2001.

Hillberg RE and Johnson DC: Noninvasive ventilation. N Engl J Med 337:1746-1752, 1997.

Keith RL and Pierson DJ: Complications of mechanical ventilation: a bedside approach. Clin Chest Med 17:439-451, 1996.

Kollef MH: The prevention of ventilator-associated pneumonia. N Engl J Med 340:627-634, 1999.

MacIntyre NR et al: Evidence-based guidelines for weaning and discontinuing ventilatory support: a collective task force facilitated by the American College of Chest Physicians; the American Association for Respiratory Care; and the American College of Critical Care Medicine. Chest 120 (Suppl):375S-395S, 2001.

McKibben AW and Ravenscraft SA: Pressure-controlled and volume-cycled mechanical ventilation. Clin Chest Med 17:395-410, 1996.

Mehta S and Hill NS: Noninvasive ventilation. Am J Respir Crit Care Med 163:540-577, 2001.

Rabatin JT and Gay PC: Noninvasive ventilation. Mayo Clin Proc 74:817-820, 1999.

Slutsky AS: Mechanical ventilation. Chest 104:1833-1859, 1993.

Tobin MJ: Mechanical ventilation. N Engl J Med 330:1056-1061, 1994.

Tobin MJ: Advances in mechanical ventilation. N Engl J Med 344:1986-1996, 2001.

Wysocki M and Antonelli M: Noninvasive mechanical ventilation in acute hypoxaemic respiratory failure. Eur Respir J 18:209-220, 2001.

Chronic Ventilatory Support

Consensus Conference Report: Clinical indications for noninvasive positive pressure ventilation in chronic respiratory failure due to restrictive lung disease, COPD, and nocturnal hypoventilation. Chest 116:521-534, 1999.

Hill NS: Clinical applications of body ventilators. Chest 90:897-905, 1986.

Make BJ et al: Mechanical ventilation beyond the intensive care unit. Report of a consensus conference of the American College of Chest Physicians. Chest 113 (Suppl):289S-344S, 1998.

Peters SG and Viggiano RW: Home mechanical ventilation. Mayo Clin Proc 63:1208-1213, 1988.

Strumpf DA, Millman RP, and Hill NS: The management of chronic hypoventilation. Chest 98:474-480, 1990.

Lung Transplantation

American Thoracic Society: International guidelines for the selection of lung transplant candidates. Am J Respir Crit Care Med 158:335-339, 1998.

Arcasoy SM and Kotloff RM: Lung transplantation. N Engl J Med 340:1081-1091, 1999.

DeMeo DL and Ginns LC: Lung transplantation at the turn of the century. Annu Rev Med 52:185-201, 2001.

Maurer J: Patient selection for lung transplantation. JAMA 286:2720-2721, 2001.

Trulock EP: Lung transplantation. Am J Respir Crit Care Med 155:789-818, 1997.

Sample Problems Using Respiratory Equations

A comatose patient with no spontaneous respiration is placed on mechanical ventilation with the following settings:

Tidal volume (V_T) = 1000 mL
Respiratory frequency (f) = 10 breaths/min
Inspired O_2 concentration = 40% (F_{IO_2} = 0.4)

The following measurements are made:

Arterial P_{CO_2} (Pa_{CO_2}) = 40 mm Hg
Mixed expired P_{CO_2} (P_{ECO_2}) = 30 mm Hg
Arterial P_{O_2} (Pa_{O_2}) = 95 mm Hg

1. Calculate minute ventilation ($\dot{V}_E$), dead space to tidal volume ratio (V_D/V_T), alveolar volume (V_A), and alveolar ventilation ($\dot{V}_A$).

2. If extra tubing with a volume of 250 mL were added to the system in a position such that it provided additional dead space, what would be the new V_D/V_T?

3. With the new system as described in Question 2, what would be the new Pa_{CO_2}?

4. Going back to the original conditions (without added extra tubing), the ventilator settings are changed to new settings:

V_T = 500 mL
f = 20 breaths/min

   a. Calculate the new $\dot{V}_E, V_A, \dot{V}_A, V_D/V_T$
   b. What would happen to Pa_{CO_2} on the new settings?
   c. What would you expect P_{ECO_2} to be if you now measured it?

5. Using the original ventilator settings and arterial blood gases as given, calculate the alveolar-arterial O_2 difference (Aa_{DO_2}).

6. Once the patient is improved, arterial blood gases, as measured with the patient breathing room air, are as follows:

P_{O_2} = 75 mm Hg
P_{CO_2} = 40 mm Hg
pH = 7.40
   Calculate the Aa_{DO_2}.

7. The next day, the patient's arterial blood gas values on room air are as follows:

P_{O_2} = 80 mm Hg
P_{CO_2} = 20 mm Hg
pH = 7.55
   What is the Aa_{DO_2}?

Answers

1. $\dot{V}E = 1000\,mL/breath \times 10\,breaths/min = 10{,}000\,mL/min = \underline{10\,L/min}$
   $V_D/V_T = (40\,mm\,Hg - 30\,mm\,Hg)/40\,mm\,Hg = \underline{0.25}$
   $V_A = V_T - V_D = 1000\,mL - (0.25 \times V_T) = 1000\,mL - 250\,mL = \underline{750\,mL}$
   $\dot{V}_A = V_A \times f = 750\,mL/breath \times 10\,breaths/min = \underline{7.5\,L/min}$

2. New $V_D = 250\,mL + 250\,mL = 500\,mL$
   New $V_D/V_T = 500\,mL/1000\,mL = \underline{0.5}$

3. Because Pa_{CO_2} is inversely proportional to $\dot{V}_A$, the new Pa_{CO_2} can be calculated from the old and the new $\dot{V}_A$ (assuming $\dot{V}_{CO_2}$ remains constant).
   As per Problem 1, old $\dot{V}_A = 7.5\,L/min$
   New $V_A = 1000\,mL - new\ V_D = 1000\,mL - 500\,mL = 500\,mL$
   New $\dot{V}_A = 500\,mL/breath \times 10\,breaths/min = 5\,L/min$
   New $\dot{V}_A = \frac{2}{3} \times old\ \dot{V}_A$
   New $Pa_{CO_2} = \frac{3}{2} \times old\ Pa_{CO_2} = \frac{3}{2} \times 40\,mm\,Hg = \underline{60\,mm\,Hg}$

4. On the basis of the new settings:
   a. $\dot{V}E = 500\,mL/breath \times 20\,breaths/min = \underline{10\,L/min}$
      $V_A = 500\,mL - 250\,mL = \underline{250\,mL}$
      $\dot{V}_A = 250\,mL/breath \times 20\,breaths/min = \underline{5\,L/min}$
      $V_D/V_T = 250\,mL/500\,mL = \underline{0.5}$
   b. New Pa_{CO_2} is inversely proportional to the ratio of the new $\dot{V}_A$ to the old $\dot{V}_A$.
      New $\dot{V}_A/old\ \dot{V}_A = (5\,L/min)/(7.5\,L/min) = \frac{2}{3}$
      New $Pa_{CO_2} = \frac{3}{2} \times old\ Pa_{CO_2} = \frac{3}{2} \times 40\,mm\,Hg = \underline{60\,mm\,Hg}$
   c. Because $V_D/V_T = (Pa_{CO_2} - P_{ECO_2})/Pa_{CO_2}$, substitute the known values and solve the equation for P_{ECO_2}.
      $0.5 = (60\,mm\,Hg - P_{ECO_2})/60\,mm\,Hg$
      $P_{ECO_2} = \underline{30\,mm\,Hg}$

5. $PA_{O_2} = (0.4 \times 713\,mm\,Hg) - (40\,mm\,Hg/0.8) = 285\,mm\,Hg - 50\,mm\,Hg = 235\,mm\,Hg$
   $AaD_{O_2} = PA_{O_2} - Pa_{O_2} = 235\,mm\,Hg - 95\,mm\,Hg = \underline{140\,mm\,Hg}$

6. $PA_{O_2} = 150\,mm\,Hg - (40\,mm\,Hg/0.8) = 100\,mm\,Hg$
   $AaD_{O_2} = 100\,mm\,Hg - 75\,mm\,Hg = \underline{25\,mm\,Hg}$

7. $PA_{O_2} = 150\,mm\,Hg - (20\,mm\,Hg/0.8) = 125\,mm\,Hg$
   $AaD_{O_2} = 125\,mm\,Hg - 80\,mm\,Hg = \underline{45\,mm\,Hg}$

Pulmonary Function Tests: Guidelines for Interpretation and Sample Problems

This appendix provides an outline of a simplified approach to the interpretation of pulmonary function tests and then gives several examples of test results presented as unknown problems. Because details of the interpretation of these tests may vary from laboratory to laboratory, the approach here focuses on the general concepts rather than the specific details, providing a step-by-step approach to analyzing pulmonary function tests. The concepts underlying this step-by-step approach are covered in the relevant section on Pulmonary Function Tests in Chapter 3.

ANALYSIS OF PULMONARY FUNCTION TESTS

1. Examination of the lung volumes:
   a. A decrease in total lung capacity (TLC) generally indicates the presence of a restrictive pattern. However, TLC measured by helium dilution may also be artificially depressed when there are poorly communicating or noncommunicating regions within the lung—for example, in bullous lung disease.
   b. Are the lung volumes symmetrically reduced, that is, are TLC, residual volume (RV), functional residual capacity (FRC), and vital capacity (VC) all decreased to approximately the same extent? If so, this suggests interstitial lung disease as the cause of the restrictive pattern. A low diffusing capacity also supports the diagnosis of interstitial lung disease as the cause of the restrictive pattern.
   c. A relatively preserved RV and a normal diffusing capacity suggest another cause of restrictive disease, such as neuromuscular or chest wall disease. Poor effort from the patient may also create this type of pattern.

2. Examination of the mechanics, that is, the flow rates measured from the forced expiratory spirogram:
   a. A decrease in the forced expiratory volume in 1 second/forced vital capacity (FEV_1/FVC) ratio indicates obstruction. In some cases of airflow obstruction, both the FEV_1 and the FVC are reduced by approximately the same extent, and the FEV_1/FVC ratio may be preserved. Clues to the presence of obstructive disease in this setting are a low forced expiratory flow from 25 percent to 75 percent of vital capacity ($FEF_{25\%-75\%}$), a normal to high TLC with a high RV/TLC ratio, and the configuration of the flow-volume curve.

b. Interpretation of $FEF_{25\%-75\%}$ (also called maximal midexpiratory flow [MMF]):

(1) $FEF_{25\%-75\%}$ is subject to more variability than most other measurements obtained during a forced expiration, so that guidelines for normal values are less well established.

(2) When lung volumes are low, $FEF_{25\%-75\%}$ can also be decreased without necessarily indicating coexisting airflow obstruction. Therefore, in the presence of decreased lung volumes, a low $FEF_{25\%-75\%}$ indicates obstruction primarily if the decrease in $FEF_{25\%-75\%}$ is out of proportion to the decrease in lung volumes.

(3) Taking into account the aforementioned qualifications, $FEF_{25\%-75\%}$ may be a relatively sensitive measurement for airway obstruction. An isolated abnormality in $FEF_{25\%-75\%}$ has sometimes been considered a marker for early or very mild airflow obstruction, theoretically reflecting "small airways disease."

3. Interpretation of diffusing capacity for carbon monoxide (D_{LCO}):

a. Make sure that the value has been corrected for the patient's hemoglobin level. If not, the value will be falsely low if the patient is anemic.

b. A decrease in the diffusing capacity reflects disease affecting the alveolar-capillary membrane (decreased surface area for gas-exchange and/or abnormal thickness of the membrane) or a decrease in pulmonary capillary blood volume.

c. An increase in the diffusing capacity can reflect increased pulmonary capillary blood volume or erythrocytes within alveolar spaces (pulmonary hemorrhage).

4. Interpretation of the flow-volume curve:

a. An obstructive pattern is reflected by decreased flow relative to lung volume, generally accompanied by a "scooped out" or "coved" appearance to the descending part of the expiratory curve (see Fig. 3-19).

b. A restrictive pattern is characterized by decreased volumes, that is, narrowing of the curve along the volume or X axis, and relatively preserved flow rates. The flow rates often appear increased relative to the small lung volumes, producing a tall, narrow curve.

Sample Pulmonary Function Test Results

1. Female 32 years of age

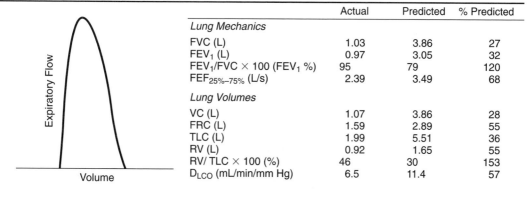

	Actual	Predicted	% Predicted
Lung Mechanics			
FVC (L)	1.03	3.86	27
FEV_1 (L)	0.97	3.05	32
FEV_1/FVC × 100 (FEV_1 %)	95	79	120
$FEF_{25\%-75\%}$ (L/s)	2.39	3.49	68
Lung Volumes			
VC (L)	1.07	3.86	28
FRC (L)	1.59	2.89	55
TLC (L)	1.99	5.51	36
RV (L)	0.92	1.65	55
RV/ TLC × 100 (%)	46	30	153
D_{LCO} (mL/min/mm Hg)	6.5	11.4	57

Flow-volume curve

2. Male 60 years of age

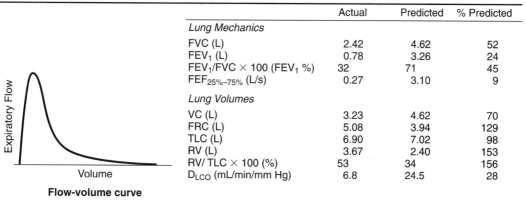

	Actual	Predicted	% Predicted
Lung Mechanics			
FVC (L)	2.42	4.62	52
FEV_1 (L)	0.78	3.26	24
FEV_1/FVC × 100 (FEV_1 %)	32	71	45
$FEF_{25\%-75\%}$ (L/s)	0.27	3.10	9
Lung Volumes			
VC (L)	3.23	4.62	70
FRC (L)	5.08	3.94	129
TLC (L)	6.90	7.02	98
RV (L)	3.67	2.40	153
RV/ TLC × 100 (%)	53	34	156
D_{LCO} (mL/min/mm Hg)	6.8	24.5	28

Flow-volume curve

3. Female 55 years of age

	Actual	Predicted	% Predicted
Lung Mechanics			
FVC (L)	0.93	2.73	34
FEV_1 (L)	0.80	2.03	39
FEV_1/FVC × 100 (FEV_1 %)	86	75	115
$FEF_{25\%-75\%}$ (L/s)	1.60	2.50	64
Lung Volumes			
VC (L)	0.90	2.73	33
FRC (L)	1.50	2.29	66
TLC (L)	2.14	4.18	51
RV (L)	1.24	1.46	85
RV/ TLC × 100 (%)	58	35	166
D_{LCO} (mL/min/mm Hg)	14	12.9	109

Flow-volume curve

Answers

1. All measurements of lung volume (TLC, VC, FRC, RV) are significantly decreased, indicative of restrictive disease. FEV_1 and FVC are decreased because of the low lung volumes, but the FEV_1/FVC ratio is preserved. This finding, along with the fact that $FEF_{25\%-75\%}$ is not decreased out of proportion to the decrease in lung volumes, indicates there is no obstruction. Diffusing capacity is decreased, suggesting that the restrictive disease is secondary to an abnormality of the pulmonary parenchyma rather than a result of chest wall or neuromuscular disease. The flow-volume curve is tall and narrow, consistent with a restrictive pattern. Diagnosis: interstitial lung disease secondary to pulmonary sarcoidosis.

2. FEV_1 and FVC are both decreased; because FEV_1 is decreased more than is FVC, the FEV_1/FVC ratio is decreased. $FEF_{25\%-75\%}$ is also decreased. These values are indicative of obstructive lung disease. TLC is normal, and RV and FRC are increased. The RV/TLC ratio is also increased. Therefore, there is no restriction, but the high RV/TLC ratio indicates there is "air trapping," as is often expected with airflow obstruction. The diffusing capacity is decreased, reflecting loss of alveolar-capillary bed. The flow-volume curve shows an obstructive pattern, characterized by a striking decrease in flow rates, well seen throughout most of the expiratory curve after the initial peak flow rate. This combination of significant airflow obstruction with normal or increased volumes and a low diffusing capacity suggests emphysema.

3. TLC and FRC are reduced, indicating restrictive disease; RV is relatively preserved. FEV_1 and FVC are both decreased, but the FEV_1/FVC ratio is preserved. There is no evidence for coexisting obstructive disease. Diffusing capacity is normal, suggesting that the alveolar-capillary bed is preserved. The flow-volume curve is relatively tall and narrow, and without any evidence for obstructive disease. Diagnosis: restrictive pattern secondary to chest wall disease (kyphoscoliosis).

Arterial Blood Gases: Guidelines for Interpretation and Sample Problems

The following guidelines are meant to expand on the material presented in Chapter 3 and to simplify the interpretation of arterial blood gas values. Because memorizing a "cookbook" approach can sometimes be counterproductive if it is not clear why the approach is used, these guidelines are meant to supplement a basic understanding of the underlying physiologic principles.

There are numerous formulas used to assess the appropriateness of compensation for a primary acid-base disorder. These formulas are particularly useful for suggesting whether a mixed acid-base disorder is present. Table C-1 lists commonly used formulas that predict the expected degree of respiratory compensation for a primary metabolic problem and metabolic compensation for a primary respiratory problem. These formulas relate arterial PCO_2 and measured HCO_3^-. However, measured values from arterial blood gases include arterial PCO_2 and pH, not serum HCO_3^-. Therefore, to use the formulas in the table, one must either measure serum HCO_3^- (as part of serum electrolyte values) or use a value calculated from PCO_2 and pH according to the Henderson-Hasselbalch equation.

Alternatively, one can use other guidelines relating PCO_2 and pH values. Because these latter guidelines are based on the direct measurements obtained with arterial blood gases—and also because they are relatively easy to remember—they are used in the method outlined here. However, these easy-to-remember formulas relating PCO_2 and pH become less accurate at the extremes of PCO_2 and pH values. Also, the formulas provide only rough guidelines; the human body does not respond to physiologic disturbances with mathematical precision.

ANALYSIS OF ACID-BASE STATUS

1. Look at the pH value to determine the *net* disturbance in acid-base balance. An alkalotic pH (>7.44) indicates the presence of a primary respiratory or metabolic alkalosis, or both. An acidotic pH (<7.36) indicates the presence of a primary respiratory or metabolic acidosis, or both. A normal pH (approximately 7.36 to 7.44) indicates normal acid-base status or a mixed disturbance (of two balancing problems).
2. Look at the PCO_2. A high PCO_2 (>44) indicates that a *respiratory acidosis* is present. A low PCO_2 (<36) indicates that a *respiratory alkalosis* is present. If the pH value moves in the appropriate direction for the PCO_2 change (i.e., ↓ pH with ↑ PCO_2; ↑ pH with ↓ PCO_2), then the respiratory disorder is the *primary* disturbance. If the pH value does not move in the

Table	C-1	

Expected Compensation For Primary Acid-Base Disorders

Primary Disorder	Compensatory Response	Expected Magnitude of Response
Metabolic acidosis	↓ P_{CO_2}	$P_{CO_2} = 1.5 \times (HCO_3^-) + 8 \pm 2$
Metabolic alkalosis	↑ P_{CO_2}	P_{CO_2} increases 6 mm Hg for each 10 mEq/L increase in HCO_3^-
Respiratory acidosis	↑ HCO_3^-	Acute: HCO_3^- increases 1 mEq/L for each 10 mm Hg increase in P_{CO_2}
		Chronic: HCO_3^- increases 3.5 mEq/L for each 10 mm Hg increase in P_{CO_2}
Respiratory alkalosis	↓ HCO_3^-	Acute: HCO_3^- falls 2 mEq/L for each 10 mm Hg decrease in P_{CO_2}
		Chronic: HCO_3^- falls 5 mEq/L for each 10 mm Hg decrease in P_{CO_2}

Adapted from Narins RG, Emmett M: Medicine 59:161-186, 1980. © by Williams & Wilkins, 1980.

appropriate direction for the P_{CO_2} change, then a metabolic disorder is the primary disorder.

3. When a primary respiratory disorder is present, the pH value should change approximately 0.08 units for each 10 mm Hg change in P_{CO_2} if the process is acute. If chronic, the kidneys compensate (by retaining or losing HCO_3^-) and blunt the pH change in response to any change in P_{CO_2}. The resulting change in pH when the respiratory disorder is chronic is slightly different for acidosis versus alkalosis. With a chronic respiratory acidosis, the expected pH decrease is approximately 0.03 for each 10 mm Hg increase in P_{CO_2}. With a chronic respiratory alkalosis, the expected pH increase is approximately 0.02 for each 10 mm Hg decrease in P_{CO_2}.

4. If a pH change cannot be explained by an alteration in P_{CO_2}, then a primary metabolic disturbance is present. A low pH value with a low P_{CO_2} indicates a *primary metabolic acidosis* with respiratory compensation. A high pH value with a high P_{CO_2} can indicate a *primary metabolic alkalosis* with secondary suppression of respiratory drive. However, in many patients the latter pattern of a high pH value with a high P_{CO_2} often represents a complex acid-base disturbance, such as a chronic compensated respiratory acidosis with a superimposed primary metabolic alkalosis (e.g., as a result of diuretics, vomiting, or nasogastric suction).

5. To determine whether there has been appropriate respiratory compensation for a primary metabolic disorder, a rough guideline is that the P_{CO_2} should approximate the last two digits of the pH value. For example, a P_{CO_2} of 25 mm Hg accompanying a pH value of 7.25 indicates appropriate respiratory compensation for a primary metabolic acidosis. However, the degree of compensatory hyperventilation (i.e., lowering of P_{CO_2}) for a metabolic acidosis tends to be more predictable than the degree of compensatory hypoventilation (i.e., CO_2 retention) accompanying a metabolic alkalosis.

ANALYSIS OF OXYGENATION

1. When analyzing the arterial P_{O_2}, first calculate the alveolar P_{O_2} according to the equation:

$$PAO_2 = (713 \times FIO_2) - \frac{PCO_2}{0.8}$$

For room air, this equation can be simplified to the following: $PAO_2 = 150 - (1.25 \times PCO_2)$. Then calculate the alveolar-arterial O_2 gradient ($AaDO_2$), which is the difference between the calculated PAO_2 and the measured PAO_2: $AaDO_2 = PAO_2 - PaO_2$.

2. If the patient is hypoxemic, the PCO_2 is elevated, and the $AaDO_2$ is normal (<15 mm Hg on room air in a young person, although it increases with age), then *hypoventilation* is the cause of the hypoxemia.

3. If the patient is hypoxemic, the PCO_2 is normal or low, and the $AaDO_2$ is increased, then either $\dot{V}/\dot{Q}$ *mismatch* or *shunting* is present. With $\dot{V}/\dot{Q}$ mismatch, there is a good response to administration of supplemental O_2; with a true shunt, PO_2 does not rise much with supplemental O_2 (even with 100 percent O_2).

4. If the patient is hypoxemic, the PCO_2 is high, and the $AaDO_2$ is increased, then the patient has both hypoventilation *and* either $\dot{V}/\dot{Q}$ mismatch or shunt as the cause of the low PO_2.

SAMPLE PROBLEMS

All blood gases are drawn with the patient breathing room air ($FIO_2 = 0.21$), except as otherwise noted.

1.	Room air:	$PO_2 = 45$ mm Hg	$PCO_2 = 30$ mm Hg	pH = 7.47
	100% O_2:	$PO_2 = 65$ mm Hg	$PCO_2 = 32$ mm Hg	pH = 7.46
2.	Room air:	$PO_2 = 45$ mm Hg	$PCO_2 = 30$ mm Hg	pH = 7.47
	100% O_2:	$PO_2 = 560$ mm Hg	$PCO_2 = 32$ mm Hg	pH = 7.46
3.		$PO_2 = 88$ mm Hg	$PCO_2 = 20$ mm Hg	pH = 7.55
4.		$PO_2 = 65$ mm Hg	$PCO_2 = 60$ mm Hg	pH = 7.35
5.		$PO_2 = 30$ mm Hg	$PCO_2 = 60$ mm Hg	pH = 7.35
6.		$PO_2 = 110$ mm Hg	$PCO_2 = 20$ mm Hg	pH = 7.30
7.		$PO_2 = 55$ mm Hg	$PCO_2 = 48$ mm Hg	pH = 7.49
8.		$PO_2 = 90$ mm Hg	$PCO_2 = 60$ mm Hg	pH = 7.20

Answers

1. Acute respiratory alkalosis. On room air, the patient's $AaDO_2 = 67.5$ mm Hg, which is elevated. The minimal elevation in PO_2 with 100% O_2 indicates that a shunt is the major cause of the hypoxemia.

2. Identical to Problem 1, except that the dramatic increase in the PO_2 with 100% O_2 indicates that ventilation-perfusion mismatch is the major cause of the hypoxemia.

3. Acute respiratory alkalosis. Even though the PO_2 appears normal, the $AaDO_2$ is elevated to 37 mm Hg, indicating the presence of a disorder impairing normal oxygenation of blood.

4. Chronic respiratory acidosis. $AaDO_2 = 10$ mm Hg, indicating that hypoxemia is due to hypoventilation.

5. Chronic respiratory acidosis, as in Problem 4. However, unlike Problem 4, $AaDO_2$ is elevated (to 45 mm Hg), indicating that both hypoventilation and either ventilation-perfusion mismatch or shunting (most likely the former) are responsible for the hypoxemia.

6. Mixed acid-base disorder with a primary metabolic acidosis complicated by a primary respiratory alkalosis. The PCO_2 is too low to represent just

compensation for the metabolic acidosis, indicating the presence of a respiratory alkalosis as well. $AaDO_2 = 15\,mm\,Hg$, the upper limit of normal for a young adult.

7. The simplest explanation of the acid-base status is a compensated metabolic alkalosis. However, this pattern probably is seen more commonly with a mixed acid-base disorder consisting of a compensated respiratory acidosis complicated by a superimposed primary metabolic alkalosis. $AaDO_2 = 35\,mm\,Hg$. Hypoxemia is therefore due partly to hypoventilation but mostly to ventilation-perfusion mismatch or shunt, probably the former.

8. Something is wrong because the $AaDO_2$ is negative ($-15\,mm\,Hg$). There are several possible explanations: (a) the patient is receiving supplemental O_2; (b) there is a laboratory error; or (c) the blood had not been collected or transported properly under anaerobic conditions.

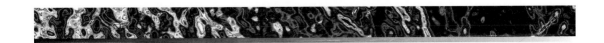

Index

Note: Page numbers followed by f refer to figures. Page numbers followed by t refer to tables.